Bone Tumors - Pathogenesis, Diagnosis, and Management

Edited by Consolato M. Sergi

Published in London, United Kingdom

Bone Tumors - Pathogenesis, Diagnosis, and Management
http://dx.doi.org/10.5772/intechopen.1006422
Edited by Consolato M. Sergi

Contributors
Changxing Liu, Consolato M. Sergi, David Wenger, Jan Beran, Jonneke Kuperus, Lizz van der Heijden, Mahnoor Hafeez, Malik Osama Tanweer, Michiel van de Sande, Mingzhu Zhai, Ruqaiya Shahid, Russel Arellanes, Shally Batham, Shraddha Srivastava, Wuping Sun, Yanni Luo

First published in London, United Kingdom, 2026 by IntechOpen
IntechOpen is the global imprint of INTECHOPEN LIMITED, registered in England and Wales, registration number: 11086078, 167-169 Great Portland Street, London, W1W 5PF, United Kingdom

For EU product safety concerns: IN TECH d.o.o., Prolaz Marije Krucifikse Kozulić 3, 51000 Rijeka, Croatia, info@intechopen.com or visit our website at intechopen.com.

British Library Cataloguing-in-Publication Data
A catalogue record for this book is available from the British Library

Bone Tumors - Pathogenesis, Diagnosis, and Management
Edited by Consolato M. Sergi
p. cm.

This title is part of the Oncology Book Series, Volume 16
Series Editor: Thomas J. FitzGerald
Topic: Cancer Diagnostics and Treatment
Topic Editor: Michael Gibson

Print ISBN 978-1-83635-977-7
Online ISBN 978-1-83635-976-0
eBook (PDF) ISBN 978-1-83635-978-4
ISSN 3049-8864

If disposing of this product, please recycle the paper responsibly.

IntechOpen Book Series

Oncology

Volume 16

Aims and Scope of the Series

The field of oncology has undergone extraordinary change and progress over the past several decades. Today, information is evolving at a rapid rate, with standards of management far different than standards of care applied during the training of most practicing oncologists. Oncology practitioners in all disciplines must remain current to optimize patient care. Basic and translational science remain critical in developing process improvements for patient care. The closer we understand the mechanism, the more we can improve targeted therapies and apply them to patient care. The pace of information is moving faster than at any previous time in history, and all oncology disciplines must remain current to provide excellent service to patients. The modern oncologist must be fluent in using big data and the volume of information generated in clinical trials. As we move closer to personalized patient care based on genomics and molecular biomarkers, the modern oncologist has to be nimble in assessing all available information and how this would be applied to each patient, balanced by the clinical status and medical co-morbidities of each patient. Targeted therapies can bring new and different sequelae, and oncology teams need to remain fluent in managing the consequences of therapy and primary management. In this book series, we will present how modern care has progressed in multiple disease areas and how modern oncology teams need to adapt in order to manage the cancer patients of today successfully. Surgery, radiation therapy, and medical oncology are practiced today with the support of exceptional modern technology, and in this series, we will review how these improvements are applied to each disease site to maintain excellence in patient care.

Meet the Series Editor

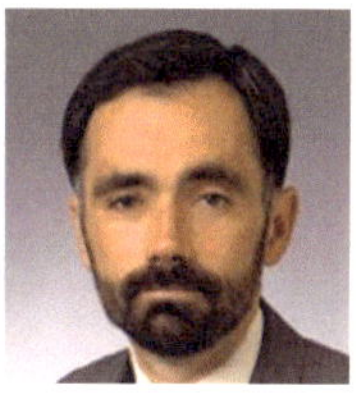

Dr. FitzGerald is the professor and chair of the Department of Radiation Oncology at UMass Chan Medical School in the USA. He serves as one of the principal investigators of the Imaging and Radiation Oncology Core (IROC) service for the National Cancer Institute clinical trials program and is directly involved in the quality assurance of clinical trials in the National Clinical Trials Network (NCTN). Dr. Fitzgerald manages NCTN clinical trials with a real-time pre-therapy review of imaging and radiation therapy treatment objects to ensure the care plan complies with study objectives and the patient stage has been assigned to the correct study. His basic science interest is in hematopoietic stem cell biology and cellular adhesion molecules as they pertain to therapeutic resistance and mitigation of injury from therapy.

Meet the Volume Editor

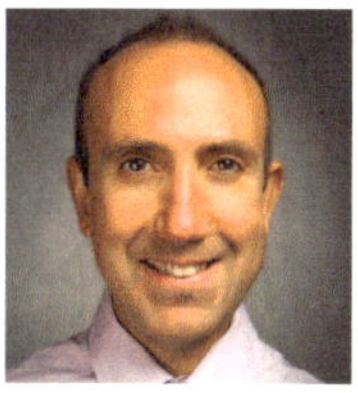

Consolato M. Sergi is the Chief of the Anatomic Pathology Division at the Children's Hospital of Eastern Ontario and a Professor of Pediatrics and Pathology at University of Alberta, and Ottawa, Canada. Dr. Sergi is Canadian, born in Rome, Italy, and holds an MD degree with honors, a qualification in Pediatrics, and a Pediatric Pathology Fellowship from the University of Genoa, Italy. Dr. Sergi obtained his qualification in Pathology at the Ruprecht Karl University of Heidelberg, Germany; the Clinical Readership at the University of Bristol, UK; a Ph.D./Habilitation at the University of Innsbruck, Austria; an MPH in Austria; and FRCPC (Pathology) from the Royal College of Physicians and Surgeons of Canada. He established his Canadian laboratory in August 2008. He welcomed more than 100 graduate MSc/Ph.D. students, fellows, undergraduates, and summer students, and continued teaching in Genetics and Pathology. Dr. Sergi is a Consultant of Carcinogenesis in Experimental Animals at the WHO/IARC, Lyon, France, and an "ad-hoc" Peer-Referee for the National Toxicology Program, NIH, USA. His areas of interest are Biology & Pathology of the Cardiovascular/Gastrointestinal System and Gut/Bile Microbiome, as well as Bone Cell Biology. Dr. Sergi has more than 450 peer-reviewed publications in PubMed (h-index: 53, RG-score: 5,960, >25,569 citations, i10-index: 253). He identified the role of apoptosis in the ductal plate malformation of the liver (Am J Pathol, 2000), a new CTL4/Neu1 gene fusion transcript in sialidosis (Hum Genet 2001, FEBS Lett 2002, J Med Genet 2003), two new genes, i. e., WDR62, which encodes a centrosome-associated protein (Nat Genet, 2010) and OTX2, mutations of which contribute to dysgnathia (J Med Genet 2012), as well as characteristics of the bile microbiome (Infect Drug Resist 2019, HPB (Oxford) 2019, J Med Microbiol 2018, Eur J Clin Microbiol Infect Dis, 2018). He is the editor-in-chief and serves on the editorial boards of prestigious medical journals and international agencies.

Contents

Preface

After the Introductory Chapter, the second chapter of this book provides a thorough presentation of bone tumors, with X-ray details. The differential diagnosis of bone tumors can be guided by the lesion's anatomical location within the bone, patient age, and radiographic features of tumor aggressiveness. The most common non-neoplastic entity is chronic osteomyelitis, which can often mimic an aggressive bone lesion on imaging. In chapter 3, the bone tumors of the head and neck are presented. Bone tumors in the head and neck can be benign (like osteomas, osteoid osteomas, osteoblastomas, chondromas, aneurysmal bone cysts) or malignant (like osteosarcoma, Ewing sarcoma, chondrosarcoma, chordoma) and involve the skull, sinuses, jaw, or neck, often causing headaches, vision/hearing changes, or swallowing/breathing issues, with treatment depending on tumor type, size, and location, usually involving surgery, radiation, and chemotherapy. In chapter 4, the radio-pathological correlation with clinical insights into bone tumors is discussed and illustrated. The majority of bone cancers are osteolytic. The most dependable criterion for assessing whether these lesions are benign or malignant is the transition zone between the lesion and the surrounding normal bone. After determining whether a bone lesion is sclerotic or osteolytic and assessing its margin definition, the next question should be: What is the patient's age? Age constitutes the fundamental clinical indicator.

Additionally, other factors must be evaluated, including the lesion's anatomical position within the skeleton and bone, any periosteal response, cortical erosion, and matrix calcifications, among others. Osteosarcoma, the most common malignant tumor of the skeletal system, will be analyzed in detail using both transmission electron microscopy and molecular biology techniques in the fifth chapter. The differential diagnosis of small round blue cell tumors is critical in pediatrics and will be highlighted, along with an update on therapeutic strategies. In the sixth chapter, the bone cancer pain (BCP) is targeted. BCP is a complex, multifactorial type of chronic pain that involves both nociceptive (tissue injury-related) and neuropathic (nerve damage-related) components. It is a common and often severe symptom, particularly in advanced or metastatic bone cancer, and can be challenging to manage effectively with conventional analgesics alone. The pain is not simply due to the physical presence of a tumor. Still, it involves dynamic interactions between cancer cells, bone cells (osteoclasts and osteoblasts), immune cells, and nerve fibers within the tumor microenvironment. Tumor cells disrupt the normal balance of bone remodeling by promoting the activity of osteoclasts (bone-resorbing cells). This process creates a highly acidic microenvironment and releases substances (such as protons and ATP) that activate acid-sensitive receptors (e.g., TRPV1 and ASIC3) on surrounding nerve endings. Tumor and immune cells release various chemical mediators, including nerve growth factor (NGF), prostaglandins, and cytokines. These factors sensitize pain-sensing neurons (nociceptors) and can cause new nerve fibers to grow abnormally (sprouting). The tumor can also directly injure existing nerve fibers, leading to the neuropathic pain component.

The constant stream of pain signals from the bone to the spinal cord and brain causes changes in the central nervous system, amplifying pain perception. In chapter 7, the role of radiotherapy in the treatment of bone tumors is addressed. Radiotherapy is rapidly evolving from primarily palliative care to an ablative, curative-intent local therapy in select cases, particularly with advances in precision techniques. Technological innovations such as SBRT and particle therapy enable higher, more targeted doses that spare healthy tissue. In the final chapter, the rotationplasty is targeted. Rorationplasty is a limb-salvage surgery, often for children with knee bone cancer, where the diseased knee and part of the thigh are removed, the lower leg is rotated 180 degrees (backwards), and the ankle is connected to the femur, allowing the ankle to function as a new, highly functional knee joint within a prosthesis. It is an alternative to above-knee amputation, offering better mobility and energy efficiency, especially for sports, by using the natural movement of the ankle within a custom socket.

Consolato M. Sergi
University of Alberta, Edmonton, Alberta,
University of Ottawa, Ontario Ottawa, ON, Canada

Section 1

Bone Tumors: Imaging and Pathology

Chapter 1

Introductory Chapter: Bone Tumors – The Way Forward

Consolato M. Sergi

1. Introduction

The diagnosis of bone cancers often presents difficulties for pathologists and doctors. This is unsurprising, as these tumors are rare, morphologically diverse, exhibit a wide range of biological behaviors, and frequently necessitate specific and intricate therapeutic approaches for a cure [1]. An accurate diagnosis necessitates a comprehensive strategy that evaluates and correlates the clinical, radiological, histological, molecular, and prognostic attributes of the tumor [2–8]. The significance of connecting histological and radiological findings of the lesion to guarantee diagnostic accuracy is paramount. In most cases, effective patient care is achieved when members of a sarcoma multidisciplinary team collaborate to identify and stage the tumor and to devise and execute an optimal treatment strategy. Bone neoplasms and the skeletal response to them frequently mirror the cells, tissue types, and biological processes that constitute the normal skeleton during growth and development. Comprehending these mechanisms and their morphological manifestations is crucial for accurately determining the type and biological potential of bone malignancies and tumor-like lesions [9–12].

The skeletal system consists of 206 bones, each formed from bone tissue, a specific form of connective tissue. This number is different for babies, who are born with around 300 bones that fuse as they grow. In detail, the axial skeleton comprises 80 bones, including the skull, spine, ribs, and sternum. In comparison, the appendicular skeleton contains 126 bones, including those of the arms, shoulders, legs, and hips. There are, obviously, variations because some people may have a slightly different number due to anatomical variations, such as extra ribs, and the total of 206 does not include tiny sesamoid bones found in tendons or the small bones in the ear [13, 14].

Bone tissue is distinctive because it comprises a biphasic combination of an inorganic mineral component (calcium hydroxyapatite) and organic elements (cells and their released proteins). The term "osteoid" denotes bone that is unmineralized *in vivo* and consists solely of organic components. Bone is the most durable and robust tissue in the body [15, 16]. It experiences continuous remodeling at fluctuating rates throughout life, facilitating growth and development, alterations in function and metabolism, and skeletal repair.

Dimensions and morphology are the criteria for classifying individual bones. The predominant category of bones is tubular, encompassing both long (appendicular) and short (acral) varieties; additional classifications include flat (bilaminar plates such as the ilium, skull, and sternum), irregular (tarsals, carpals, and vertebrae), and

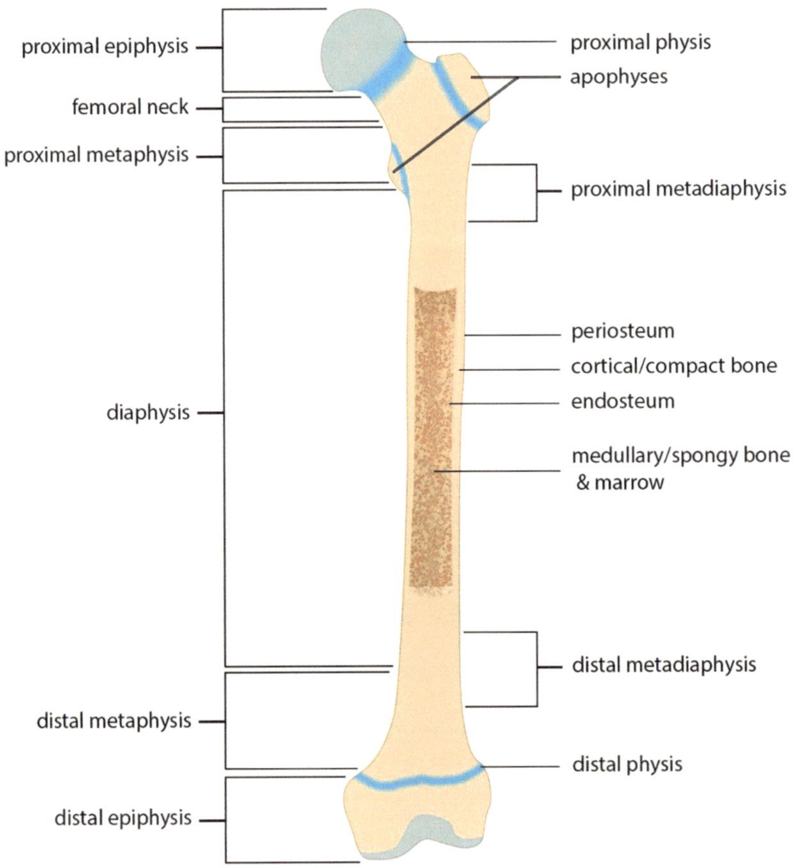

Figure 1.
Anatomy of long bones. A long bone (here: the femur) consists of epiphyses, metaphysis (metaphyses in plural), and a diaphysis (shaft). The epiphyseal plate has closed in this bone. It has become the epiphyseal line after puberty [print reproduction: "Radiopaedia – drawing anatomy of long bones (femur) – English labels" at AnatomyTool.org by Matt Skalski, license: creative commons attribution-non-commercial-no derivatives; digital reproduction: "Radiopaedia – drawing anatomy of long bones (femur) – English labels" by Matt Skalski, license: CC BY–NC–ND].

sesamoid bones. Tubular bones are anatomically categorized into regions: epiphysis, metaphysis, and diaphysis (see **Figure 1**).

The epiphysis extends from the base of the articular surface to the growth plate. The metaphysis is the area of bone that has a notable reduction in diameter and extends from the growth plate or its scar to the location where the bone diameter is constricted. The diaphysis, or shaft, stretches from the base of one metaphysis, where the reduction in bone diameter concludes, to the base of the opposite metaphysis. Throughout growth and development, the metaphysis primarily consists of a cartilaginous growth plate, called the physis, along with the primary and secondary spongiosa [17–23]. Apophysis, or epiphyseal equivalent, is a natural bony protrusion for tendon or ligament attachment, including the greater and lesser trochanters and the iliac crest. A correlation exists between skeletal position and the specific anatomical site, particularly in long bones and vertebrae, and distinct forms of bone cancer. Beginning in the embryo and continuing until adult height is reached, the bones of the body experience considerable growth in size, enhancement of shape, and alteration of contour. Due to its rigidity, bone does not undergo interstitial growth and only increases in size through the apposition of new bone onto old surfaces. Conversely, cartilage possesses the ability for both appositional and interstitial growth; it augments its mass and expands in all dimensions by incorporating new cells that produce extracellular matrix both internally and on its surfaces. The attributes of bone and cartilage underpin the two principal processes of bone production and growth, termed enchondral and intramembranous ossification. In enchondral ossification, a cartilage model is substituted by bone, but in intramembranous ossification, bone tissue is directly generated by precursor cells located within a membranous layer of fibrous tissue. The elongation of tubular bones in embryos and prepubertal children transpires as developing cartilage is substituted by bone, namely by enchondral ossification, with most of the development originating from the cartilage anlage and growth plate. The cartilage anlage initially arises during early embryogenesis from mesenchymal cells that form cellular condensations at the sites of prospective bones.

These mesenchymal cells differentiate into chondrocytes that generate a cartilage model, or anlage, of the impending bone [19, 24]. The process begins at a designated period for each bone, and the chronological order of anlage development is consistent across individuals. Mesenchymal cells encircle the newly developed cartilage anlage, constituting the perichondrium. The perichondrium converts into the periosteum upon the commencement of ossification. This process initially occurs in the central region of the cartilaginous shaft, where mesenchymal stem cells within the perichondrium begin to produce a layer of osteoblasts that deposit a collar of woven mineralized bone on the cartilage model's surface. This signifies the conversion of the perichondrium into the periosteum, and this anatomical area in the central portion of the diaphysis, consisting of several tissue types, is referred to as the principal center of ossification. Subsequently, the chondrocytes within the cartilaginous shaft, enclosed by the periosteal bone shell, commence hypertrophy and swelling. Subsequently, these cells experience apoptosis, and the adjacent matrix undergoes mineralization [25–29]. Simultaneously, the periosteal vessels generate a capillary network. Facilitated by osteoclastic resorption, it infiltrates the woven bone of the primary ossification center into the mineralized cartilage. Osteoclasts persist in excavating the cartilaginous core of the bone, resulting in the formation of residual, longitudinally aligned matrix struts. The cartilage struts serve as a framework for the freshly created bone produced by osteoblasts derived from mesenchymal stem cells. The initial trabeculae consist of a central cartilaginous core encased in a layer of woven bone, constituting the main spongiosa. A persistent degradation of cartilage generates voids that merge to establish the medullary cavity. The intricate process of cartilage substitution by bone, accompanied by the formation of a marrow cavity, advances toward both extremities, simultaneously with the elongation of the bone. In most long bones, a comparable process subsequently occurs in the epiphyses, which serve as the secondary center of ossification. The maturation and replacement of the cartilage anlage in the secondary ossification center mirror the process in the diaphysis, with maturation advancing centrifugally from the center to the periphery. The ongoing expansion of the primary and secondary ossification centers ultimately leads to their amalgamation. Currently, a plate of bone delineating the secondary center from the primary center is established, resulting in a hemispheric centrifugal expansion of the epiphysis. Upon the formation of the bony plate that distinguishes the secondary from the major center of ossification, the definitive structure of the growth plate is achieved. Growth plates primarily facilitate the longitudinal growth of bones and, by endochondral ossification, contribute to the formation of the initial cancellous bone in the skeleton. In the growth plate, chondrocytes are organized in overlapping zones that reflect various stages of chondrocyte proliferation and maturation. As cells progress through several stages of their lifecycle, they do not physically relocate inside the matrix but rather mature in their initial positions upon formation.

The stages of maturation are evident in their morphology, which underpins their classification into distinct zones: (1) a region of resting or reserve chondrocytes situated closest to the bone ends, (2) a region of proliferating chondrocytes organized in spiral columns, (3) a region of chondrocyte hypertrophy, (4) a region of chondrocyte apoptosis and matrix mineralization, and (5) a region of cartilage resorption by osteoclasts [1, 30]. The chondrocytes in the reserve zone are diminutive, round or oval, and encased in a copious matrix; those located at the base generate the chondrocytes that constitute the zone of proliferation. The chondrocytes in the proliferative zone are flattened, undergo mitosis, align in spiral columns, and produce extracellular matrix. Within the hypertrophic zone, chondrocytes undergo significant enlargement, with cytoplasmic volume increasing tenfold as they simultaneously remodel the surrounding matrix. Within the mineralization zone, or calcifying cartilage – occasionally seen as a subregion of the hypertrophic zone – chondrocytes release matrix vesicles originating from the cell membrane, which regulate the mineralization of the adjacent extracellular matrix. As the matrix mineralizes, the chondrocytes experience fast apoptosis in the final row of lacunae preceding the ossification front. This process involves the secretion of cytokines that recruit endothelial-lined blood vessels and osteoclasts, which penetrate the mineralized matrix, degrading the transverse septa that separate the chondrocytes. Consequently, vertically aligned intercolumnar struts of mineralized cartilage persist; their orientation is dictated by the previous columnar configuration of the chondrocytes in the proliferative and hypertrophic zones, aligning with the long axis of the bone. The cartilage struts serve as the framework for freshly formed bone. Cartilage undergoing enchondral ossification, resembling growth plate cartilage, is present in all benign and malignant bone tumors, including cartilage, as well as in non-neoplastic situations such as fracture callus. Intramembranous ossification arises from mesenchymal condensations in the embryo and the periosteum in the fetus, child, and adult [31]. The osteoprogenitor cells in the condensations and periosteum generate progeny that differentiate into mature osteoblasts, which deposit bone matrix. The extensive sections of the flat bones of the skull, comprising the frontal, parietal, occipital, and temporal bones, develop exclusively through this mechanism. All bone cortices are predominantly formed by osteoblasts originating from the periosteum, indicating that all bones undergo intramembranous ossification to some extent. Regardless of whether bone tissue arises from enchondral or intramembranous ossification, or whether it is cortical or cancellous, and irrespective of its normal or pathological nature, it is classified into woven and lamellar types based on the arrangement of its type I collagen fibers, the principal structural proteins of bone tissue. In woven bone, the collagen fibers are organized into an apparently random network, whereas in lamellar bone, they are arranged in parallel configurations. Neoplastic bone typically has a braided and trabecular architecture rather than a cortical appearance. Reactive bone can be classified as either woven or lamellar and may exhibit trabecular or cortical patterns.

Bone tumors are classified as primary (starting in bone) or secondary/metastatic (spreading from elsewhere), and further as benign (non-cancerous) or malignant (cancerous). Common types include osteoid osteoma, osteoblastoma, osteosarcoma, Ewing sarcoma, chondrosarcoma, osteochondroma, enchondroma, and giant cell tumors. Classification relies on cell origin, location, and histological appearance (such as World Health Organization [WHO] grades) [32, 33]. Benign tumors are more common than malignant ones. Osteochondroma is the most common benign bone tumor, originating from cartilage/bone, whereas enchondroma originates in cartilage within the bone. Osteoid osteoma/osteoblastoma produces new bone, while the giant cell tumor is locally aggressive but usually benign. The three most common malignant bone tumors include osteosarcoma, the most common primary bone cancer that produces bone matrix; Ewing sarcoma, which affects young people and is composed of small round blue cells; and chondrosarcoma, which usually affects adults and is a malignant cartilage tumor, graded I–III. Secondary (metastatic) bone tumors are neoplastic processes that originate in other organs (such as the breast, prostate, lung, or kidney) and spread to the bone. The WHO classification provides a detailed, updated system for these diverse tumors that integrates genetics and histology.

Author details

Consolato M. Sergi[1,2]

1 University of Alberta, Edmonton, Alberta

2 University of Ottawa, Ottawa, Canada

*Address all correspondence to: csergi@cheo.on.ca

References

[1] Sergi CM. Pathology of Childhood and Adolescence Heidelberg: Springer; 2020b

[2] AA. (2025). Introduction to Bone Tumors. Available from: https://www.nankodo.co.jp/foreign/AFIP/img/book_sample/attupc08.pdf

[3] Adin ME, Woolf G, Hegde R, Elsamadicy AA, Mendel E, Zucconi WB, Pucar D, Aygun N. Sacral tumors: A comprehensive review of imaging, diagnostic challenges, and tumor mimics. Skeletal Radiology. 2025;**54**(8):1581–1606. DOI: 10.1007/s00256-024-04862-6

[4] Alston ELJ, Ecklund K, Al-Ibraheemi A. Pediatric Bone Tumors. Surgical Pathology Clinics. 2025;**18**(3):581–595. DOI: 10.1016/j.path.2025.01.003

[5] Grieser T, Hirsch E, Todtmann N. Bone Tumors of the Jaw-the "Blind Spot" for Radiologists Experienced with Tumors?-Part I. RöFo-Fortschritte Auf Dem Gebiet der Röntgenstrahlen Und der Bildgebenden Verfahren. 2025;**197**(4):397–415. DOI: 10.1055/a-2415-8880. Original work published Kiefertumoren-der "blinde Fleck" des tumorversierten Radiologen?-Teil I

[6] Grieser T, Hirsch E, Todtmann N. Bone Tumors of the Jaw-the "Blind Spot" for Radiologists Experienced with Tumors?-Part II. RöFo-Fortschritte Auf Dem Gebiet der Röntgenstrahlen Und der Bildgebenden Verfahren. 2025;**197**(6):621–637. DOI: 10.1055/a-2416-1282. Original work published Kiefertumoren-der "blinde Fleck" des tumorversierten Radiologen?-Teil II

[7] Ruiz Santiago F, Orellana Gonzalez C, Moraleda Cabrera B, Lainez Ramos-Bossini AJ. Accuracy of clinical diagnosis, imaging methods, and biopsy in tumours and pseudo-tumours of the hand. Quantitative Imaging in Medicine and Surgery. 2024;**14**(11):7803–7816. DOI: 10.21037/qims-24-347

[8] Zhang AB, Zhao JR, Wang S, Xue J, Zhang JY, Sun ZP, Sun LS, Li TJ. CT-based radiomics analysis of different machine learning models for differentiating gnathic fibrous dysplasia and ossifying fibroma. Oral Diseases. 2024;**30**(8):5243–5254. DOI: 10.1111/odi.14984

[9] Sergi CM. Pediatric cancer-pathology and microenvironment influence: A perspective into osteosarcoma and non-osteogenic mesenchymal malignant neoplasms. Discover Oncology. 2024;**15**(1):358. DOI: 10.1007/s12672-024-01240-5

[10] Sergi CM, Burnett M, Jantuan E, Hakoum M, Beug ST, Leng R, Shen F. Digging Through the Complexities of Immunological Approaches in Emerging Osteosarcoma Therapeutics: A Comprehensive Narrative Review with Updated Clinical Trials. Biomedicines. 2025;**13**(3):664.DOI: 10.3390/biomedicines13030664

[11] Taylor AM, Sheng J, Ng PKS, Harder JM, Kumar P, Ahn JY, Cao Y, Dzis AM, Jillette NL, Goodspeed A, Bodlak A, Wu Q, Isakoff MS, George J, Grassmann JDS, Luo D, Flynn WF, Courtois ET, Robson P, Lau CC. Immunosuppressive Tumor Microenvironment of Osteosarcoma.

Cancers (Basel). 2025;**17**(13):2117. DOI: 10.3390/cancers17132117

[12] Vitale I, Pietrocola F, Guilbaud E, Aaronson SA, Abrams JM, Adam D, Agostini M, Agostinis P, Alnemri ES, Altucci L, Amelio I, Andrews DW, Aqeilan RI, Arama E, Baehrecke EH, Balachandran S, Bano D, Barlev NA, Bartek J, Galluzzi L. Apoptotic cell death in disease-Current understanding of the NCCD 2023. Cell Death and Differentiation. 2023;**30**(5):1097–1154. DOI: 10.1038/s41418-023-01153-w

[13] Ricci V, Chang KV, Nanka O, Ozcakar L. Superficial retrocalcaneal bursae and nerves: From anatomy to ultrasound-guided procedures. Clinical Anatomy. 2025;**38**(1):29–34. DOI: 10.1002/ca.24193

[14] Testut L. Traité D'anatomie Humaine. Vol. **I & II**. Paris: Doin; 1899

[15] Gross JM, Hameed M. Osteosarcoma. Surgical Pathology Clinics. 2025;**18**(3):449–470. DOI: 10.1016/j.path.2025.01.009

[16] McHugh KE, Reith JD, Kilpatrick SE. Benign bone forming (Osteoblastic) tumors. Surgical Pathology Clinics. 2025;**18**(3): 471–488. DOI: 10.1016/j. path.2025.01.006

[17] Ballabriga A. Morphological and physiological changes during growth: An update. European Journal of Clinical Nutrition. 2000;**54**(1):S1–6

[18] Chang CY, Rosenthal DI, Mitchell DM, Handa A, Kattapuram SV, Huang AJ. Imaging Findings of Metabolic Bone Disease. Radiographics. 2016;**36**(6):1871–1887. DOI: 10.1148/ rg.2016160004

[19] Chang X, Ma Z, Zhu G, Lu Y, Yang J. New perspective into mesenchymal stem cells: Molecular mechanisms regulating osteosarcoma. Journal of Bone Oncology. 2021;**29**:100372. DOI: 10.1016/j. jbo.2021.100372

[20] Gat-Yablonski G, De Luca F. Effect of Nutrition on Statural Growth. Hormone Research in Paediatrics. 2017;**88**(1):46–62. DOI: 10.1159/ 000456547

[21] Lira Dos Santos EJ, Mohamed FF, Kramer K, Foster BL. Dental manifestations of hypophosphatasia: Translational and clinical advances. JBMR Plus. 2025;**9**(2):ziae180. DOI: 10.1093/jbmrpl/ziae180

[22] St-Arnaud R. The direct role of vitamin D on bone homeostasis. Archives of Biochemistry and Biophysics. 2008;**473**(2):225–230. DOI: 10.1016/j.abb.2008.03.038

[23] Yakar S, Werner H, Rosen CJ. Insulin-like growth factors: Actions on the skeleton. Journal of Molecular Endocrinology. 2018;**61**(1):T115–T137. DOI: 10.1530/JME-17-0298

[24] de Azevedo JWV, de Medeiros Fernandes TAA, Fernandes Jr JV, de Azevedo JCV, Lanza DCF, Bezerra CM, Andrade VS, de Araujo JMG, Fernandes JV. Biology and pathogenesis of human osteosarcoma. Oncology Letters. 2020;**19**(2):1099–1116. DOI: 10.3892/ol.2019.11229

[25] Baumgartner-Sigl S, Haberlandt E, Mumm S, Scholl-Burgi S, Sergi C, Ryan L, Ericson KL, Whyte MP, Hogler W. Pyridoxine-responsive seizures as the first symptom of infantile hypophosphatasia caused by two novel missense mutations (c.677T>C,

p.M226T; c.1112C>T, p.T371I) of the tissue-nonspecific alkaline phosphatase gene. Bone. 2007;**40**(6):1655–1661. DOI: 10.1016/j.bone.2007.01.020

[26] Sergi C, Mornet E, Troeger J, Voigtlaender T. Perinatal hypophosphatasia: Radiology, pathology and molecular biology studies in a family harboring a splicing mutation (648+1A) and a novel missense mutation (N400S) in the tissue-nonspecific alkaline phosphatase (TNSALP) gene. American Journal of Medical Genetics. 2001;**103**(3):235–240

[27] Sergi CM. Hypophosphatasia: The Unusual Presentation. Journal of Clinical Research in Pediatric Endocrinology. 2020a;**12**(4):450–451. DOI: 10.4274/jcrpe.galenos. 2020.2020.0094

[28] Stonich D, Su Y, Dad S, Reddy S, Mostofi Y, Russell D, Chung TDY, Hedrick NM, Rascon J, Garcia X, Sergienko E, Millan JL, Stonich D, Cosford N. The Role of PHOSPHO1 in the Initiation of Skeletal Calcification. In Probe Reports from the NIH Molecular Libraries Program. 2010

[29] Zhang M, Shen F, Petryk A, Tang J, Chen X, Sergi C. "English disease": Historical notes on rickets,the bone-lung link and child neglect issues. Nutrients. 2016;**8**(11):722. DOI: 10.3390/nu8110722

[30] Dunkel L, Wickman S. Novel treatment of short stature with aromatase inhibitors. The Journal of Steroid Biochemistry and Molecular Biology. 2003;**86**(3-5):345–356

[31] Seino Y. Cytokines and growth factors which regulate bone cell function. Acta Astronautica. 1994;**33**:131–136

[32] Board WCOTE. World Health Organization Classification of Tumours: Soft Tissue and Bone Tumours. 5th ed., Vol. **3**. Lyon, France: IARC Press; 2020

[33] Sbaraglia M, Bellan E, Dei Tos AP. The 2020 WHO Classification of Soft Tissue Tumours: News and perspectives. Pathologica. 2021;**113** (2):70–84. DOI: 10.32074/1591-951X-213

Chapter 2

Xray Imaging of Bone Tumors

Jan Beran

Abstract

The newest, updated World Health Organization (WHO) classification of bone tumors was released in 2020. In my publication, I will emphasize Xray imaging, as it is the first choice in diagnosing every bone disease or suspicion of it. Primary bone tumors are rare, with a frequency of 0.2% of all tumors in the human body, and their etiology remains unknown. The fifth edition of the WHO classification, published in April 2020, follows the same system based on the tissues from which the tumors originate, as seen in the previous classification from 2013. There are significant changes in histological and molecular classification, along with an increased number of subtypes for certain tumors. The group "Tumor-like affections" has been removed, and all such conditions have been redistributed to other groups based on their histology.

Keywords: WHO classification, bone tumors, Xray imaging, benign tumors, malignant tumors

1. Introduction

Primary bone tumors are relatively rare, accounting for 0.2% of all neoplasms. Their etiology remains largely unknown. In April 2020, the fifth edition of the World Health Organization (WHO) classification of soft tissue and bone tumors was published (**Table 1**), incorporating advances in molecular biology as well as modifications in histological classification. This edition introduced several new entities and subtypes. The WHO classification constitutes the foundation for the accurate diagnosis of bone tumors [1].

Tumor grading is divided into three levels. Low grade (Grade I) denotes very slow, circumscribed growth. Intermediate grade (Grade II) is characterized by a higher number of atypical nuclei, with nuclei of larger size. High grade (Grade III) demonstrates an increased proportion of necrosis and more pronounced nuclear alterations compared to Grade II.

Given the relatively low incidence of bone tumors in the human population, the initial clinical manifestations are often atypical, and the first detection of a tumor is frequently achieved through radiographic imaging. Such imaging subsequently becomes a crucial element in guiding the further management of patients [2, 3].

Chondrogenic tumors

- *Benign*
  - Subungual exostosis
  - Bizarre parosteal osteochondromatous proliferation
  - Periosteal chondroma
  - Enchondroma
  - Osteochondroma
  - Chondroblastoma, NOS
  - Chondromyxoid fibroma
  - Osteochondromyxoma
- *Intermediate (locally aggressive)*
  - Chondromatosis, NOS
  - Atypical cartilaginous tumor (ACT)
- *Malignant*
  - Chondrosarcoma, Grade I
  - Chondrosarcoma, Grade II
  - Chondrosarcoma, Grade III
  - Periosteal chondrosarcoma
  - Clear cell chondrosarcoma
  - Mesenchymal chondrosarcoma
  - Dedifferentiated chondrosarcoma

Osteogenic tumors

- *Benign*
  - Osteoma, NOS
  - Osteoid osteoma, NOS
- *Intermediate (locally aggressive)*
  - Osteoblastoma, NOS
- *Malignant*
  - Low-grade central osteosarcoma
  - Osteosarcoma, NOS
    - Conventional osteosarcoma
    - Telangiectatic osteosarcoma
    - Small cell osteosarcoma
  - Parosteal osteosarcoma
  - Periosteal osteosarcoma
  - High-grade surface osteosarcoma
  - Secondary osteosarcoma

Fibrogenic tumors

- *Intermediate (locally aggressive)*
  - Desmoplastic fibroma
- *Malignant*
  - Fibrosarcoma, NOS

Vascular tumors of bone

- *Benign*
  - Hemangioma, NOS
- *Intermediate (locally aggressive)*
  - Epithelioid hemangioma
- *Malignant*
  - Epithelioid hemangioendothelioma, NOS
  - Angiosarcoma

Osteoclastic giant-cell-rich tumors

- *Benign*
  - Aneurysmal bone cyst
  - Nonossifying fibroma
- *Intermediate (locally aggressive, rarely metastasizing)*
  - Giant cell tumor of bone, NOS
- *Malignant*
  - Giant cell tumor of bone, malignant

Notochordal tumors

- *Benign*
  - Benign notochordal cell tumor
- *Malignant*
  - Chordoma, NOS
    - Chondroid chordoma
  - Poorly differentiated chordoma
  - Dedifferentiated chordoma

Other mesenchymal tumors of bone

- *Benign*
  - Chondromesenchymal hamartoma of the chest wall
  - Simple bone cyst
  - Fibrous dysplasia
  - Osteofibrous dysplasia
  - Lipoma, NOS
  - Hibemoma
- *Intermediate (locally aggressive)*
  - Osteofibrous dysplasia-like adamantinoma
  - Mesenchymoma, NOS
- *Malignant*
  - Adamantinoma of long bones
    - Dedifferentiated adamantinoma
  - Leiomyosarcoma, NOS
  - Pleomorphic sarcoma, undifferentiated
  - Bone metastases

Hematopoietic neoplasms of bone

- Plasmacytoma of bone
- Malignant lymphoma, non-Hodgkin, NOS
- Hodgkin disease, NOS
- Diffuse large B-cell lymphoma, NOS
- Follicular lymphoma, NOS
- Marginal zone B-cell lymphoma, NOS
- T-cell lymphoma, NOS
- Anaplastic large cell lymphoma, NOS
- Malignant lymphoma, lymphoblastic, NOS
- Burkitt lymphoma, NOS
- Langerhans cell histiocytosis, NOS
- Langerhans cell histiocytosis, disseminated
- Erdheim–Chester disease
- Rosai–Dorfman disease

NOS, not otherwise specified.

Table 1.
WHO classification of bone tumors (reprinted from reference [1]).

2. General remarks

The foundation of accurate diagnosis lies in the correct description of the pathological lesion on radiographic imaging, where it is essential to differentiate benign from malignant lesions. This requires a thorough analysis of individual lesions, including a description of the affected structures, an evaluation of the size and delineation of the lesion, possible extension into surrounding structures, and the nature of any periosteal reaction to the tumor.

Certain tumors exhibit a predilection for specific anatomical locations within the bone.

Another important criterion is the age of the patient, as some lesions predominantly occur in younger individuals, while others present at a more advanced age. The classification is commonly divided into three groups: under 20 years, 20–40 years, and 40 years and above.

2.1 Lesion delineation

This parameter reflects both the growth rate and aggressiveness of the tumor [4]. In benign lesions, which grow more slowly, the bone has sufficient capacity for repair; the margins are well defined, with a sclerotic rim demarcating the lesion from healthy tissue (Grade 1a). In semimalignant lesions, growth is more aggressive, and the lesion margins are indistinct (Grade 1b). When there is penetration into adjacent structures accompanied by a periosteal reaction, the lesion is considered malignant (Grade 1c).

Lesions may infiltrate the surrounding bone in different patterns. In solitary lesions, the adjacent bone displays an irregular structure with a broad transition zone into normal tissue (Grade 2). In cases of permeative spread, the bone structure within a given area is interspersed with numerous small, ill-defined foci, producing an appearance classically described as "moth-eaten" (Grade 3) (**Figure 1**).

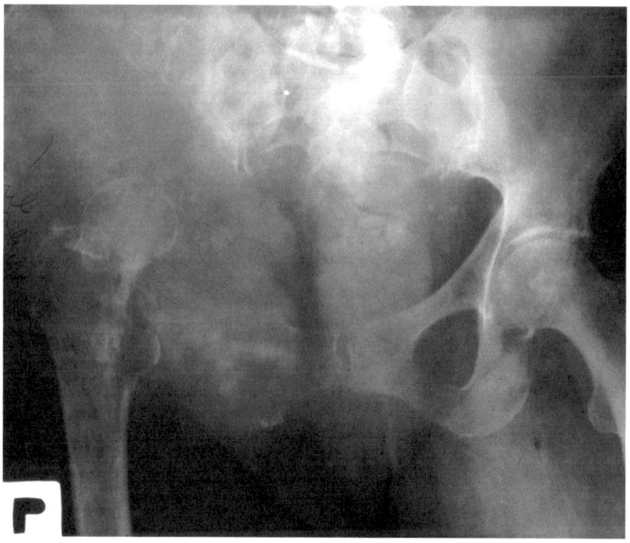

Figure 1.
Right pelvic chondrosarcoma with moth-eaten spread in the proximal femur.

2.2 Periosteal reaction

Periosteal reactions arise as a response of bone to various stimuli, not only malignant ones (e.g., inflammation, metabolic and congenital diseases, infections, or venous involvement) [5]. A feature suggestive of benignity is a solid periostosis with smooth contours and without disruption of its internal architecture. Conversely, malignant periostoses often display irregular structures, frequently with separation of internal components into individual lamellae (the so-called onion-skin periostosis) or with a spiculated surface of the entire periostosis (resembling "hair-on-end" [**Figure 2**] or "sunburst" patterns). In this latter type, the differential diagnosis may also include chronic osteomyelitis, in which the above-described appearance is produced by long-term inflammatory irritation of the bone. When the lesion penetrates the periosteum, a clearly malignant appearance emerges in the form of Codman's triangle (**Figure 3**), where the periosteum is elevated from the bone at the margin of the lesion.

2.3 Age

Primary bone tumors occur more frequently at a younger age, while metastases are more common in individuals over 40 years of age. In adolescent patients, the most common findings are Ewing sarcoma and osteosarcoma, with lymphomas and neuroblastomas occurring less frequently. Benign lesions in young individuals are

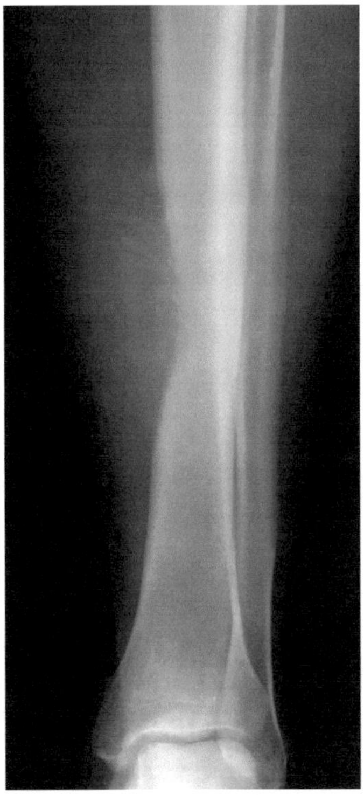

Figure 2.
Metastasis of colorectal carcinoma: "sunburst" periostosis.

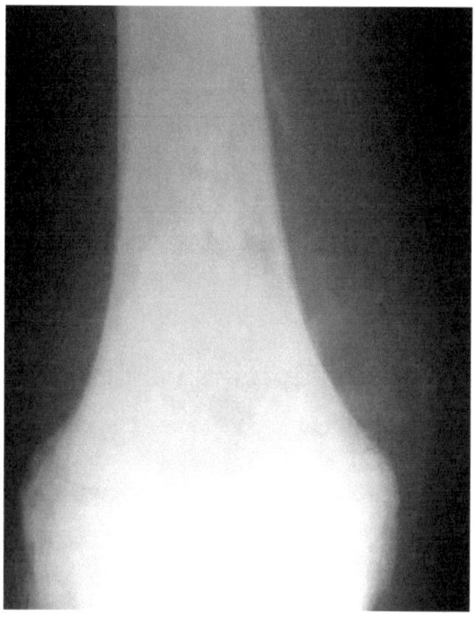

Figure 3.
Ewing sarcoma, Codman's triangle and malignant periostosis.

often incidental findings or manifest only following trauma, such as nonossifying fibroma or bone cysts [6]. Between the ages of 20 and 40, enchondromas, chondroblastomas, osteoid osteomas, and osteoblastomas are more common, while giant cell tumors represent the predominant malignant lesions. In individuals over 40 years of age, metastases are the most frequent, followed among primary tumors by multiple myeloma and, less often, osteosarcoma and chondrosarcoma. Among benign findings, fibrous dysplasia is the most common.

2.4 Localization

Giant cell tumors are typically situated in the epiphyses of long bones, with differential diagnoses including osteomyelitis and subchondral cysts (geodes) in osteoarthritis. At the epiphyseal–metaphyseal junction, aneurysmal bone cysts (ABCs) and osteosarcomas are found. In the metaphyses, enchondromas, nonossifying fibromas, and osteochondromas are most common. Within the diaphyses, in the medullary cavity, metastases, multiple myeloma, and lymphoma predominate, whereas among benign lesions, fibrous dysplasia is typical. In the cortical bone, osteoid osteoma and Ewing's sarcoma are most frequently observed.

When classified by specific skeletal sites, metastases and multiple myeloma occur in the skull; bone cysts in the proximal humerus; and in the vertebrae, multiple myeloma, metastases, hemangiomas, osteoblastomas, chordomas, and osteoid osteomas. In the pelvis, osteosarcoma, chondrosarcoma, lymphoma, and Ewing's sarcoma are encountered. In the proximal femur, fibrous dysplasia and Ewing's sarcoma are characteristic, while around the knee joint, osteosarcoma and Ewing's sarcoma are most common. In this region, particular attention should be paid to nontraumatic knee pain in children. In the tibia, osteoid osteoma, fibrous dysplasia, and nonossifying fibroma are frequently found; in the calcaneus, bone cysts, lipomas, osteoblastomas, and chondroblastomas; and in the phalanges of the hand and foot, enchondromas.

2.5 Tumor structure

Well-demarcated bone tumors include bone cysts, osteoid osteoma, osteoblastoma, fibrous dysplasia, and nonossifying fibroma. Poorly demarcated tumors include osteosarcoma, Ewing sarcoma, chondrosarcoma, and giant cell tumor. Osteosclerotic tumors comprise osteoid osteoma, osteoblastoma, osteoma, and certain subtypes of osteosarcoma. Metastatic lesions may present with all structural patterns; for instance, sclerotic metastases are commonly observed in prostate carcinoma.

3. Most common types of bone tumors (benign, intermediate and malignant entities)

According to WHO classification of bone tumors version 2020 [7, 8].

3.1 Tumors from cartilaginous origin

Tumors coming out of cartilaginous tissue [9, 10].

3.1.1 Enchondroma

Enchondroma is a benign, intramedullary neoplasm composed of hyaline cartilage, most frequently localized in the phalanges of the hands and feet, particularly in the proximal phalanges. Other common sites include the femur, tibia, humerus, pelvis, ribs, and scapula. It typically originates from the growth plate, where cartilage cells are present, and extends toward the diaphysis.

Radiographically, enchondroma presents as a well-circumscribed, osteolytic lesion with fine, punctate, or serpiginous calcifications, which are particularly characteristic in the phalanges. Minor endosteal scalloping of the inner cortex may occur, involving

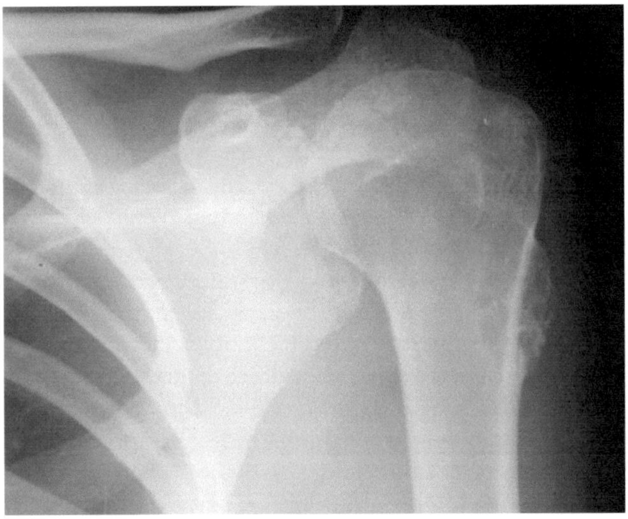

Figure 4.
Left humerus, periosteal chondroma (histologically verified), 21 woman.

up to one-third of its thickness, usually without periosteal reaction (**Figure 4**). A definitive sign of malignant transformation is accelerated tumor growth on follow-up imaging or more pronounced cortical disruption accompanied by possible periosteal reaction. Malignant transformation occurs in approximately 4.2% of cases. Enchondroma may occur as part of Ollier disease and Maffucci syndrome.

3.1.2 Osteochondroma

Osteochondroma represents one of the more frequent bone tumors (accounting for 10–15% of cases). It is typically asymptomatic, benign, and most often detected incidentally during skeletal imaging performed for other reasons. The lesion develops at a young age and may enlarge during childhood but ceases to grow thereafter. Osteochondromas may occur as part of multiple cartilaginous exostoses (**Figure 5**). In solitary osteochondromas, malignant transformation is exceedingly rare and, when present, usually arises from the cartilaginous cap (**Figure 6**).

The most common sites of occurrence include the distal femur (up to 30%), proximal tibia (15–20%), and humerus (10–20%). The radiographic appearance is generally pathognomonic, showing a sessile or pedunculated outgrowth. The cartilaginous cap is usually indistinguishable on imaging; however, in larger lesions,

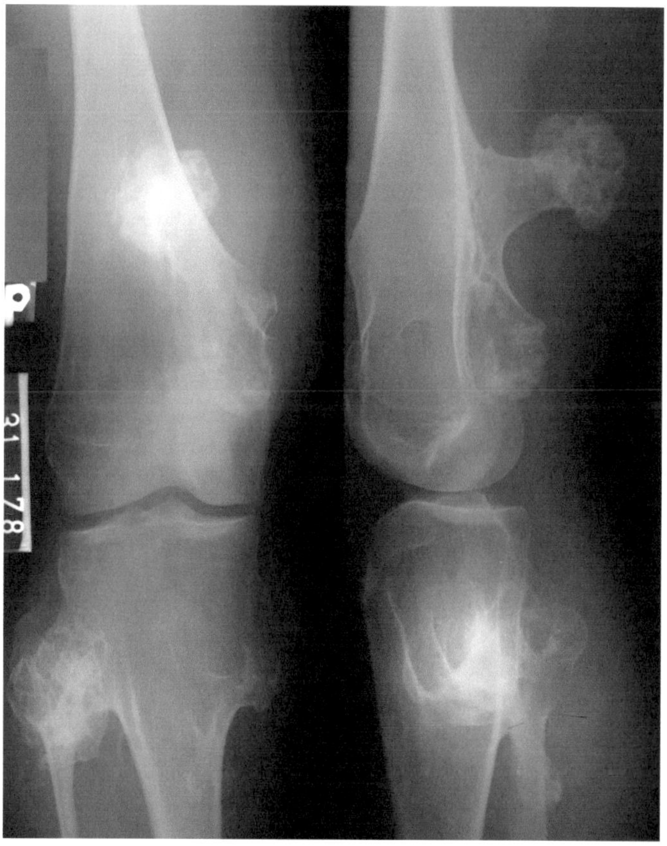

Figure 5.
Multiple cartilaginous exostoses in a 21-year-old man.

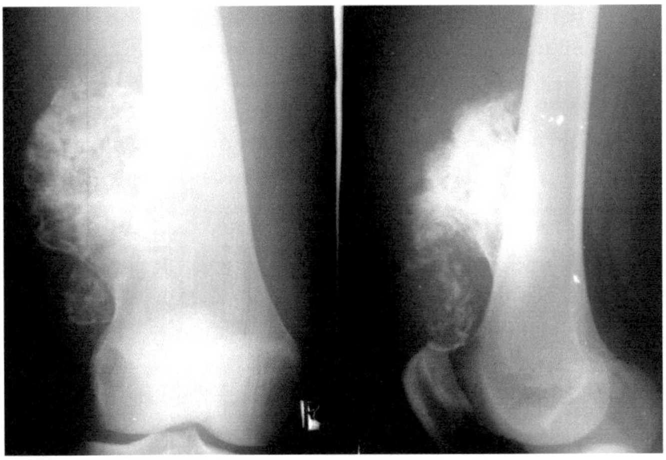

Figure 6.
Malignant transformation of osteochondroma in a 20-year-old man.

it may display fine calcifications. The origin of osteochondromas is most likely related to aberrant ossification pathways, which explains why their size does not increase once skeletal growth is completed.

3.1.3 Chondrosarcoma

Chondrosarcoma is a malignant bone tumor. According to the WHO, this entity is classified into eight subtypes, with particular distinction given to central ACT, replacing the earlier designation of Grade 1 chondrosarcoma (CS1-3). ACT has been introduced as a category of central atypical and secondary peripheral cartilaginous neoplasms in order to emphasize their predominantly locally aggressive behavior and low proliferative activity while maintaining well-differentiated histological features.

Other subgroups include central Grade 2 and Grade 3 chondrosarcomas, secondary peripheral Grade 2 and Grade 3 chondrosarcomas, periosteal chondrosarcoma, clear cell chondrosarcoma, mesenchymal chondrosarcoma, and dedifferentiated chondrosarcoma.

The most frequent sites of involvement are the femur (20–35%), pelvis (20%), proximal humerus (10–20%), and tibia (5%). Radiographically, the tumor most commonly presents as a lytic lesion with calcifications in up to 70% of cases (**Figure** 7), ranging from punctate or lamellar patterns to the so-called popcorn appearance. Cortical thinning of more than two-thirds may occur, and the lesion often demonstrates a "moth-eaten" or permeative pattern of bone destruction with extension into surrounding tissue. Periosteal reaction is often present.

3.2 Osteogenic tumors

Tumors coming out of bony tissue [11].

3.2.1 Osteoma

A benign neoplasm most commonly located in the skull consists of compact bone and is therefore usually well differentiated on plain radiographs. Typical sites

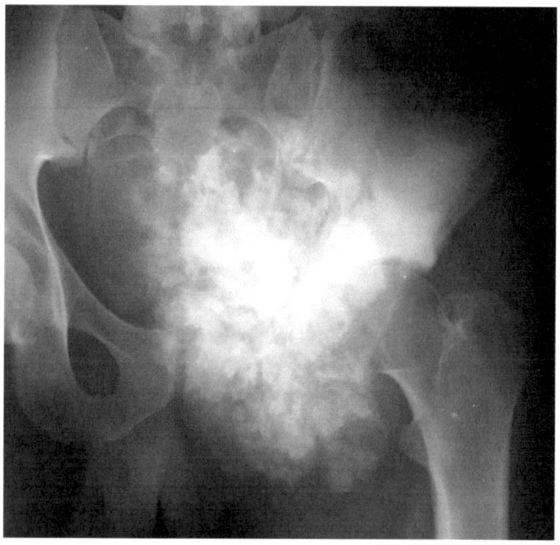

Figure 7.
Pelvic chondrosarcoma in a 26-year-old man.

include the paranasal sinuses – most frequently the frontal sinus – as well as the calvaria and nasal bone. Osteomas arise from the bone surface, on the calvaria predominantly along the outer contour, and are usually asymptomatic.

3.2.2 Osteoid osteoma

A benign tumor primarily affects children. On radiographs, it presents with a central radiolucency (**Figure 8**), although this may not always be detectable due to its small size. The lesion typically measures up to 15–20 mm and is located in the cortical bone. Clinically, the tumor is characterized by nocturnal pain, which subsides following the administration of nonsteroidal anti-inflammatory drugs or acetylsalicylic acid (the latter contraindicated in children under 12 years). The nidus corresponds to the tumor tissue and contains dilated vessels, osteoblasts, and osteoid; the surrounding area shows reactive trabecular bone formation. The most common locations are the femoral neck and proximal diaphysis, phalanges, and lumbar or thoracic vertebrae. Historically, treatment was primarily surgical, but currently, percutaneous radiofrequency or microwave ablation is the preferred approach.

3.2.3 Osteoblastoma

An intermediate, locally aggressive lesion, histologically resembling osteoid osteoma but with irregular margins and a lytic character, is described. The most frequent sites are the vertebral bodies of the cervical spine and the sacrum. A more aggressive, malignant variant is termed epithelioid osteoblastoma.

3.2.4 Osteosarcoma

A malignant bone tumor with six recognized subtypes: low-grade central osteosarcoma, osteosarcoma not otherwise specified (NOS), parosteal osteosarcoma,

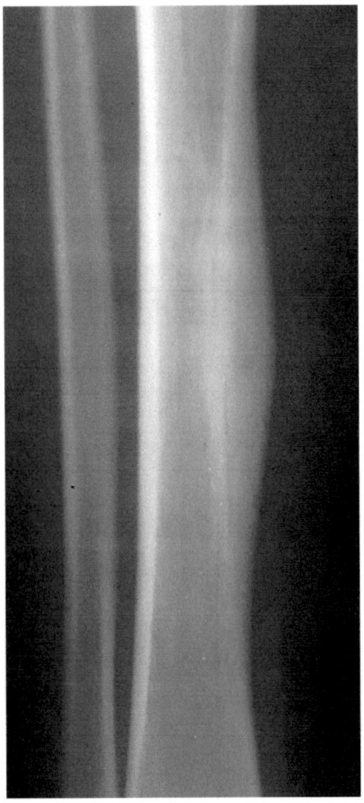

Figure 8.
Osteoid osteoma of the tibia in a 16-year-old male.

periosteal osteosarcoma, high-grade surface osteosarcoma, and secondary osteosarcoma. Other subgroups previously distinguished – such as central, telangiectatic, and small-cell osteosarcomas – are now classified under osteosarcoma NOS.

Osteosarcoma is the second most common primary malignant bone tumor after multiple myeloma. Approximately 75% of cases occur in individuals under 20 years of age. In patients over 40, the disease is most often secondary (associated with Paget's disease or postradiation changes). The typical sites of occurrence are the metaphyseal–diaphyseal regions of long bones: femur (40%), tibia (15%), and humerus (14%), with other locations being less frequent.

Radiographically, the tumor demonstrates destruction of both the medullary cavity and cortical bone, with a broad transition zone to adjacent normal bone (**Figure 9**). Features include a "moth-eaten" pattern of bone destruction and extensive spread into surrounding tissues. The periosteum is disrupted, often showing an aggressive periosteal reaction with Codman's triangle formation. Both central and peripheral lesions frequently extend into adjacent soft tissues. Pulmonary metastases, as well as affected lymph nodes, may exhibit ossification. A pathological fracture may represent both a complication and the initial clinical manifestation.

3.3 Fibrogenic tumors

This group remains unchanged in classification.

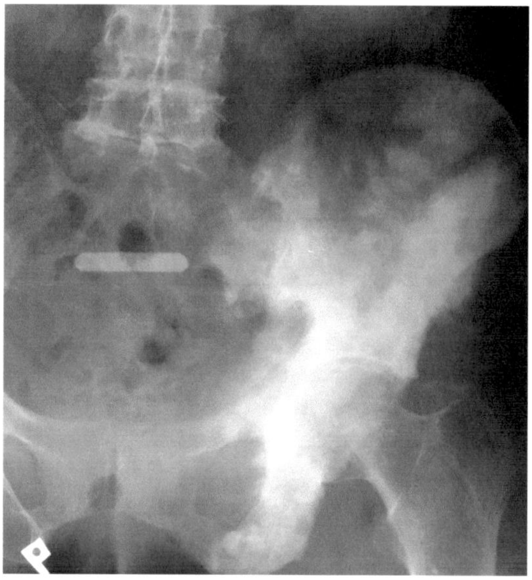

Figure 9.
Left pelvis osteosarcoma in a 67-year-old woman.

3.3.1 Bone fibrosarcoma, NOS

A rare tumor occurs between the ages of 30 and 60 years. It is highly destructive, with a broad transition zone, typically lacking a periosteal reaction, and often extending into adjacent soft tissues.

3.4 Vascular tumors of bone

3.4.1 Hemangioma, NOS

A primary intraosseous hemangioma most commonly arises in the vertebral bodies and the calvaria. It generally demonstrates a lytic pattern with an internal striated architecture, often described as resembling a "corduroy cloth" or a "spoked wheel."

3.4.2 Epithelioid hemangioma

An intermediate, locally aggressive lesion. Approximately 18–25% of cases present with multifocal distribution, predominantly in long bones (up to 40%). Radiographically, it appears as a lytic to cystic lesion with a narrow transition zone and cortical thinning. A malignant variant has also been described.

3.4.3 Angiosarcoma

A very rare neoplasm of bone, most frequently affecting the femur (23%), tibia (18%), and humerus (13%). Lesions may be solitary or multifocal. The process is purely osteolytic, highly aggressive, and lacks periosteal reaction.

3.5 Osteoclastic giant-cell-rich tumors

3.5.1 Aneurysmal bone cyst

A benign but expansile lesion is characterized by multiple cystic cavities, the walls of which are composed of fibroblasts, osteoclastic giant cells, and hemosiderin deposits [12]. Fluid–fluid levels may be detected by certain imaging modalities. Clinical presentation may include local pain, acute swelling, or pathological fracture. Approximately 50–60% of lesions occur in long bones – most often the femur, proximal tibia and fibula, and humerus – predominantly in the metaphyses, usually in an eccentric location.

Radiographically, ABC presents as an expansile, lytic lesion with internal septations. Treatment is most often surgical, although recurrence occurs in 15–30% of cases. Alternative approaches include percutaneous injection of sclerosing agents or arterial embolization; however, most lesions are hypovascular.

3.5.2 Nonossifying fibroma

A benign lesion is most often discovered incidentally during imaging performed for unrelated reasons [13]. Histologically, it is composed of bone tissue rich in osteoclastic giant cells and is typically located in the metaphyses of long bones. Formerly used terms – such as *fibrous cortical defect*, *metaphyseal bone defect*, and *benign fibrous histiocytoma* – are no longer recommended.

On radiographs, it appears as a multilocular, asymmetrically distributed lesion aligned with the long axis of the bone and surrounded by a sclerotic margin (**Figure 10**). With skeletal growth, the lesion tends to migrate toward the diaphysis. Small lesions may completely regress in adulthood. A more detailed classification, proposed by Ritschl, distinguishes four groups based on the lesion's relationship to the growth plate and the extent of sclerotic margin formation.

3.5.3 Giant cell tumor of bone, NOS

An intermediate, locally aggressive, and relatively rare neoplasm typically arises after the closure of the growth plates, most frequently between 20 and 50 years of age. The most common sites are the epiphyses of the distal femur and proximal tibia (50–65%) and the distal radius (10–12%).

Radiographically, a giant cell tumor appears as an osteolytic lesion, usually lacking a sclerotic rim (**Figure 11**). A frequent complication is pathological fracture. In a small proportion of cases, malignant transformation may occur, with possible pulmonary metastases.

3.6 Notochordal tumors

3.6.1 Chordoma

A malignant neoplasm arising from embryonic remnants of the notochord exhibits slow but aggressive growth. The most frequent locations are the sacrum (30–50%), the spheno-occipital region (30–35%), and the mobile spine (15–30%), most typically the C2 vertebra.

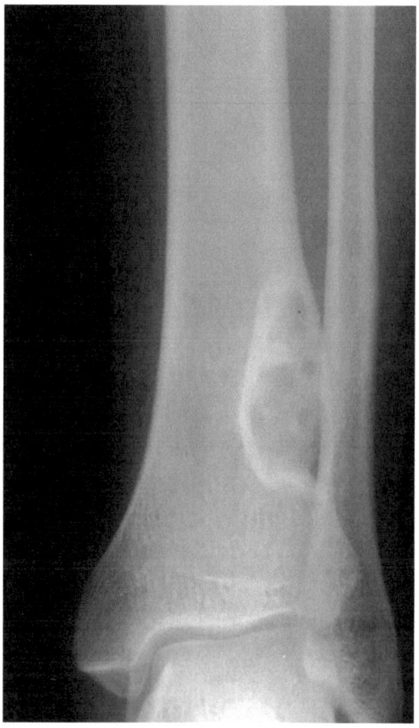

Figure 10.
Distal tibia nonossifying fibroma in a 16-year-old girl.

In spinal locations, extension into the epidural space may occur, leading to neurological symptoms. Magnetic resonance imaging (MRI) is the most valuable modality for diagnosis. The treatment of choice is surgical resection, although recurrence is common.

3.7 Other mesenchymal bone tumors

3.7.1 Simple bone cyst

A benign condition typically diagnosed during childhood or adolescence (up to 20 years of age) is usually asymptomatic and often detected only following a pathological fracture. The most common locations are the proximal humerus (50–60%) and the proximal femur (30%). Diagnosis is readily established from radiographic imaging (**Figure 12**). The differential diagnosis includes intraosseous lipoma (especially in the calcaneus) and intraosseous ganglion.

3.7.2 Fibrous dysplasia

Fibrous dysplasia is a benign bone lesion most frequently located in the diaphyses of long bones of the extremities [14]. Most cases involve monostotic disease, whereas polyostotic forms are less common. Malignant transformation is extremely rare (approximately 0.5%). Radiographically, lesions appear lytic or lytic–sclerotic with a characteristic "ground-glass" appearance; lytic areas are typically homogeneous or

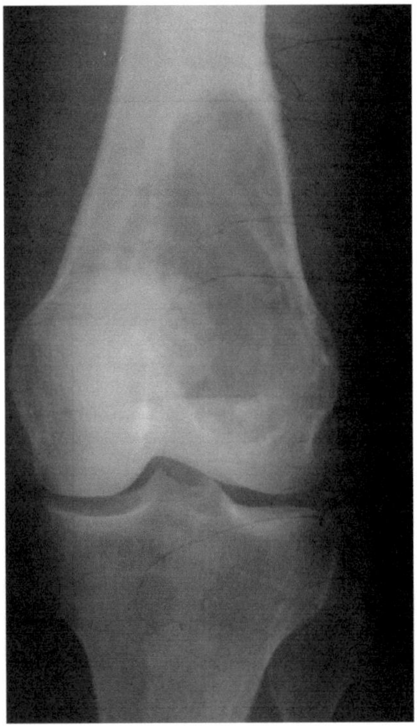

Figure 11.
Distal femur giant cell tumor in a 33-year-old woman.

bubble-like (**Figure 13**). In long bones, the lesion is situated within the medullary cavity and is surrounded by a sclerotic margin. No periosteal reaction is observed. Involvement of the femoral neck may lead to bowing due to bone weakening, producing a "shepherd's hook" deformity. Lesion distribution includes the ribs (28%), proximal femur (23%), calvarium (20%), tibia (8%), and pelvis and humerus (5%). Fibrous dysplasia may occur as part of McCune–Albright syndrome or Mazabraud syndrome.

3.7.3 Bone lipoma

A rare benign bone tumor, most commonly located in the calcaneus (32%), but also in the intertrochanteric region of the femur (20%) and the tibia (13%), is typically identified radiographically as a lytic lesion, with MRI providing superior visualization. In the calcaneus, central calcifications may be present, supporting the diagnosis.

3.8 Leiomyosarcoma

Primary leiomyosarcoma of the bone is extremely rare.

3.9 Bone metastases

Bones represent the third most common site of metastases after the lungs and liver, spreading primarily via the hematogenous route to the bone marrow [15]. The most frequent sites include the vertebrae (with a predominance in the lumbar region over the thoracic or cervical), followed by the pelvis, proximal femur and

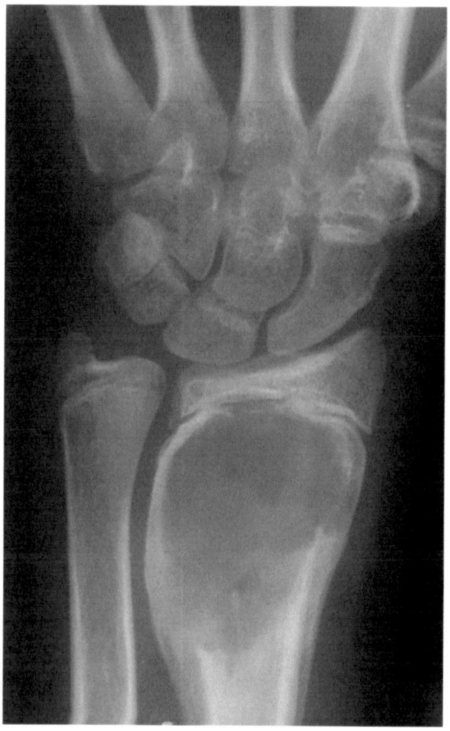

Figure 12.
Distal radius bone cyst in a 16-year-old girl.

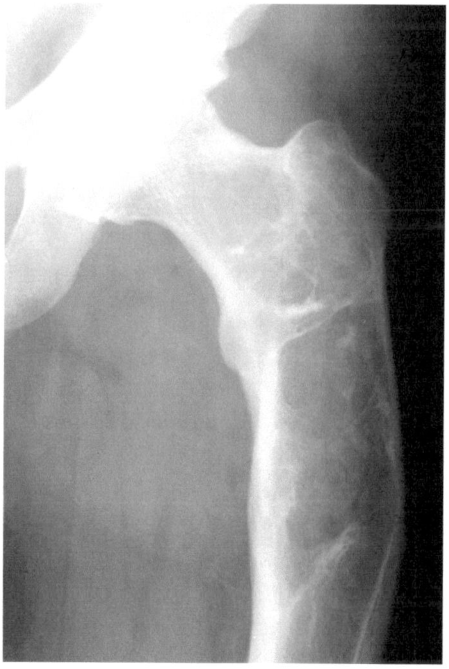

Figure 13.
Proximal femur fibrous dysplasia.

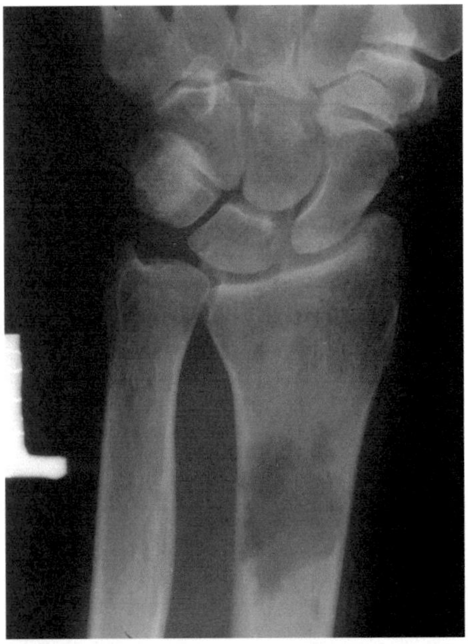

Figure 14.
Distal radius metastasis, pulmonary carcinoma in a 63-year-old man.

humerus, and skull. Depending on the tumor type, metastases can be classified as osteolytic (**Figure 14**) or osteoblastic. Osteolytic lesions are typical of renal cell carcinoma, non-small-cell lung carcinoma, and thyroid carcinoma, whereas osteoblastic lesions are commonly associated with prostate cancer, breast cancer, neural tumors, and other pulmonary malignancies. Mixed lesions can occur in prostate, breast, lung, testicular, and uterine cancers. Confirmation by conventional radiography is not always definitive, even in cases of pathological fracture or vertebral body compression; skeletal scintigraphy and MRI are the methods of choice.

3.10 Hematopoietic bone tumors

3.10.1 Solitary bone plasmacytoma

Solitary bone plasmacytoma is a rare neoplasm of plasma cells, most frequently occurring in bones containing red marrow. The typical age of onset ranges from 40 to 80 years, with a higher prevalence among older individuals. The spine, predominantly the thoracic region, is the most common site of involvement. Radiographically, the lesion appears as a lytic, expansile mass with a bubbly or lamellar structure. Pathological fractures and vertebral compression are frequently observed.

3.10.2 Malignant non-Hodgkin bone lymphoma, NOS

This malignancy can occur at any age, with a peak incidence between 50 and 60 years. Solitary involvement is more common than multifocal disease. The pelvis and vertebrae are the most frequently affected sites. Radiographic findings may be normal, but lytic lesions are usually observed.

3.10.3 Hodgkin lymphoma, NOS

Hodgkin lymphoma spreads via hematogenous or lymphatic routes, with the possibility of direct extension from an involved lymph node. The spine is most commonly affected, often presenting with erosions of the anterior vertebral margins. In cases of solitary involvement of a single vertebral body, the structure may appear diffusely sclerotic, producing the classic "ivory vertebra" appearance.

3.10.4 Langerhans cell histiocytosis (LCH)

Langerhans cell histiocytosis is a multisystem disorder, with the skeleton being the most frequently affected organ, usually manifesting as solitary bone lesions. The disease is often asymptomatic, with incidental detection. The most commonly involved sites are the skull (50%), pelvis (23%), femur (17%), and spine (15%). In the skull, lesions may be solitary or multiple, sharply demarcated, nonsclerotic, and occasionally exhibit double contours resulting from disruption of the inner and outer cortical plates; central sequestra may also be present. In long bones, lesions are typically permeative, with aggressive osteolysis, cortical thinning, and periosteal reaction. Vertebra plana is observed in spinal involvement. Historically, the disease was referred to as "histiocytosis X."

3.10.5 Erdheim–Chester disease

Erdheim–Chester disease is a systemic non-Langerhans cell histiocytosis characterized by inflammation and fibrosis [16]. The condition is relatively rare, though its reported incidence has increased recently. Skeletal involvement is present in most cases, typically causing pain. Other manifestations include pulmonary involvement, diabetes insipidus, retroperitoneal fibrosis, and neurological symptoms. Bone lesions are usually symmetrical and bilateral, with diaphyseal–metaphyseal sclerosis and cortical thickening, in contrast to LCH, which produces lytic lesions.

3.11 Undifferentiated small round cell tumors of bone and soft tissue

These are highly aggressive neoplasms composed of undifferentiated small, round cells, occurring in both bone and soft tissues. They are characterized by rapid growth, destructive local behavior, and a high potential for metastasis, necessitating early and accurate diagnosis.

3.11.1 Ewing sarcoma

Ewing sarcoma represents the second most common malignant tumor in the pediatric population, following osteosarcoma [17]. It originates within the medullary cavity and extends into the compact bone, typically demonstrating permeative osteolysis with potential invasion into adjacent soft tissues. The tumor is associated with a malignant periosteal reaction. Radiographically, it often presents as a large

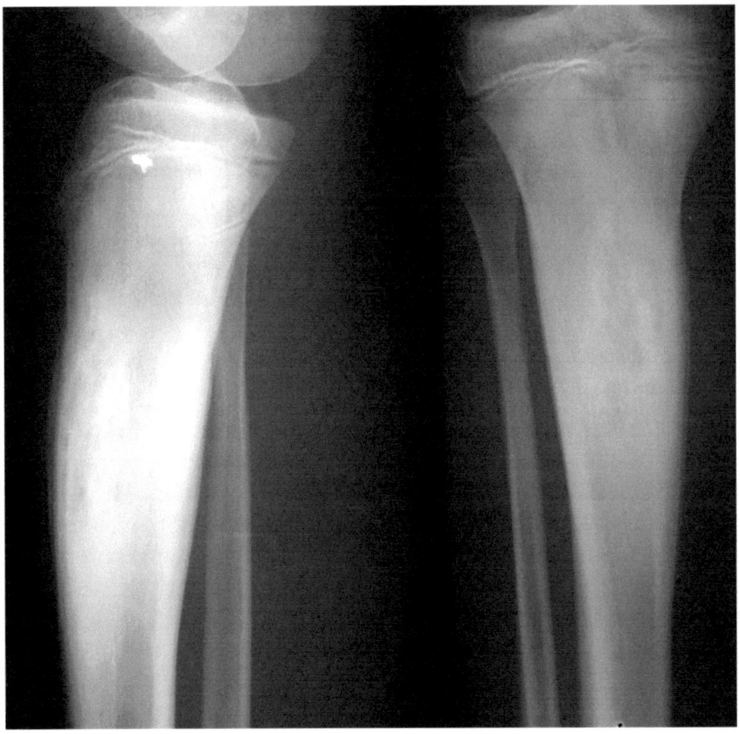

Figure 15.
Tibia Ewing sarcoma "onion skin" periostosis in a 14-year-old boy.

osteolytic lesion with a wide zone of transition to the surrounding bone and may be complicated by a pathological fracture; however, the radiographic appearance of the tumor is highly variable (**Figure 15**). Accurate interpretation of imaging findings is critical to prevent delays in diagnosis. The tumor most frequently involves the metaphysis-diaphysis and diaphysis, with the highest incidence in the femur (25%), pelvis (14%), tibia (11%), and humerus (10%). Metastatic spread is relatively common, primarily to the lungs and bones, with the spine being the most frequently affected skeletal site.

4. Differential diagnosis

The differential diagnosis of bone tumors can be guided by the lesion's anatomical location within the bone, the patient's age, and the radiographic features of tumor aggressiveness. The most common nonneoplastic entity is chronic osteomyelitis, which can often mimic an aggressive bone lesion on imaging [18, 19].

5. Conclusion

Bone tumors represent a diverse group of musculoskeletal disorders. Although their incidence is relatively low, it is important to recognize that malignant forms can also affect the pediatric population, where early and, above all, accurate diagnosis is essential. A comprehensive skeletal radiograph often serves as the initial – and, in some cases, definitive – diagnostic tool for detecting neoplastic lesions of the human skeleton.

Author details

Jan Beran
Department of Radiology and Interventional Radiology, Institute for Clinical and Experimental Medicine (IKEM), Prague, Czech Republic

*Address all correspondence to: jan.beran@ikem.cz

References

[1] Choi JH, Ro JY. the 2020 classification of tumors of bone: An updated review. Advances in Anatomic Pathology. 2021;**28**(3):119–138

[2] Matějovský Z, Povýšil C, Kostní Nádory KJ, Avicenum 1988

[3] Davies AM, Sundaram M, and James SLJ. Imaging of Bone Tumors and Tumor-Like Lesions. Berlin: Springer; 2009

[4] Miller TT. Bone tumors and tumor-like conditions: Analysis with conventional radiography. Radiology. 2008, **246** (3), 662–674

[5] Rana RS, Wu JS. Periosteal reaction. American Journal of Roentgenology 2009, **193**(4), 259–272

[6] Davies M, Lalam R, Woertler K, Bloem J. Aström G ten commandments for the diagnosis of bone tumors. Seminars in Musculoskeletal Radiology. 2020;**24**:203–213

[7] Resnick D, and Kransdorf MJ. Bone and Joint Imaging, 3rd ed. Philadelphia: Elsevier Saunders, 1989:1120–1264

[8] Greenspan A, Beltran J. Orthopedic Imaging, A Practical Approach, 6th ed. Wolters Kluwer, 2015:1333–1987

[9] Radiopaedia. Cartilaginous lesions. 2019. Available from: radiopaedia .org//articles/cartilaginous-lesions.

[10] Haygood TM, Amini B. Chondroid tumors of bone. Seminars in Ultrasound, CT and MRI. 2021;**42**:123–133

[11] Amini B, Valenzuela RF, Bird JE, Haygood TM. Osteoid tumors of bone. Seminars in Ultrasound, CT and MRI. 2021;**42**:134–149

[12] Radiopaedia. Aneurysmal bone cyst. 2025. Available from: radio paedia.org//articles/aneurysmal-bone/-cyst.

[13] Radiopaedia. Non-ossifying fibroma. 2025. Available from: radio paedia.org//articles/non-ossifying/-fibroma/-1

[14] Beran J, Beran T. Fibrózní dysplazie v rtg obrazu (X-ray image of fibrous dysplasia). Ceská Radiologie. 2024;**78**(3):164–169

[15] Costelloe CM, Lin PP, Chuang HH, Amini B, Chainitikun S, et al. Bone metastasis: Mechanism of the metastatic process, imaging and therapy. Seminars in Ultrasound, CT and MRI. 2020;**42**:164–183

[16] Řezáčová R, Kvasnička T, Dvořák P, Slezák O, Tilšer J. Erdheimova-chesterova choroba – Radiologické nálezy u vzácného multisystémového onemocnění (erdheim-chester disease – Radiologic findings of the rare multisystemic disease). Ceská Radiologie. 2024;**78** (4):219–224

[17] Weber MA, Papakonstantinou O, Nikodinovska VV, Vanhoenacker FM. Ewing´s sarcoma and primary osseous lymphoma: Spectrum of imaging appearances. Seminars in Musculoskeletal Radiology. 2019;**23**:36–57

[18] Mehta K, McBee MP, Mihal DC, England EB. Radiographic analysis of bone tumors: A systematic approach. Seminars in Roentgenology. 2017;**52** (4):194–208

[19] Umer M, Hasan OHA, Khan D, Uddin N, Noordin S. Systematic approach to musculoskeletal benign tumors. International Journal of Surgery Oncology. 2017;**2**(11):e46–e46

Chapter 3

Bone Tumors of the Head and Neck

David Wenger, Russell Arellanes and Changxing Liu

Abstract

Head and neck bone tumors are a group of distinct entities, primarily due to the unique and complex anatomy and function of the head and neck region. The correct management of head and neck bone tumors requires multidisciplinary approaches, with surgical management often being the main approach. This chapter will discuss the general management of head and neck bone tumors, including both benign and malignant lesions. We have also included the surgical principles in managing head and neck bone tumors, such as surgical resection and reconstruction. This chapter will cover all types of reconstructions. The goal is to provide insight into managing head and neck bone tumors for head and neck surgeons, oncologists, physical therapists, and speech pathologists.

Keywords: head and neck bone tumor, head and neck oncology, head and neck surgery, head and neck reconstruction, free tissue transfer

1. Introduction

Bone tumors and lesions of the head and neck represent a heterogeneous and diagnostically challenging group of neoplasms arising within the highly specialized craniofacial skeleton, which contains and protects critical neurosensory structures. These lesions encompass a broad spectrum of entities, including primary benign and malignant neoplasms, as well as tumor-like conditions related to developmental, metabolic, and reactive abnormalities. The craniofacial region demonstrates unique biological behavior compared to peripheral skeletal sites, likely attributable to the distinct embryological development of these bones. While primary bone cancers overall account for only approximately 0.2% of all malignancies, their clinical heterogeneity and potential for significant morbidity necessitate accurate diagnosis through a multidisciplinary approach involving pathologists, radiologists, oncologists, and head and neck surgeons. Here, we outline the most common malignant and benign neoplasms that can be found in the bony craniofacial skeleton, along with their common presentations, diagnostic challenges, and management strategies.

2. Ameloblastoma

Ameloblastoma is a rare, benign odontogenic tumor that originates from remnants of the dental enamel and is characterized by its aggressive local behavior and high recurrence rates. Although histologically benign, ameloblastomas exhibit a propensity for cortical bone expansion, infiltration into surrounding soft tissues, and significant facial deformity if left untreated. The tumor most commonly affects the mandible, accounting for approximately 80% of cases, particularly the posterior region, including the ramus and molar area. Maxillary ameloblastomas, though less frequent, tend to be more clinically aggressive due to the thinner cortical bone and proximity to the sinus, orbit, and cranial base [1, 2].

Histologically, ameloblastomas mimic the enamel organ, with neoplastic epithelial cells resembling preameloblasts surrounding a loosely arranged, spiculated formation of reticulum-like cells. Several histologic patterns are recognized, including follicular, plexiform, acanthomatous, desmoplastic, and granular cell variants. The follicular and plexiform patterns are the most common and demonstrate characteristic palisading of columnar basal cells with reverse nuclear polarity and central stellate areas [2, 3]. Additionally, the WHO classifies ameloblastoma into several histological subtypes, including conventional (solid and multicystic) ameloblastoma, unicystic ameloblastoma, peripheral ameloblastoma, and desmoplastic ameloblastoma. Conventional ameloblastoma is the most common subtype, with a high associated recurrence risk. Unicystic ameloblastoma often affects younger patients and may be amenable to conservative treatment depending on mural invasion. The peripheral ameloblastoma subtype is a rare, extraosseous lesion involving the gingiva. The desmoplastic ameloblastoma is radiographically mixed radiolucent—radiopaque with aggressive growth.

At the molecular level, significant advancements have elucidated the genetic underpinnings of ameloblastoma pathogenesis. Notably, BRAF V600E mutations are identified in over 60% of mandibular ameloblastomas, driving persistent activation of the MAPK pathway, thus promoting tumor proliferation and survival [4, 5]. In contrast, maxillary ameloblastomas more commonly harbor mutations in SMO, FGFR2, and RAS, implicating the hedgehog and tyrosine kinase signaling pathways in tumorigenesis [6]. These discoveries have fostered interest in targeted therapies, particularly for recurrent or unresectable cases.

Clinically, patients with ameloblastoma often present with a slow-growing, painless swelling of the jaw, which may progress to facial asymmetry, tooth displacement, malocclusion, or paresthesia. Ulceration and pain are typically late findings. In the maxilla, tumors may cause nasal obstruction or sinus-related symptoms. Diagnostic evaluation begins with imaging studies. Panoramic radiography (orthopantomogram) often reveals a multilocular radiolucent lesion with a classic "soap bubble" or "honeycomb" appearance, though unilocular variants are possible and may mimic odontogenic cysts [7] (**Figure 1**). Computed tomography (CT) is essential for assessing bony destruction, cortical perforation, and extension into adjacent anatomical structures. Magnetic resonance imaging (MRI) is capable of providing superior soft tissue resolution, useful for delineating cystic from solid tumor components and evaluating proximity to the orbit or intracranial space [8]. Biopsy remains necessary for histopathologic confirmation. Intraoral incisional biopsy is typically preferred, and care should be taken to avoid contamination of uninvolved bone to prevent tumor cell seeding.

Surgical excision remains the gold standard for treatment due to the tumor's invasive nature and high recurrence rate following conservative approaches such as curettage or enucleation. In conventional (solid/multicystic) ameloblastomas, wide

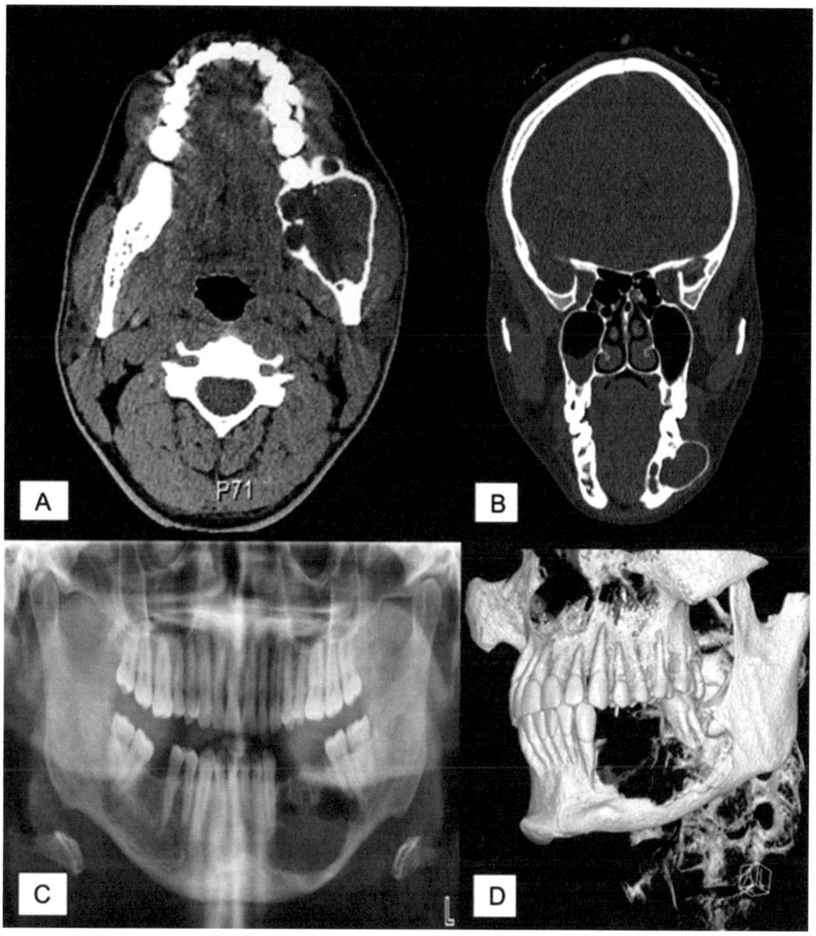

Figure 1.
Ameloblastoma of the mandible. (A) Axial CT imaging of an ameloblastoma of the left angle of the mandible. (B) Coronal section of the same lesion. (C) Panorex of an ameloblastoma of the left mandibular body. (D) 3D reconstruction of an ameloblastoma of the left mandibular body [1–4].

local excision with 1 to 1.5 cm margins is recommended to ensure complete tumor clearance. This typically necessitates a segmental mandibulectomy for mandibular lesions or partial maxillectomy for maxillary tumors [9]. Marginal (rim) resections or simple curettage carry recurrence rates as high as 50–90%, especially for tumors with mural or soft tissue involvement [10]. In unicystic ameloblastomas, which predominantly affect younger patients, treatment may vary depending on the histologic subtype. Luminal and intraluminal variants may be amenable to enucleation and peripheral ostectomy, whereas those with mural invasion require more aggressive resection due to higher recurrence risk [11].

Reconstruction following ablative surgery poses both functional and aesthetic challenges, especially in extensive mandibular or midface defects. Vascularized free tissue transfer is the current standard for mandibular reconstruction, with the fibula free flap offering the advantages of adequate bone length, the possibility for dental implant placement, and a dual-skin paddle for intraoral and cutaneous resurfacing [11, 12]. Alternative options include scapular or iliac crest free flaps, selected based on the specific contour and volume requirements of the defect. In cases where free flap reconstruction is not feasible, titanium reconstruction plates may be employed as a temporary or definitive solution, though long-term stability and exposure remain concerns. Maxillary defects often require obturators or osseous flaps, particularly when the orbital floor or nasal cavity is involved.

Adjunctive therapy for ameloblastoma has historically been limited. The tumor is overall considered to be radio-resistant, and radiotherapy is reserved for unresectable, recurrent, or residual disease when complete re-excision is not feasible [13, 14]. However, with the advent of targeted molecular therapy, agents such as BRAF inhibitors (vemurafenib, dabrafenib) and MEK inhibitors have shown clinical benefit in BRAF-mutated ameloblastomas, achieving tumor volume reduction and, in some cases, enabling less extensive surgery [14]. Clinical trials and case series continue to explore their role, particularly in the neoadjuvant setting.

Long-term surveillance is imperative, given the tumor's notorious propensity for late recurrence. Recurrence has been reported decades after initial treatment, necessitating a follow-up period extending beyond 10 years. Annual imaging, preferably CT or MRI, is advisable for early detection, especially in the first five postoperative years when recurrence is most likely [15].

Although most ameloblastomas are benign, two malignant entities must be recognized: malignant ameloblastoma and ameloblastic carcinoma. Malignant ameloblastoma exhibits benign histology but metastasizes, most often to the lungs or lymph nodes. Ameloblastic carcinoma displays overt cytologic atypia, mitotic activity, and architectural disarray, with a more aggressive clinical course and poorer prognosis. These rare variants warrant more aggressive multimodal treatment, including wide excision, neck dissection, and consideration of adjuvant radiation or chemotherapy [15, 16].

3. Osteoma, osteoid osteoma, and osteoblastoma

Benign osteogenic tumors of the craniofacial region, though relatively rare, are of significant clinical relevance to otolaryngologists and oral and maxillofacial surgeons. Osteoma, osteoid osteoma, and osteoblastoma represent a spectrum of benign bone-forming tumors characterized by varying patterns of pain, growth, and anatomical location. While histologically nonmalignant, these lesions may produce substantial functional and aesthetic impairment due to their proximity to critical craniofacial structures.

Osteogenic tumors arise from osteoblast-lineage cells responsible for bone matrix production. They are classified based on their clinical behavior, radiologic appearance, and histological architecture. Osteomas are composed of mature lamellar bone and are most frequently encountered in the craniofacial skeleton, particularly within the paranasal sinuses. They are considered hamartomatous growths rather than true neoplasms [17]. In contrast, osteoid osteoma and osteoblastoma are true neoplastic entities. Osteoid osteoma is typically a small, painful lesion that responds to nonsteroidal anti-inflammatory drugs (NSAIDs), while osteoblastoma is larger, exhibits less reactive sclerosis, and may demonstrate locally aggressive behavior [18, 19].

4. Osteoma

Osteomas most commonly present in young to middle-aged adults and exhibit a slight male predominance. They may occur sporadically or as part of Gardner syndrome, an autosomal dominant condition characterized by familial adenomatous polyposis, epidermoid cysts, and multiple craniofacial osteomas [20]. The pathogenesis of osteomas remains under investigation. Peripheral osteomas are hypothesized to arise as reactive processes to chronic inflammation or trauma, whereas central osteomas may represent developmental anomalies or true neoplastic growths [21].

Craniofacial osteomas are most frequently located in the frontal sinus, followed by the ethmoid, maxillary, and sphenoid sinuses. Many lesions are asymptomatic and identified incidentally on imaging. When symptoms do arise, patients may experience headache, facial pain or pressure, recurrent sinusitis, nasal obstruction, or, in cases of orbital extension, proptosis and diplopia. Larger lesions can obstruct sinus drainage pathways or invade adjacent anatomical compartments, leading to visual disturbances or intracranial pressure effects [22].

High-resolution CT is the diagnostic modality of choice, revealing a well-demarcated, hyperdense lesion composed of compact or cancellous bone (**Figure 2**). CT imaging provides excellent visualization of lesion margins and potential

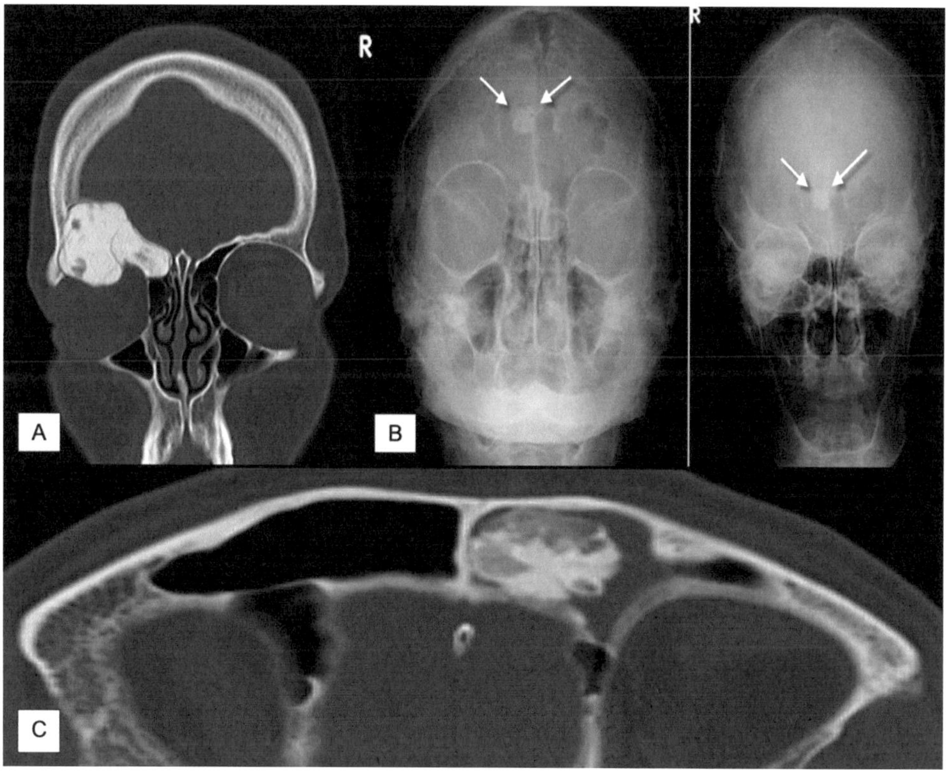

Figure 2.
Osteoma of the frontal sinus. (A) Coronal CT reconstruction of an osteoma of the right posterior table of the frontal sinus. (B) Xray of an osteoma of the right frontal sinus. (C) Axial CT of an osteoma of the left frontal sinus [5–7].

anatomical distortion. MRI is reserved for cases in which soft tissue involvement, intracranial extension, or periorbital displacement is suspected. Histologically, osteomas consist of dense, lamellar bone with limited cellularity and an absence of atypia.

Asymptomatic and small osteomas may be safely observed with periodic radiologic surveillance. Surgical excision is indicated in patients with symptomatic lesions, functional impairment (e.g., sinus obstruction or proptosis), significant cosmetic deformity, or suspicion of Gardner syndrome. Endonasal endoscopic approaches are preferred for paranasal sinus osteomas due to reduced morbidity and excellent visualization. Larger lesions or those involving the skull base or lateral facial skeleton may necessitate external or transfacial approaches for adequate exposure. Complete resection is curative, and recurrence is rare following total excision [23].

5. Osteoid osteoma

Osteoid osteoma is a benign bone-forming neoplasm consisting of a central nidus of immature osteoid and woven bone surrounded by reactive sclerotic bone. This tumor primarily affects males between 10 and 30 years of age and is uncommon in the craniofacial region, although isolated cases involving the mandible, maxilla, and temporal bone have been described [24]. Unlike osteomas, osteoid osteomas are associated with intense, localized pain that is characteristically worse at night and dramatically responsive to NSAIDs. This pain is believed to result from elevated prostaglandin levels within the vascular stroma of the nidus [25].

Craniofacial osteoid osteomas typically present with persistent localized pain, often described as nocturnal and severe. Depending on the location, patients may also experience swelling or tenderness in the affected area, restricted jaw movement or trismus when the mandibular condyle is involved, and hearing loss or otalgia in cases involving the temporal bone. The clinical presentation often mimics that of odontogenic infections or temporomandibular joint disorders, contributing to diagnostic delay.

CT imaging is highly sensitive in detecting the characteristic radiolucent nidus of osteoid osteoma, usually less than 1.5 cm in diameter, often surrounded by a halo of dense reactive sclerosis (**Figure 3**). The nidus may demonstrate central mineralization. MRI is less specific but may show surrounding marrow edema and soft tissue reaction. Histologically, the lesion consists of irregular osteoid trabeculae lined by osteoblasts in a highly vascular stroma.

Although NSAIDs provide temporary symptom relief, definitive management requires complete surgical excision of the nidus. Accurate preoperative localization is critical to ensure complete resection and prevent recurrence. In the craniofacial skeleton, en bloc resection or precise curettage is typically employed. CT-guided radiofrequency ablation (RFA) has emerged as a minimally invasive alternative in other skeletal regions, but its use in the head and neck is limited by proximity to neurovascular structures and the potential for collateral damage [26]. Prognosis is excellent with complete resection, and recurrence is uncommon.

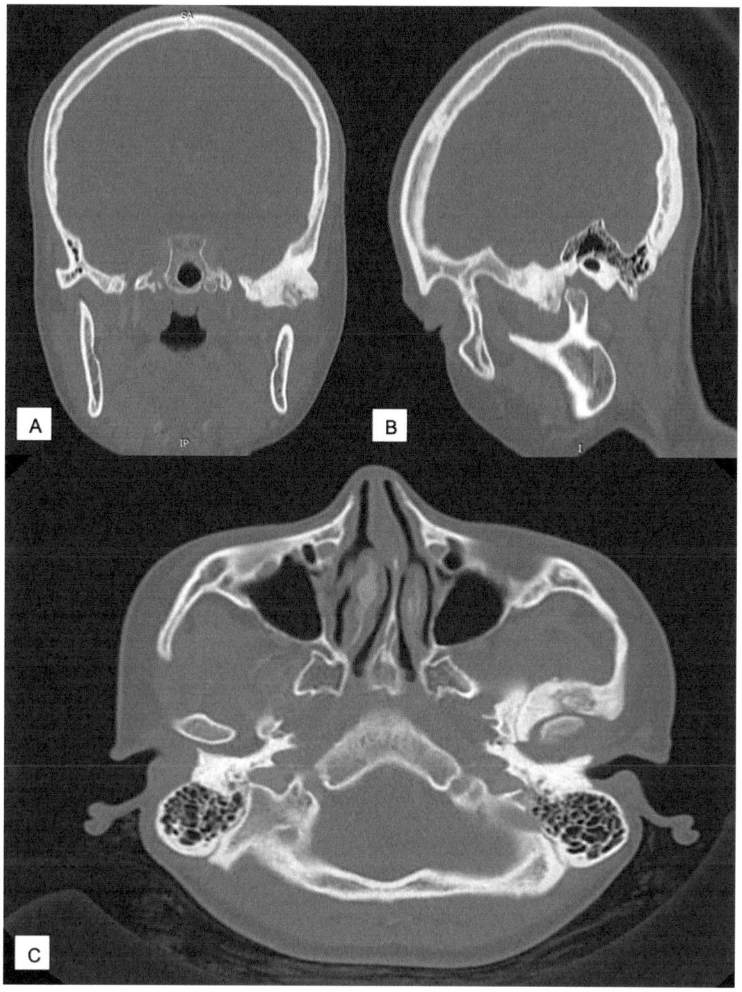

Figure 3.
Osteoid osteoma of the left temporal bone. (A) Coronal CT reconstruction. (B) Sagittal CT reconstruction. (C) Axial CT [8].

6. Osteoblastoma

Osteoblastoma is a rare, benign but potentially aggressive bone-forming tumor that shares histological features with osteoid osteoma but is distinguished by its larger size (usually >1.5–2 cm), reduced reactive sclerosis, and greater tendency for local expansion. Like osteoid osteoma, osteoblastoma typically affects young adults between the ages of 10 and 30 and shows a slight male predilection [27]. Though more frequently found in the spine and long bones, osteoblastoma may also affect the craniofacial skeleton, particularly the mandible, maxilla, orbit, or temporal bone. Pain associated with osteoblastoma is often dull, persistent, and less responsive to NSAIDs, distinguishing it from the classic presentation of osteoid osteoma.

The clinical presentation varies by anatomical location and tumor size. Patients may present with facial swelling, persistent pain, or facial asymmetry. When located in the jaw, the tumor may impair mandibular function or cause trismus. In cases involving the temporal bone, symptoms such as hearing loss, tinnitus, or otalgia may arise. Lesions affecting the skull base or orbit may produce neurological signs or visual disturbances due to mass effect. While histologically benign, some osteoblastomas demonstrate local invasiveness, particularly those classified as "aggressive osteoblastomas."

Radiologic evaluation typically reveals a well-circumscribed, radiolucent or mixed-density lesion, often with internal mineralization and lacking the dense sclerotic rim seen in osteoid osteoma. CT imaging delineates bony involvement, while MRI is helpful in evaluating soft tissue extension (**Figure 4**). Histologically, osteoblastomas display trabeculae of osteoid and woven bone lined by prominent osteoblasts in a richly vascularized stroma. The presence of mitotic figures may be noted, but nuclear atypia is minimal, distinguishing the lesion from osteosarcoma.

Surgical resection is the mainstay of treatment for osteoblastoma. Depending on the tumor's location and extent, options include curettage, marginal resection, or en bloc excision. In the craniofacial skeleton, preservation of neurovascular structures and facial aesthetics must be balanced with the goal of achieving complete tumor removal. Aggressive variants of osteoblastoma may recur or exhibit atypical growth, necessitating wider margins and closer postoperative follow-up [28]. Radiation therapy is generally avoided due to the theoretical risk of sarcomatous transformation. Recurrence rates vary from 10% to 20% in cases of incomplete excision [29].

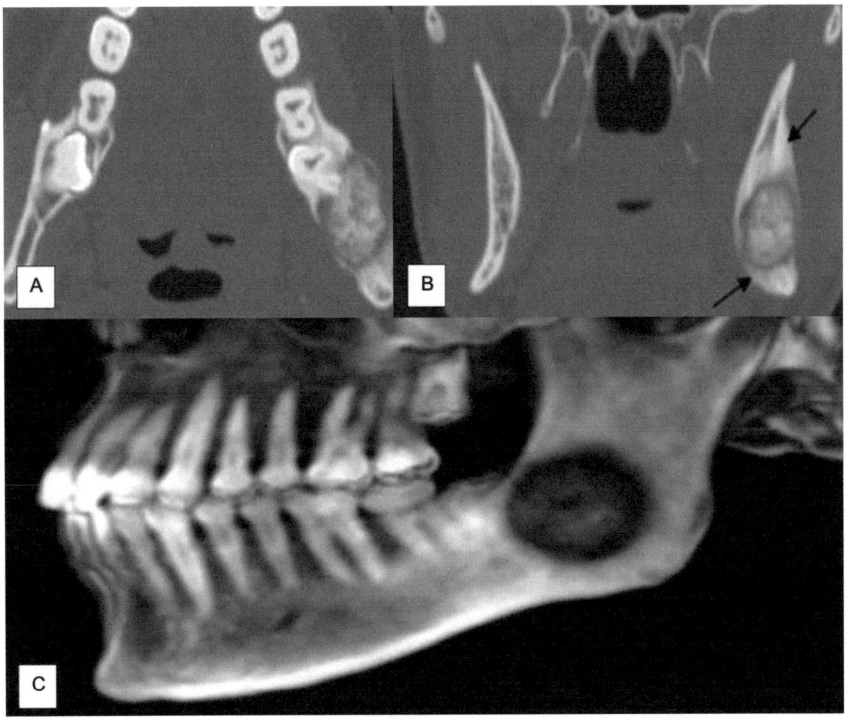

Figure 4.
Osteoblastoma of the left mandibular angle. (A) Axial CT section. (B) Coronal CT reconstruction of the same lesion. (C) Lateral radiograph of the same lesion [9].

7. Fibrous dysplasia

Fibrous dysplasia (FD) is a benign, noninherited developmental anomaly of bone characterized by the replacement of normal lamellar bone with fibro-osseous connective tissue. This condition results from a postzygotic activating mutation in the *GNAS* gene, which encodes the α-subunit of the stimulatory G protein (Gsα). This mutation leads to constitutive activation of adenylate cyclase and overproduction of cyclic AMP, promoting the proliferation of fibroblasts and defective osteoblastic differentiation. Consequently, normal bone is replaced by poorly organized, immature woven bone embedded in a fibrous stroma, leading to weakened and expansile lesions of affected bones [30, 31].

FD can present in a monostotic form, involving a single bone, or a polyostotic form, affecting multiple bones. When associated with endocrinopathies (e.g., precocious puberty, hyperthyroidism) and café-au-lait skin pigmentation, it is part of McCune-Albright syndrome. In the head and neck region, FD most commonly involves the maxilla, followed by the mandible, frontal, sphenoid, ethmoid, and temporal bones. Craniofacial FD typically presents during childhood or adolescence and may manifest as painless facial swelling, deformity, dental malocclusion, nasal obstruction, or cranial neuropathies, depending on the involved anatomical structures [32, 33].

Radiographically, FD classically demonstrates a "ground-glass" appearance on CT (**Figure 5**), which reflects the mixture of fibrous and osseous components. The lesion is usually ill-defined, expansile, and can exhibit thinning of the cortical bone while maintaining the overall bony contour. Three radiographic patterns have been described: ground-glass, homogeneously radiopaque, and cystic. CT is the imaging modality of choice for assessing the extent of craniofacial involvement, anatomical distortion, and potential complications such as sinus obstruction or orbital displacement. MRI is generally less specific but can be helpful in evaluating soft tissue or optic nerve compression [34].

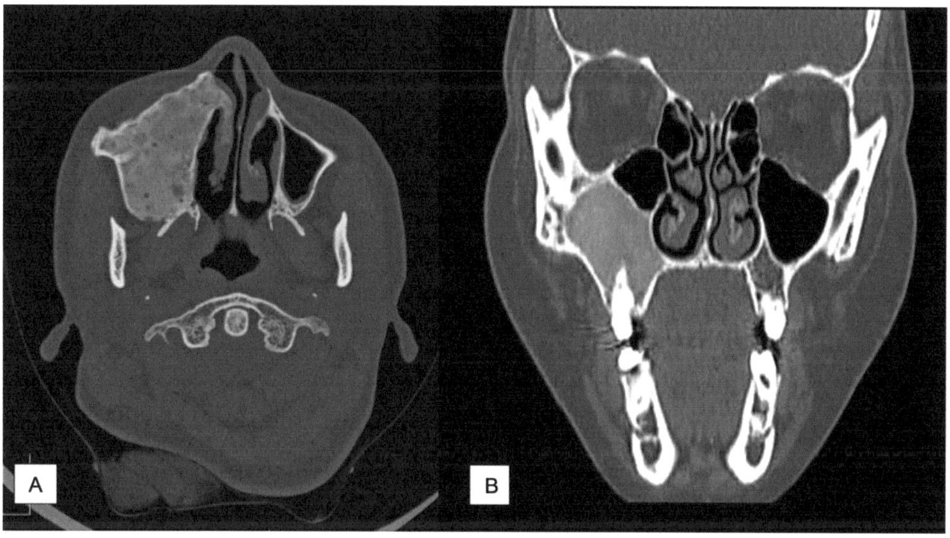

Figure 5.
FD of the right maxilla. (A) Axial CT section. (B) Coronal CT reconstruction [10, 11].

The management of FD in the head and neck depends on the extent of the disease, symptoms, anatomical distortion, and risk of complications. Observation with periodic imaging is appropriate for asymptomatic, stable lesions. Surgical intervention is reserved for patients with functional impairment, progressive deformity, or cosmetic concerns. Conservative recontouring (shaving) may suffice for mild cases, whereas radical excision with reconstruction is considered in aggressive or recurrent disease. Complete resection is often not feasible due to the lesion's diffuse and poorly defined borders, particularly in skull base involvement. Bisphosphonates have been used to reduce bone pain and suppress bone turnover, although their efficacy in altering disease progression is limited. Malignant transformation, although rare (<1%), has been reported, especially in polyostotic disease or previously irradiated lesions [34–36].

8. Ossifying fibroma

Ossifying fibromas of the head and neck are benign, well-demarcated fibro-osseous neoplasms that most commonly arise from the periodontal ligament, with a predilection for the mandible, maxilla, and paranasal sinuses. Pathophysiologically, these lesions are characterized by the replacement of normal bone with cellular fibrous tissue containing varying degrees of mineralized material, including bone and cementum-like deposits. Two main subtypes are recognized: juvenile ossifying fibroma (JOF), which includes trabecular and psammomatoid variants, and cemento-ossifying fibroma (COF), with JOF tending to be more locally aggressive and occurring in younger patients [37–39].

The diagnostic workup involves a combination of clinical, radiographic, and histopathological assessments. Clinically, patients present with painless, slow-growing swelling, facial asymmetry, or symptoms related to mass effect, such as nasal obstruction and proptosis. Radiographically, ossifying fibromas typically appear as well-circumscribed, expansible lesions with mixed radiodensity, often unilocular, and may cause displacement of adjacent teeth or bone expansion without cortical perforation (**Figure 6**) [37–41]. Definitive diagnosis requires

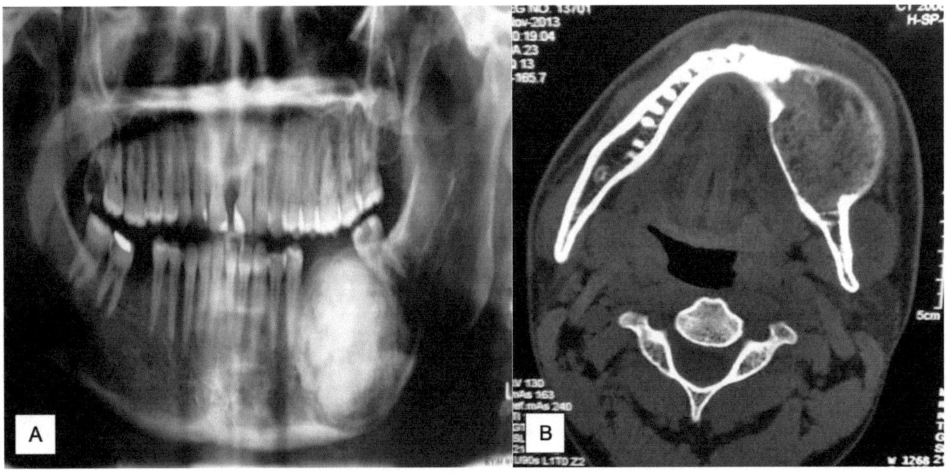

Figure 6.
Ossifying fibroma of the left mandibular body. (A) Panorex imaging. (B) Axial CT section [12, 13].

histopathological confirmation, with JOF showing either trabecular or psammomatoid ossicles in a cellular stroma [38, 42].

Management of ossifying fibromas is primarily surgical. For JOF, enucleation followed by curettage or peripheral osteotomy is recommended to minimize morbidity, as simple curettage alone is associated with higher recurrence rates. More extensive resection is reserved for large, recurrent, or skull base-involving lesions but carries greater risk of functional and cosmetic sequelae [37–39, 43, 44]. For adult COF, asymptomatic lesions may be managed with observation, such as "wait and scan," while symptomatic or enlarging lesions warrant surgical excision, which can often be performed endoscopically for paranasal sinus involvement [45]. Long-term follow-up is essential due to the risk of recurrence, particularly in juvenile variants [38, 39].

9. Giant cell tumor of bone

Giant cell tumor of bone (GCTB) is classified as an intermediate, locally aggressive neoplasm, with a predilection for skeletally mature individuals. In the head and neck, GCTB most commonly involves the sphenoid, temporal, and maxillofacial bones [46, 47]. The tumor is characterized by neoplastic mononuclear stromal cells that overexpress RANKL, driving the recruitment and proliferation of osteoclast-like multinucleated giant cells, which mediate bone resorption and local destruction [48, 49]. The presence of the H3F3A (G34W) mutation is highly specific for GCTB and can be detected by immunohistochemistry, facilitating differentiation from other giant cell-rich lesions such as aneurysmal bone cysts, tenosynovial giant cell tumors, and giant cell reparative granulomas [50]. The cumulative risk of malignant transformation is estimated at approximately 4%, with secondary malignancy most often following radiotherapy.

A comprehensive diagnostic approach is essential for accurate identification and management. Initial evaluation should include high-resolution CT and MRI to delineate the extent of osseous and soft tissue involvement, particularly in complex skull base or temporomandibular joint cases [49, 51]. Radiographically, GCTB often presents as an eccentric, lytic lesion with cortical thinning or destruction and may show soft tissue extension [49]. MRI is valuable for assessing extraosseous spread and distinguishing GCTB from other entities; for example, fluid-fluid levels on MRI suggest an aneurysmal bone cyst [46]. Histopathological confirmation is mandatory, with strong p63 positivity in mononuclear stromal cells and H3.3-G34W immunohistostaining supporting the diagnosis [50]. Core biopsy is preferred for definitive diagnosis and subclassification [46]. PD–L1 expression may be associated with higher recurrence risk and is under investigation as a prognostic marker.

The cornerstone of GCTB management in the head and neck is complete surgical excision with negative margins, which offers the best chance for cure and minimizes recurrence risk [46, 49]. In anatomically challenging locations, such as the skull base, endoscopic or nerve-sparing approaches may be considered to reduce morbidity [51]. Extended intralesional curettage with local adjuvants (e.g., phenol, PMMA, cryosurgery) is preferred when joint or critical structure preservation is feasible, though recurrence rates remain significant [49, 52]. En bloc resection is reserved for highly aggressive lesions or when joint salvage is not possible, but may result in poorer functional outcomes [52].

For unresectable, recurrent, or borderline resectable tumors, denosumab – a monoclonal antibody targeting RANKL – is FDA-approved and increasingly utilized [48–52]. Denosumab is typically administered at 120 mg subcutaneously every 4 weeks, with loading doses on Days 8 and 15 of the first cycle [51]. Neoadjuvant denosumab can reduce tumor size and facilitate less morbid surgery but may increase local recurrence rates if used preoperatively, and its optimal duration is under investigation [48]. Long-term denosumab may be considered for unresectable or metastatic disease, with ongoing monitoring for adverse effects and malignant transformation [49, 52]. Bisphosphonates, such as zoledronic acid, have shown activity in controlling tumor growth and may be considered as adjuncts, though direct comparative trials are ongoing [48, 50]. Radiotherapy is reserved for cases where surgery and RANKL inhibitors are contraindicated due to the risk of malignant transformation [49, 52].

Long-term follow-up with serial imaging is recommended due to the risk of local recurrence and rare malignant transformation [49]. Multidisciplinary collaboration is essential for optimal outcomes, particularly in complex cases of the head and neck.

10. Chondromas

Chondromas of the head and neck are rare, benign cartilaginous tumors that may arise in soft tissue or bone, including sites such as the nasal septum, tongue, larynx, jaw, chin, masticatory space, and temporomandibular joint [53–59]. Their pathophysiology is characterized by the proliferation of mature hyaline cartilage, often with focal calcification. The etiology is unclear, but repeated microtrauma has been suggested as a possible factor in some cases [55].

Clinical presentation depends on tumor location and size. Common symptoms include painless, slow-growing submucosal or subcutaneous masses, speech impairment, swallowing disturbances, nasal obstruction, epistaxis, hoarseness, stridor, dyspnea, and cranial nerve palsies if the cranial base is involved [53, 54, 56–58, 60, 61]. Lesions may remain asymptomatic until they reach a size that causes functional impairment or cosmetic concerns.

Diagnostic workup begins with a thorough clinical examination and imaging. MRI is preferred for soft tissue localization and extent, while CT is valuable for assessing calcification, bone involvement, and surgical planning (**Figure** 7) [53–56, 58, 60, 61]. Definitive diagnosis requires histopathological examination, which demonstrates mature cartilage without atypia. Distinguishing chondroma from low-grade chondrosarcoma can be challenging; correlation of clinical, radiologic, and histologic features, along with close follow-up, is essential [61, 62].

Management is primarily surgical excision with clear margins, which is curative in most cases [53–56, 58–61]. Endoscopic approaches are favored for accessible lesions, such as the nasal septum [54]. There is no established role for radiotherapy or chemotherapy in benign chondromas. Long-term follow-up is recommended to monitor for recurrence or rare malignant transformation, especially in syndromic cases (e.g., Ollier disease) [63]. Multidisciplinary management is indicated for complex cases involving the cranial base or TMJ [57, 60].

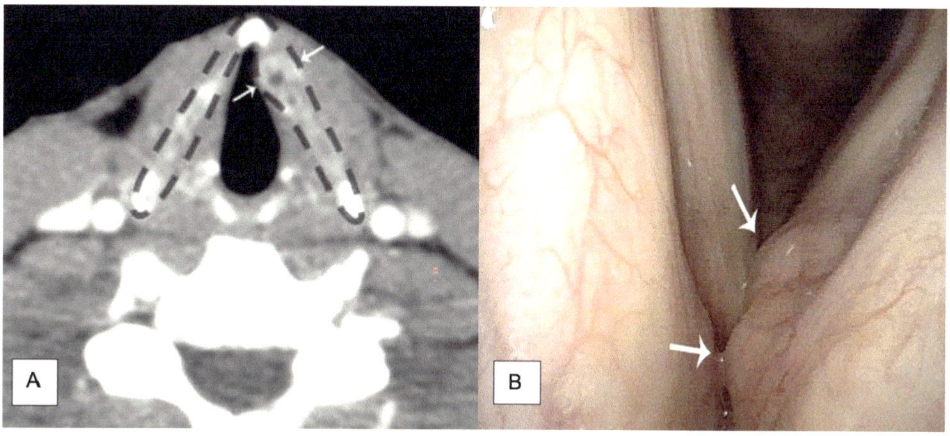

Figure 7.
Chondroma of the thyroid cartilage. (A) CT soft tissue neck with contrast showing a chondroma of the left hemilarynx. (B) Endoscopic view of the same lesion [14].

11. Osteosarcoma

Osteosarcoma of the head and neck (OSHN) is an uncommon, aggressive malignant bone tumor that accounts for less than 10% of all osteosarcomas and fewer than 1% of head and neck malignancies [64, 65]. Unlike appendicular osteosarcoma, which typically presents in adolescents, OSHN is more often diagnosed in adults in the third to fifth decades of life [64, 66]. The pathophysiology is characterized by malignant mesenchymal cells that produce an osteoid matrix, with histologic subtypes including osteoblastic, chondroblastic, and fibroblastic patterns. Risk factors include prior radiation exposure, Paget's disease, and inherited syndromes such as Li-Fraumeni [64, 67]. While distant metastasis is less common than in long-bone osteosarcoma, OSHN demonstrates a higher propensity for local recurrence, making margin-negative resection critical [65, 68].

Patients frequently present with nonspecific or insidious symptoms. Common mandibular findings include painless or painful swelling, cortical expansion, facial asymmetry, tooth mobility, or ill-fitting dentures [65, 69]. Involvement of the inferior alveolar nerve may lead to paresthesia. Maxillary tumors may manifest as nasal obstruction, epistaxis, or orbital symptoms such as proptosis [64, 69]. Pathologic fractures, common in appendicular disease, are less typical in gnathic osteosarcomas. Diagnostic delay is frequent because of overlapping features with odontogenic or inflammatory lesions [69].

Work-up relies on multimodality imaging. CT scanning delineates cortical destruction, ossified soft-tissue extension, and occasionally a sunburst periosteal reaction, while MRI better defines marrow invasion, perineural spread, and soft-tissue extension (**Figure 8**) [66]. PET/CT or bone scintigraphy can assist in staging, and chest CT is indicated for pulmonary metastasis screening [67]. Histopathologic confirmation via incisional biopsy remains essential, but the biopsy tract should be carefully planned to avoid compromising future surgical margins [66]. Staging generally follows AJCC bone sarcoma TNM and grade (G) systems, although craniofacial disease has unique prognostic behavior [67].

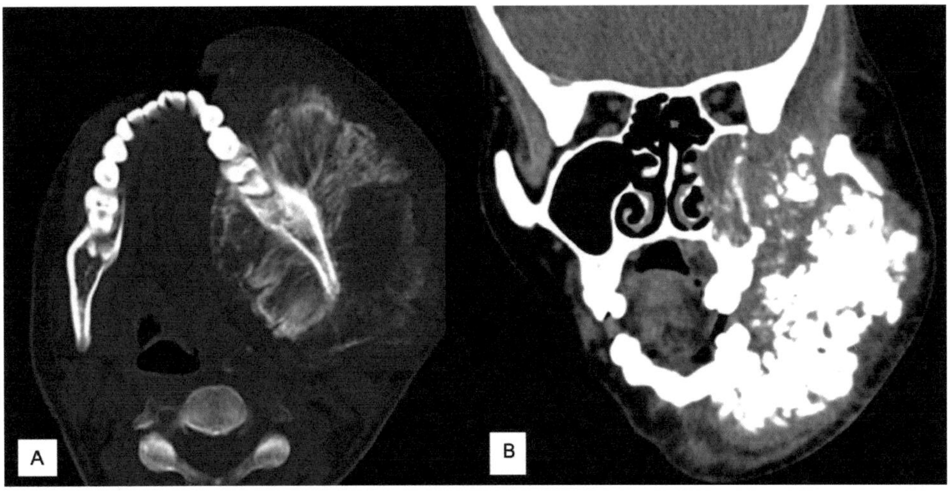

Figure 8.
Osteosarcoma of the mandible. (A) Axial CT of an osteosarcoma of the left mandibular angle. (B) Coronal CT reconstruction of an osteosarcoma of the left mandible with invasion of the left maxilla [15].

Management is centered on surgical resection with wide margins, which remains the single most important prognostic factor [65, 68]. Many centers aim for ≥2 cm of bony clearance and ≥5 mm of soft-tissue clearance when feasible, with worse outcomes observed when margins are <1 cm. Achieving adequate resection is often challenging due to proximity to critical neurovascular structures. Reconstructive planning, frequently employing vascularized free bone flaps, is integral for the restoration of form, function, and aesthetics[65, 69].

The role of adjuvant therapy in OSHN is more controversial than in appendicular disease. While systemic chemotherapy is standard in long-bone osteosarcoma, its survival benefit in OSHN is inconsistent; it may be considered in high-grade lesions or when metastatic potential is suspected [68, 70]. Postoperative radiotherapy can improve local control in the setting of positive or close margins, unresectable disease, or when surgical clearance is anatomically limited. Advanced delivery methods, including IMRT or particle therapy, may optimize local disease control while sparing adjacent critical structures [68, 71]. Long-term surveillance is essential, as most recurrences occur within the first 2–3 years, with both local recurrence and pulmonary metastasis requiring vigilance [70].

12. Chondrosarcoma

Chondrosarcoma (CS) is a malignant neoplasm of cartilage-producing cells that uncommonly affects the head and neck, accounting for a small fraction of craniofacial tumors, with the skull base, nasal–paranasal region, larynx, and mandible among the typical sites [72, 73]. Most head and neck CS are conventional (hyaline) chondrosarcomas that grow slowly and are graded histologically (Grade 1–3), with higher-grade and dedifferentiated or mesenchymal subtypes showing more aggressive clinical biology and worse outcomes [73, 74]. Molecularly, cranial/skull-base CS frequently harbor IDH1/2 mutations and other cartilaginous-tumor alterations, whereas mesenchymal chondrosarcoma shows distinct gene fusions (and behaves more like a high-grade small-round-cell sarcoma), a distinction that carries therapeutic and prognostic implications [74, 75].

Presentation is anatomic-site dependent but often indolent, producing symptoms from mass effect rather than early systemic spread. Skull-base lesions classically present with cranial neuropathies, diplopia, headaches, or trigeminal/optic pathway symptoms; paranasal/nasal tumors cause obstruction, epistaxis, or facial fullness; laryngeal CS presents with hoarseness, airway symptoms, or a submucosal neck mass; mandibular lesions may present with localized swelling, tooth mobility, or alveolar paresthesia [72, 76]. Because low-grade CS can mimic benign cartilaginous lesions radiographically and symptomatically, a high index of suspicion is required for progressive or atypical presentations, and biopsy should be pursued in concert with imaging and multidisciplinary planning [72, 77].

Cross-sectional imaging is mandatory: thin-slice CT best defines cortical destruction and calcified chondroid matrix (ring-and-arc calcifications), while MRI delineates marrow, dural, cavernous sinus, and perineural extension and helps with surgical planning (**Figure 9**) [77, 78]. PET/CT and bone scintigraphy have limited sensitivity for low-grade CS but can be useful for higher-grade or dedifferentiated lesions and systemic staging; chest CT is recommended because the lung is the most common site of distant spread in higher-grade disease [78, 79]. Biopsy (endoscopic, open, or image-guided) must be planned along a definitive resection corridor to avoid contamination; because grade drives management, pathologic assessment should include grading and ancillary molecular testing (e.g., IDH1/2, where available) when results may influence systemic or radiation decisions [74, 75].

Surgery aiming for maximal safe resection with negative margins remains the principal curative therapy for resectable head and neck CS; in skull-base disease, gross total resection, when feasible, improves local control but must be balanced against neurologic risk [76, 78]. Conventional low-grade CS are generally managed with surgery alone when wide/radical resection is achieved; adjuvant radiation is considered for subtotal resection, positive margins, higher-grade or dedifferentiated tumors, or when anatomy precludes complete resection. Modern high-dose conformal photon therapy, proton therapy, and carbon-ion therapy have been used effectively at skull-base sites to optimize local control while limiting dose to critical structures – particle therapy shows particular promise for radioresistant or surgically constrained lesions in several series and meta-analyses [74, 75, 79, 80]. Systemic chemotherapy has a limited role for conventional low- to intermediate-grade CS but is indicated for mesenchymal and dedifferentiated subtypes or metastatic/high-grade disease, often following regimens used for other high-grade bone sarcomas; enrollment in sarcoma multidisciplinary centers and clinical trials is recommended for rare histologies [74, 80]. Long-term surveillance must be prolonged (years to decades) because of the potential for late recurrence – routine interval clinical exams and periodic MRI of the primary site, plus chest imaging, are standard components of follow-up, with intensity tailored to grade and margin status [76, 78].

Given the anatomical complexity of craniofacial CS, coordinate care early with skull-base neurosurgery, radiation oncology (including particle therapy programs), head and neck reconstructive teams, and sarcoma pathology/genomics services. Plan biopsies strategically to preserve future reconstructive options and definitive surgical corridors. For skull-base or

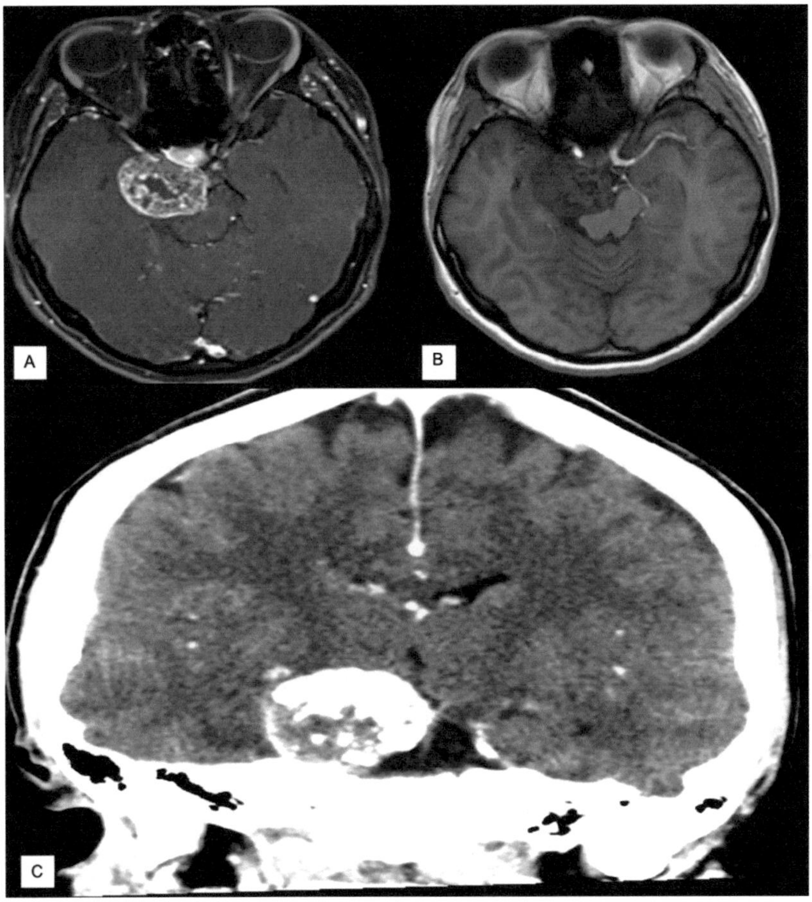

Figure 9.
Chondrosarcoma of the skull base. (A) Axial T1-weighted MRI of an osteosarcoma of the right sphenoid sinus. (B) T1-weighted MRI postcontrast with fat suppression section of the same lesion. (C) Coronal reconstruction CT brain with contrast of the same lesion [16].

cavernous sinus–adjacent lesions, discuss upfront whether near-total resection followed by high-dose conformal or particle radiotherapy offers a better overall risk–benefit than attempted radical resection with high neurologic morbidity [76, 79].

13. Ewing sarcoma

Ewing sarcoma (ES) is a highly aggressive "small-round-blue-cell" malignancy of bone and soft tissue, defined by characteristic FET-ETS gene fusions – most commonly EWSR1-FLI1 – driving an oncogenic transcriptional program and chemosensitivity profile that distinguish it from other small-round-cell tumors [81, 82]. In the head and neck, ES may arise from gnathic bones, the skull base, or as extraskeletal soft-tissue tumors; histologic variants (including adamantinoma-like or primitive neuroectodermal tumor patterns) are recognized, and cytogenetic or molecular confirmation of an EWSR1 rearrangement is essential for definitive diagnosis and for informing systemic therapy decisions [82, 83].

Clinical presentation depends on the anatomic site but is typically driven by a rapidly enlarging mass with local pain, swelling, and functional deficits. Mandibular or maxillary primaries commonly cause facial swelling, tooth mobility, malocclusion, or alveolar/IAN paresthesia; skull-base lesions more often produce cranial neuropathies, headache, or diplopia; soft-tissue (extraskeletal) lesions can present as submucosal or cutaneous masses [84, 85]. Because ES most often affects children, adolescents, and young adults, new or rapidly progressive osseous or soft-tissue lesions in these age groups – especially when imaging suggests permeative bone destruction or a heterogeneous soft-tissue component – should prompt early biopsy and molecular workup to avoid diagnostic delay. In the head and neck, case series emphasize that presentations can be misattributed to benign odontogenic, inflammatory, or other neoplastic processes, so a high index of suspicion is required.

Initial evaluation mirrors general ES protocols: high-resolution MRI of the primary site to define marrow and soft-tissue extent (including perineural or dural involvement for skull-base tumors), contrast-enhanced CT to assess cortical destruction and surgical anatomy, and chest CT to screen for pulmonary metastases (**Figure 10**). Whole-body staging with 18 F-FDG PET/CT (or bone scan where PET is unavailable) is recommended to detect osseous or soft-tissue metastatic disease and to aid baseline response assessment [81, 85]. Tissue diagnosis should be obtained by a core or incisional biopsy planned along a future resection or radiotherapy corridor; pathology should include immunohistochemistry and molecular testing (FISH/RT-PCR or next-generation sequencing) for EWSR1 rearrangements to confirm ES and exclude mimics. Staging and risk stratification follow contemporary bone-sarcoma guidelines and influence local-therapy selection (surgery vs. radiotherapy vs. combined) and systemic chemotherapy regimens.

Treatment is multimodal. For localized disease, the backbone is multiagent systemic chemotherapy (induction, local therapy, and adjuvant cycles), using regimens established in pediatric and young-adult cooperative group trials (e.g.,

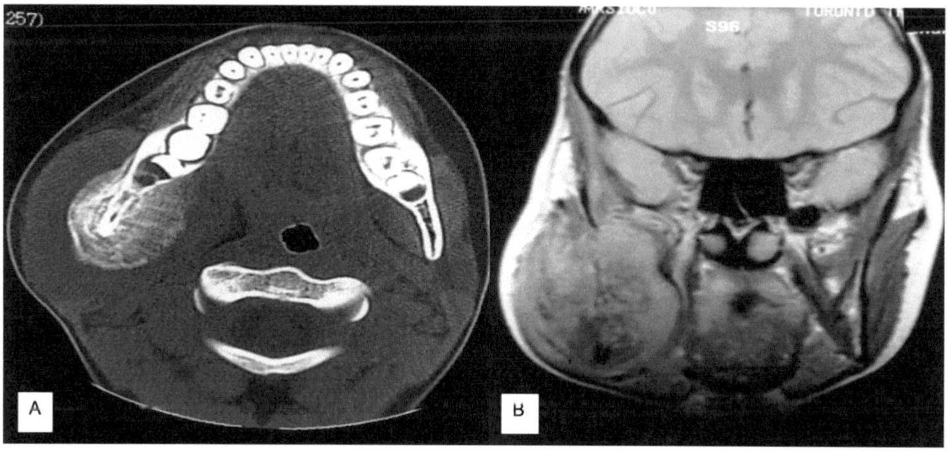

Figure 10.
Ewing sarcoma of the right mandibular angle. (A) Axial CT section. (B) T2-weighted MRI coronal reconstruction [17].

vincristine-doxorubicin-cyclophosphamide alternating with ifosfamide-etoposide or analogous protocols), because systemic therapy substantially improves event-free and overall survival compared with local therapy alone [81, 83]. Local control is achieved with surgery, radiotherapy, or both; whenever anatomically and functionally feasible, complete surgical resection with negative margins is preferred for craniofacial primaries because it can offer superior local control and histologic response assessment, but definitive or adjuvant radiotherapy is a well-established alternative or complement when resection would carry prohibitive morbidity or when margins are positive [64, 81]. Skull-base tumors commonly require multidisciplinary planning (neurosurgery + skull-base ENT/OMFS + radiation oncology) and may be managed with subtotal resection followed by high-dose conformal radiotherapy or particle therapy when radical resection risks unacceptable neurologic deficit [85]. For unresectable, metastatic, or relapsed disease, treatment options include intensified systemic therapy, targeted agents/trials where available, and metastasis-directed therapies per consensus guidance. Timely referral to specialized sarcoma centers and inclusion in clinical trials are advised given the rarity and therapeutic complexity of head-and-neck ES [86].

Prognosis is driven primarily by metastatic status at diagnosis and response to induction chemotherapy. Localized head-and-neck ES treated with multiagent chemotherapy and effective local control can have outcomes comparable to ES at other sites when managed in multidisciplinary centers, but presentation with metastatic disease portends substantially worse long-term survival [64, 81]. Surveillance after completion of therapy includes interval clinical exams, MRI of the primary site to detect local recurrence, and chest CT to survey for pulmonary metastases; the exact frequency follows trial-based or guideline recommendations and is tailored to initial stage and treatment response. For relapsed disease, consensus documents recommend individualized local and systemic approaches and, when appropriate, enrollment in trials of novel agents or metastasis-directed strategies [87].

14. Multiple myeloma

Multiple myeloma is a clonal plasma-cell malignancy characterized by the proliferation of monoclonal plasma cells in the bone marrow, with the production of a monoclonal immunoglobulin (M protein) and end-organ effects (CRAB features: hypercalcemia, renal dysfunction, anemia, bone lesions) or myeloma-defining biomarkers. Solitary plasmacytoma represents a localized collection of clonal plasma cells either in bone (solitary bone plasmacytoma, SBP) or soft tissue (extramedullary plasmacytoma, EMP) and may be a precursor to systemic MM [88, 89]. In the head and neck, plasmacytic lesions most commonly involve the sinonasal tract, nasopharynx, larynx, and gnathic bones (mandible > maxilla), and lesions may represent either isolated plasmacytoma or the first manifestation of systemic myeloma [90].

Head-and-neck manifestations reflect local mass effect or bone destruction: gnathic involvement frequently presents with jaw pain, swelling, mobile teeth, ill-fitting dentures, nonhealing extraction sockets, or alveolar/mental nerve paresthesia; sinonasal or nasopharyngeal disease may cause obstruction, epistaxis, or cranial neuropathies; laryngeal EMP can present with hoarseness or airway compromise [91]. Systemic symptoms (fatigue, recurrent infections, bone pain at other sites) or laboratory abnormalities (anemia, hypercalcemia, renal impairment) suggest disseminated MM rather than isolated plasmacytoma and should prompt a bone-marrow and systemic work-up [88, 89].

ENT/OMFS teams should coordinate diagnostic steps with hematology/oncology. Basic initial testing includes CBC, serum calcium and creatinine, serum protein electrophoresis (SPEP) with immunofixation, urine protein electrophoresis (UPEP) or urine immunofixation, and serum free light-chain assay to detect a monoclonal protein or light-chain disease [88, 90]. Cross-sectional imaging of the local site (contrast CT for bony detail and surgical planning; MRI for marrow/perineural/soft-tissue extent) is essential; whole-body assessment for skeletal disease uses low-dose whole-body CT or FDG-PET/CT (and whole-body or spine/pelvis MRI when indicated) per IMWG/NCCN recommendations (**Figure 11**) [89, 92, 93]. Tissue diagnosis (core/incisional biopsy) is required to establish plasmacytic histology and to exclude mimics; biopsy tracts should be planned to permit wide resection or radiotherapy without contaminating future definitive fields [90]. For suspected solitary plasmacytoma, bone-marrow biopsy and systemic imaging are mandatory to exclude occult MM before labeling the lesion "solitary" [89, 93].

Therapy diverges based on whether the disease is solitary (SBP/EMP) or systemic MM. Definitive external-beam radiotherapy (typically 40–50 Gy in conventional fractionation) is the standard of care for most solitary plasmacytomas of bone or soft tissue in the head and neck and achieves high rates of local control; surgery is reserved for diagnostic purposes, resection of small, well-circumscribed lesions when morbidity is low, or management of pathologic fractures or structural

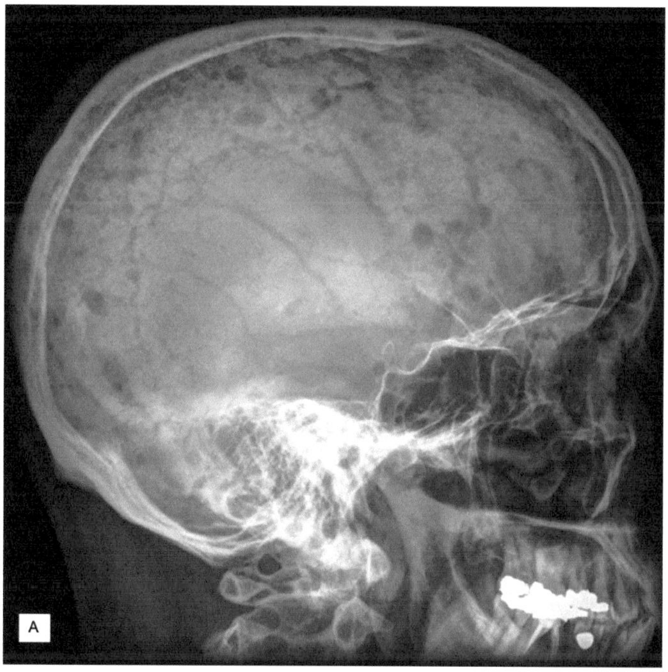

Figure 11.
Moth-eaten lesions of multiple myeloma involving the cranial vault. (A) Lateral plain film [18].

instability [90, 94]. If systemic MM is present, treatment involves systemic therapy (triplet regimens based on proteasome inhibitors, immunomodulatory drugs, and anti-CD38 antibodies for transplant-eligible and ineligible patients), often with local radiotherapy for symptomatic head-and-neck lesions; autologous stem cell transplant remains a consolidation option in eligible patients per contemporary guidelines [88, 95]. Close collaboration with medical oncology/sarcoma centers ensures appropriate systemic staging and access to MM-directed regimens.

Be alert to the risk of progression: a substantial minority of patients with SBP will progress to MM over time, so long-term hematology follow-up with serial SPEP/serum free light chains and interval imaging is required [90, 94]. For MM patients, early dental evaluation is necessary before initiating intravenous bisphosphonates or denosumab (agents that reduce skeletal-related events but increase the risk of medication-related osteonecrosis of the jaw); invasive dental work should ideally be completed prior to antiresorptive therapy, and MRONJ precautions should be applied during follow-up [95, 96]. In the head and neck, indications for surgery are limited (biopsy, decompression, stabilization, or resection when appropriate), while radiotherapy provides an effective organ-preserving local therapy for most EMP/SBP cases [90]. Multidisciplinary planning (ENT/OMFS, hematology/oncology, radiation oncology, dental/maxillofacial prosthetics, radiology, and pathology) is essential for optimal oncologic, functional, and dental outcomes.

Author details

David Wenger[1], Russell Arellanes[1] and Changxing Liu[2]*

1 DO – Department of Otolaryngology and Head and Neck Surgery, Oklahoma State University, Tulsa, United States

2 Department of Otolaryngology – Head and Neck Surgery, Ascension St. John Medical Center, Tulsa, United States

*Address all correspondence to: changxing.Liu@Ascension.org

References

[1] Reichart PA, Philipsen HP, Sonner S. Ameloblastoma: Biological profile of 3677 cases. European Journal of Cancer Part B: Oral Oncology. 1995;**31B**:86–99

[2] Kieserman SP, Baker P, Eberle R. Ameloblastoma of the maxilla: A series of three cases. Otolaryngology–Head and Neck Surgery. 1997;**116**:395–398

[3] World Health Organization. International Agency for Research on Cancer. Pathology and Genetics of Head and Neck Tumours. Iarc. 2005;**9**:296–300

[4] Brown NA, Rolland D, McHugh JB, Weigelin HC, Zhao L, Lim MS, et al. Activating FGFR2–RAS–BRAF mutations in ameloblastoma. Clinical Cancer Research. 2014;**20**:5517–5526

[5] Kurppa KJ, Catón J, Morgan PR, Ristimäki A, Ruhin B, Kellokoski J, et al. High frequency of BRAF V600E mutations in ameloblastoma. The Journal of Pathology. 2014;**232**: 492–498

[6] Sweeney RT, McClary AC, Myers BR, Biscocho J, Neahring L, Kwei KA, et al. Identification of recurrent SMO and BRAF mutations in ameloblastomas. Nature Genetics. 2014;**46**:722–725

[7] Speight PM, Takata T. New tumour entities in the 4th edition of the World Health Organization Classification of Head and Neck tumours: Odontogenic and maxillofacial bone tumours. Virchows Archiv. 2018;**472**:331–339

[8] More C, Tailor M, Patel HJ, Asrani M, Thakkar K, Adalja C. Radiographic analysis of ameloblastoma: A retrospective study. Indian Journal of Dental Research. 2012;**23**:698

[9] Carlson ER, Marx RE. The ameloblastoma: Primary, curative surgical management. Journal of Oral and Maxillofacial Surgery. 2006;**64**:484–494

[10] Lau SL, Samman N. Recurrence related to treatment modalities of unicystic ameloblastoma: A systematic review. International Journal of Oral and Maxillofacial Surgery. 2006;**35**: 681–690

[11] Ackermann GL, Altini M, Shear M. The unicystic ameloblastoma: A clinicopathological study of 57 cases. Journal of Oral Pathology & Medicine. 1988;**17**:541–546

[12] Hidalgo DA. Fibula free flap: A new method of mandible reconstruction. Plastic and Reconstructive Surgery. 1989;**84**:71–79

[13] Broudic-Guibert M, Blay J-Y, Vazquez L, Evrard A, Karanian M, Taïeb S, et al. Persistent response to vemurafenib in metastatic ameloblastoma with BRAF mutation: A case report. Journal of Medical Case Reports. 2019;**13**:245

[14] Fernandes GS, Girardi DM, Bernardes JPG, Fonseca FP, Fregnani ER. Clinical benefit and radiological response with BRAF inhibitor in a patient with recurrent ameloblastoma harboring V600E mutation. BMC Cancer. 2018;**18**:887

[15] Olaitan AA, Arole G, Adekeye EO. Recurrent ameloblastoma of the jaws. A

follow-up study. International Journal of Oral and Maxillofacial Surgery. 1998;**27**:456–460

[16] Corio RL, Goldblatt LI, Edwards PA, Hartman KS. Ameloblastic carcinoma: A clinicopathologic study and assessment of eight cases. Oral Surgery, Oral Medicine, Oral Pathology. 1987;**64**:570–576

[17] Sayan NB, Uçok C, Karasu HA, Günhan Ö. Peripheral osteoma of the oral and maxillofacial region: A study of 35 new cases. Journal of Oral and Maxillofacial Surgery. 2002;**60**: 1299–1301

[18] Greenspan A. Benign bone-forming lesions: Osteoma, osteoid osteoma, and osteoblastoma. Clinical, imaging, pathologic, and differential considerations. Skeletal Radiology. 1993;**22**:485–500

[19] Atesok KI, Alman BA, Schemitsch EH, Peyser A, Mankin H. Osteoid osteoma and osteoblastoma. American Academy of Orthopaedic Surgeons. 2011;**19**:678–689

[20] Gardner EJ, Richards RC. Multiple cutaneous and subcutaneous lesions occurring simultaneously with hereditary polyposis and osteomatosis. American Journal of Human Genetics. 1953;**5**:139–147

[21] Longo F, Califano L, De Maria G, Ciccarelli R. Solitary osteoma of the mandibular ramus: Report of a case. Journal of Oral and Maxillofacial Surgery. 2001;**59**:698–700

[22] Chiu AG, Schipor I, Cohen NA, Kennedy DW, Palmer JN. Surgical decisions in the management of frontal sinus osteomas. American Journal of Rhinology. 2005;**19**:191–197

[23] Sofokleous V, Maragoudakis P, Kyrodimos E, Giotakis E. Management of paranasal sinus osteomas: A comprehensive narrative review of the literature and an up-to-date grading system. American Journal of Otolaryngology. 2021;**42**:102644

[24] Singh A, Solomon MC. Osteoid osteoma of the mandible: A case report with review of the literature. Journal of Dental Sciences. 2017;**12**:185–189

[25] Tepelenis K, Skandalakis GP, Papathanakos G, Kefala MA, Kitsouli A, Barbouti A, et al. Osteoid osteoma: An updated review of epidemiology, pathogenesis, clinical presentation, radiological features, and treatment option. In Vivo. 2021;**35**:1929–1938

[26] Rosenthal DI, Hornicek FJ, Wolfe MW, Jennings LC, Gebhardt MC, Mankin HJ. Percutaneous radiofrequency coagulation of osteoid osteoma compared with operative treatment. The Journal of Bone & Joint Surgery. 1998;**80**:815–821

[27] Lucas DR, Unni KK, McLeod RA, O'Connor MI, Sim FH. Osteoblastoma: Clinicopathologic study of 306 cases. Human Pathology. 1994;**25**:117–134

[28] Lypka MA, Goos RR, Yamashita - D-DR, Melrose R. Aggressive osteoblastoma of the mandible. International Journal of Oral and Maxillofacial Surgery. 2008;**37**:675–678

[29] Alvares Capelozza AL, Gião Dezotti MS, Casati Alvares L, Negrão Fleury R, Sant'Ana E. Osteoblastoma of the mandible: Systematic review of the literature and report of a case. Dentomaxillofacial Radiology. 2005;**34**:1–8

[30] Weinstein LS, Shenker A, Gejman PV, Merino MJ, Friedman E, Spiegel AM. Activating mutations of the stimulatory G protein in the McCune-Albright syndrome. New England Journal of Medicine. 1991;**325**:1688–1695

[31] Dumitrescu CE, Collins MT. McCune-Albright syndrome. Orphanet Journal of Rare Diseases. 2008;**3**:1–12

[32] MacDonald-Jankowski D. Fibrous dysplasia: A systematic review. Dentomaxillofacial Radiology. 2009;**38**:196–215

[33] Lee JS, FitzGibbon EJ, Chen YR, Kim HJ, Lustig LR, Akintoye SO, et al. Clinical guidelines for the management of craniofacial fibrous dysplasia. Orphanet Journal of Rare Diseases 2012;**7**:S2

[34] Fitzpatrick KA, Taljanovic MS, Speer DP, Graham AR, Jacobson JA, Barnes GR, et al. Imaging findings of fibrous dysplasia with histopathologic and intraoperative correlation. American Journal of Roentgenology. 2004;**182**:1389–1398

[35] DiCaprio MR, Enneking WF. Fibrous dysplasia. Pathophysiology, evaluation, and treatment. The Journal of Bone and Joint Surgery. American Volume. 2005;**87**:1848–1864

[36] Valentini V, Cassoni A, Marianetti TM, Terenzi V, Fadda MT, Iannetti G. Craniomaxillofacial fibrous dysplasia: Conservative treatment or radical surgery? A retrospective study on 68 patients. Plastic and Reconstructive Surgery. 2009;**123**: 653–660

[37] Titinchi F. Juvenile ossifying fibroma of the maxillofacial region: Analysis of clinico-pathological features and management. Medicina Oral Patología Oral Y Cirugia Bucal. 2021;**26**: e590–e597

[38] Chrcanovic BR, Gomez RS. Juvenile ossifying fibroma of the jaws and paranasal sinuses: A systematic review of the cases reported in the literature. International Journal of Oral and Maxillofacial Surgery. 2020;**49**:28–37

[39] Wenig BM, Vinh TN, Smirniotopoulos JG, Fowler CB, Houston GD, Heffner DK. Aggressive psammomatoid ossifying fibromas of the sinonasal region: A clinicopathologic study of a distinct group of fibro-osseous lesions. Cancer. 1995;**76**:1155–1165

[40] Akcam T, Altug HA, Karakoc O, Sencimen M, Ozkan A, Bayar GR, et al. Synchronous ossifying fibromas of the jaws: A review. Oral Surgery, Oral Medicine, Oral Pathology and Oral Radiology. 2012;**114**:S120–5

[41] Gondivkar SM, Gadbail AR, Chole R, Parikh RV, Balsaraf S. Ossifying fibroma of the jaws: Report of two cases and literature review. Oral Oncology. 2011;**47**:804–809

[42] Sarode SC, Sarode GS, Waknis P, Patil A, Jashika M. Juvenile psammomatoid ossifying fibroma: A review. Oral Oncology. 2011;**47**: 1110–1116

[43] Ganesh P, Raut RP, Boyina KK, Shetty S, Salins PC. Le fort I disassembly for the management of juvenile ossifying fibroma extending to the skull base. Journal of Craniofacial Surgery. 2016;**27**:e595–e598

[44] Salge-Arrieta FJ, Vior-Fernández C, Lee P, Reguero-Callejas ME,

Pian-Arias HG, Martínez-San Millán JS, et al. Giant fronto-spheno-orbitary juvenile psammomatoid ossifying fibroma: Case report and literature review. Child's Nervous System. 2024;**40**:939–945

[45] Ledderose GJ, Stelter K, Becker S, Leunig A. Paranasal ossifying fibroma: Endoscopic resection or wait and scan? European Archives of Oto-Rhino-Laryngology. 2011;**268**:999–1004

[46] van der Heijden L, Lipplaa A, van Langevelde K, Jvmg B, van de Sande Maj, Gelderblom H. Updated concepts in treatment of giant cell tumor of bone. Current Opinion in Oncology. 2022;**34**:371–378

[47] van der Heijden L, Dijkstra PDS, van de Sande Maj, Kroep JR, Nout RA, van Rijswijk Csp, et al. The clinical approach toward giant cell tumor of bone. The Oncologist. 2014;**19**:550–561

[48] Gao X, Wang S, Zhan X, Liu Y, Chen L, Sun J, et al. Case Report: Giant cell lesions in the Maxillofacial region: Diagnostic points and treatment strategies. Frontiers in Oncology. 2025;**15**:1572560

[49] Goto Y, Furuno Y, Kawabe T, Ohwada K, Tatsuzawa K, Sasajima H, et al. Treatment of a skull-base giant cell tumor with endoscopic endonasal resection and denosumab: Case report. Journal of Neurosurgery. 2017;**126**: 431–434

[50] Tsukamoto S, Mavrogenis AF, Kido A, Errani C. Current Concepts in the Treatment of Giant Cell Tumors of Bone. Cancers (Basel). 2021;13. DOI: 10.3390/cancers13153647

[51] Brochu BM, Mirsky NA, Nayak VV, Witek L, Thaller SR, Carlini JL, et al. Exploring denosumab in the treatment of giant cell tumors: Clinical evidence and controversies. Journal of Craniofacial Surgery. 2025;**36**: 1220–1225

[52] Borkowska AM, Szumera-Ciećkiewicz A, Szostakowski B, Pieńkowski A, Rutkowski PL. Denosumab in giant cell tumor of bone: Multidisciplinary medical management based on pathophysiological mechanisms and real-world evidence. Cancers (Basel). 2022;14. DOI: 10.3390/cancers14092290

[53] Dimitrijevic MV, Sopta J, Ivisevic TB, Dudvarski Z. Chondroma of the tongue. Journal of Craniofacial Surgery. 2019;**30**:e315–e317

[54] Demir M, Bahadir O, Çobanoğlu HB. Endoscopic resection of nasal septal chondroma. Journal of Craniofacial Surgery. 2024; **35**:1852–1854. DOI: 10.1097/SCS.0000000000010180

[55] Kim SR, An S, Lee JY. Soft tissue chondroma of the chin. Journal of Craniofacial Surgery. 2023;**34**: e501–e503

[56] de Jong Rj B, van Lent S, Hogendoorn PCW. Chondroma and chondrosarcoma of the larynx. Current Opinion in Otolaryngology & Head and Neck Surgery. 2004;**12**:98–105

[57] Gross AJ, Houston KR, Hudson J-W, McCoy JM. A multidisciplinary approach to synovial chondromatosis of the temporomandibular joint with cranial base involvement: A brief review of the literature and case report. Journal of Oral and Maxillofacial Surgery. 2020;**78**:1759–1765

[58] RA Jr F, Singh B, Har-El G. Laryngeal chondroma. Journal of Voice. 2002;**16**:92–95

[59] De Riu G, Meloni SM, Gobbi R, Contini M, Tullio A. Soft-tissue chondroma of the masticatory space. International Journal of Oral and Maxillofacial Surgery. 2007;**36**:174–176

[60] Geng S, Zhang J, L-W Z, Wu Z, Jia G, Xiao X, et al. Diagnosis and microsurgical treatment of chondromas and chondrosarcomas of the cranial base. Oncology Letters. 2014;**8**:301–304

[61] Tan Z, Yao M, Liu T, Wang S, Xu J, Zhang Y, et al. Chondroma of laryngeal cartilage mimicking thyroid tumor: A case report. Medicine (Baltimore). 2019;**98**:e15005

[62] Almansoori AA, Kim H-Y, Kim B, Kim S-M, Lee J-H. Chondrosarcoma of the jaw: A retrospective series. Oral Surgery, Oral Medicine, Oral Pathology and Oral Radiology. 2019;**128**:106–111

[63] Jacobi CMC, Hiranya ES, Gay A, Holzmann D, Kollias S, Soyka MB. Enchondroma of the nasal septum due to Ollier disease: A case report and review of the literature. Head & Neck. 2015;**37**:E30–3

[64] Kobayashi K, Hanai N, Yoshimoto S, Saito Y, Homma A. Current topics and management of head and neck sarcomas. Japanese Journal of Clinical Oncology. 2023;**53**:743–756

[65] Sandeep KS, Rathod P, Dalvi R, Pawar A, Thottiyen S, Pandya S, et al. Osteosarcoma of head and neck region: Tertiary cancer care center experience. Indian Journal of Otolaryngology and Head & Neck Surgery. 2024;**76**:581–586

[66] Grier HE. National Cancer Institute (US). Osteosarcoma and Undifferentiated Pleomorphic Sarcoma of Bone Treatment (PDQ®). PDQ Cancer Information Summaries [Internet]; 2024

[67] Osteosarcoma Stages. Available from: https://www.cancer.org/cancer/types/osteosarcoma/detection-diagnosis-staging/staging.html [Accessed: 2025-August-31]

[68] Biermann JS, Hirbe A, Ahlawat S, Bernthal NM, Binitie O, Boles S, et al. Bone Cancer, Version 2.2025, NCCN Clinical Practice Guidelines In Oncology. Journal of the National Comprehensive Cancer Network. 2025;**23**. DOI: 10.6004/jnccn.2025.0017

[69] Rodriguez-Molinero J, Pozo-Kreilinger JJ, Ruiz-Roca JA, Lopez-Sanchez AF, Cebrian-Carretero JL. Clinical and pathological features of osteosarcomas of the jaws: A retrospective study. Clinics and Practice. 2024;**14**:965–979

[70] Weber V, Stigler R, Lutz R, Kesting M, Weber M. Systematic review of craniofacial osteosarcoma regarding different clinical, therapeutic and prognostic parameters. Frontiers in Oncology. 2023;**13**:1006622

[71] Medscape. Osteosarcoma Guidelines. 2025. Available: https://emedicine.medscape.com/article/1256857-guidelines#:~:text=ESMO%2DPaedCan%2DEURACAN%20guidelines%20recommend,chemotherapy%2C%20resection%2C%20or%20both. [Accessed: 2025-August-31]

[72] Mireștean CC, Simionescu CE, Iancu RI, Stan MC, Iancu DPT, Bădulescu F. Head and neck low grade chondrosarcoma-A rare entity.

Diagnostics (Basel). 2023;13. DOI: 10.3390/diagnostics13193026

[73] Ravindran PK, Keizer ME, Kunst HPM, Compter I, Van Aalst J, Eekers DBP, et al. Skull-base chondrosarcoma: A systematic review of the role of postoperative radiotherapy. Cancers (Basel). 2024;**16**. DOI: 10.3390/cancers16050856

[74] Agosti E, Zeppieri M, Antonietti S, Ius T, Fontanella MM, Panciani PP. Advancing the management of skull base chondrosarcomas: A systematic review of targeted therapies. Journal of Personalized Medicine. 2024;14. DOI: 10.3390/jpm14030261

[75] El Beaino M, Roszik J, Livingston JA, Wang W-L, Lazar AJ, Amini B, et al. Mesenchymal chondrosarcoma: A review with emphasis on its fusion-driven biology. Current Oncology Reports. 2018;**20**:37

[76] Lee SY, Lim YC, Song MH, Seok JY, Lee WS, Choi EC. Chondrosarcoma of the head and neck. Yonsei Medical Journal. 2005;**46**:228–232

[77] Yeom KW, Lober RM, Mobley BC, Harsh G, Vogel H, Allagio R, et al. Diffusion-weighted MRI: Distinction of skull base chordoma from chondrosarcoma. American Journal of Neuroradiology. 2013;**34**:1056–61,S1

[78] Liu H, Li Z, Xue Y, Zhao T, Wu Y. A multicenter retrospective analysis of clinical outcomes of intracranial chondrosarcoma in 26 patients. Scientific Reports. 2023;**13**:14647

[79] Medscape. Chondrosarcoma Guidelines. 2025. Available: https://emedicine.medscape.com/article/1258236-guidelines?form=fpf [Accessed: 2025-August-31]

[80] Nakamura M, Mizumoto M, Saito T, Shimizu S, Li Y, Oshiro Y, et al. A systematic review and meta-analysis of radiotherapy and particle beam therapy for skull base chondrosarcoma: TRP-chondrosarcoma 2024. Frontiers in Oncology. 2024;**14**:1380716

[81] National Cancer Institute (.gov). 2025. Available: https://www.cancer.gov/types/bone/hp/ewing-treatment-pdq [Accessed: 2025-August-31]

[82] Carpentieri DF, Qualman SJ, Bowen J, Krausz T, Marchevsky A, Dickman PS, et al. Protocol for the examination of specimens from pediatric and adult patients with osseous and extraosseous ewing sarcoma family of tumors, including peripheral primitive neuroectodermal tumor and ewing sarcoma. Archives of Pathology & Laboratory Medicine. 2005;**129**:866–873

[83] Mata Fernández C, Sebio A, Orcajo Rincón J, Martín BJ, Martín Benlloch A, Marcilla Plaza D, et al. Clinical practice guidelines for the treatment of Ewing sarcoma (Spanish Sarcoma Research Group-GEIS). Clinical and Translational Oncology. 2025;**27**:824–836

[84] Spiguel MH, Schuch LF, Kovalski LN, Ribeiro JT, Só BB, Silveira FM, et al. Ewing's sarcoma of the head and neck: A systematic review. Oral Diseases. 2024;**30**:1784–1792

[85] Zöllner SK, Amatruda JF, Bauer S, Collaud S, de Álava E, DuBois SG, et al. Ewing sarcoma-diagnosis, treatment, clinical challenges and future perspectives. Journal of Clinical Medicine. 2021;10. DOI: 10.3390/jcm10081685

[86] Almohaisen GA, Alhuwairini SF, Aljrayed MA, Alenezi MM, Alsaab F.

Extraskeletal Ewing's sarcoma of the head and neck region in pediatric patients: A case report and literature review. International Journal of Surgery Case Reports. 2023;**106**:108142

[87] Shah C, Campbell SR, Murphy E, Braunstein S, Dietz MS, Binitie O, et al. Consensus recommendations regarding local and metastasis-directed therapies in the management of relapsed/ recurrent Ewing sarcoma. Cancer. 2025;**131**:e35858

[88] Kumar SK, Callander NS, Adekola K, LD Jr A, Baljevic M, Baz R, et al. Multiple myeloma, version 2.2024, NCCN clinical practice guidelines in oncology. Journal of the National Comprehensive Cancer Network. 2023;**21**:1281–1301

[89] Hillengass J, Usmani S, Rajkumar SV, Durie BGM, Mateos M-V, Lonial S, et al. International myeloma working group consensus recommendations on imaging in monoclonal plasma cell disorders. The Lancet Oncology. 2019;**20**:e302–e312

[90] Caers J, Paiva B, Zamagni E, Leleu X, Bladé J, Kristinsson SY, et al. Diagnosis, treatment, and response assessment in solitary plasmacytoma: Updated recommendations from a European Expert Panel. Journal of Hematology & Oncology. 2018;**11**:10

[91] Suryavanshi H, Patankar S, Dhumal S, Choudhari S. Solitary plasmacytoma of jaw bone: A case report and systematic review of fifty cases from literature. Journal of Oral and Maxillofacial Pathology. 2021;**25**:205

[92] Wilkinson S, Jawad S, Kowa X-Y. Head and neck manifestations of extramedullary plasmacytomas and their differential diagnoses: A pictorial review. British Journal of Radiology. 2025;**98**:640–649

[93] Fouquet G, Guidez S, Herbaux C, Van de Wyngaert Z, Bonnet S, Beauvais D, et al. Impact of initial FDG-PET/CT and serum-free light chain on transformation of conventionally defined solitary plasmacytoma to multiple myeloma. Clinical Cancer Research. 2014;**20**:3254–3260

[94] Goyal G, Bartley AC, Funni S, Inselman J, Shah ND, Marshall AL, et al. Treatment approaches and outcomes in plasmacytomas: Analysis using a national dataset. Leukemia. 2018;**32**:1414–1420

[95] Mikhael J, Ismaila N, Martin T. Treatment of multiple myeloma: ASCO and CCO joint clinical practice guideline summary. Journal of Oncology Practice. 2019;**15**:279–286

[96] Ruggiero SL, Dodson TB, Aghaloo T, Carlson ER, Ward BB, Kademani D. American association of oral and maxillofacial surgeons' position paper on medication-related osteonecrosis of the jaws-2022 update. Journal of Oral and Maxillofacial Surgery: Official Journal of the American Association of Oral and Maxillofacial Surgeons. 2022;**80**: 920–943

Chapter 4

Clinical and Radio-pathological Spectrum of Bone Tumors: Review and Update

Mahnoor Hafeez, Ruqaiya Shahid and Malik Osama Tanweer

Abstract

Bone tumors (BTs) range from benign to malignant and differ in pathogenesis according to the origin of the skeletal tissue, that is, osteogenic, chondrogenic, fibrogenic, vascular, osteoclastic giant cell-rich, hematopoietic neoplasm, notochordal, and other mesenchymal tumors of bone. The location, site, and type of BT vary according to the age of the patient. The confirmatory diagnosis for malignant ones involves the combined radiological and histopathological approach, that is, radiograph, MRI, bone scan, tissue biopsy with gross specimen, microscopy, molecular biology, and immunohistochemistry (IHC). MRI is useful to assess the local extent and staging, recurrent/residual disease, and post-operative complications. CT is indicated to evaluate only few BT because of the ionizing radiation. Contrast CT chest and bone scans are indicated for metastatic work-up. Management ranges from a conservative approach, wide local excision, en bloc resection, limb salvage surgery/amputation to chemotherapy depending upon molecular markers and radiotherapy. In this chapter, authors shed the spotlight on BT, based on multi-modality and multidisciplinary collaborative pragmatic approach, with updates from current literature.

Keywords: radiograph, CT, MRI, histopathology, wide local excisionchemotherapy

1. Introduction

Bone tumors (BTs) can be found incidentally or may present with clinical symptoms (**Figures 1** and **2**). Malignant BTs usually present with fever, pain, swelling, anemia, elevated inflammatory markers (i.e., ESR, CRP), raised alkaline phosphatase levels, and/or pathologic fractures.

Radiologically, tumors can be classified into benign and aggressive types based on Xray imaging, depending upon the radiographic features, for example, margins, lesion type (sclerotic or lytic), pattern (permeative, geographic, moth-eaten), type of matrix, zone of transition (narrow/wide), periosteal reaction (smooth, irregular), site within the bone (cortical, medullary, epi-/metaphyseal, diaphyseal), and within the skeleton (axial vs. appendicular; endochondral vs. membranous); these features help in narrowing the differential diagnosis.

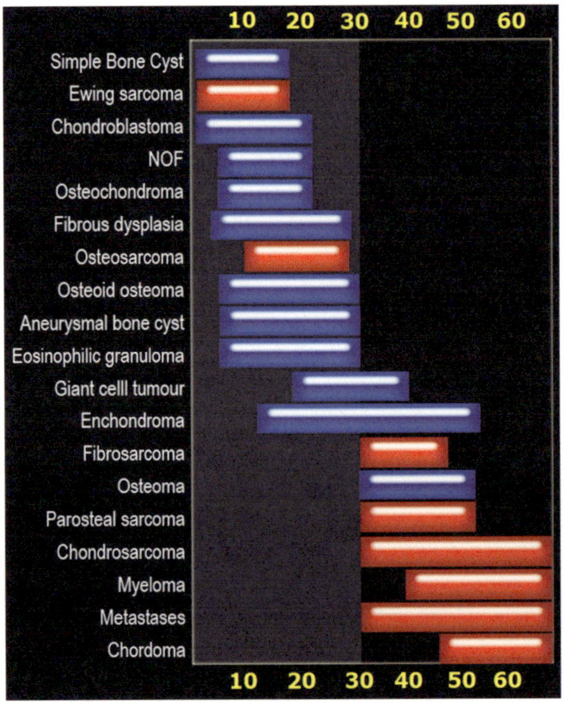

Figure 1.
Age distribution of various kinds of bony tumors (Reproduced with kind permission from author Dr. Robin Smithuis, Radiology Assistant – educational site of the Radiological Society of the Netherlands).

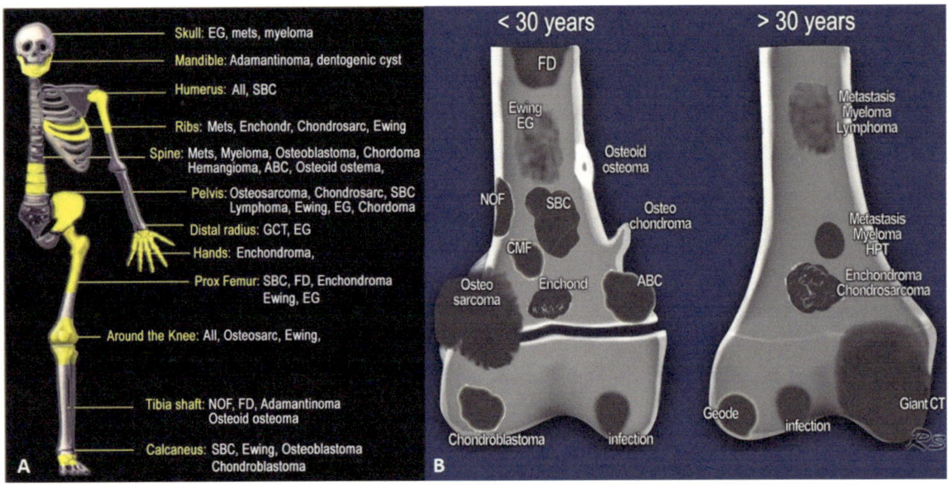

Figure 2.
A: age distribution of various kinds of bony tumors. B: the location of bone lesions according to age (Reproduced with kind permission from author Dr. Robin Smithuis, Radiology Assistant – educational site of the Radiological Society of the Netherlands).

Radiographic imaging appearance of a benign bony lesion is a lytic/sclerotic lesion with well-defined margins, a narrow zone of transition, a possible benign single-layered periosteal reaction, and no cortical break, whereas an aggressive/malignant BT is a lesion with a wide zone of transition, bony expansion, remodeling, cortical destruction, ± pathologic fracture, and an extra osseous soft tissue mass with displaced fat planes.

2. Lodwick classification of lytic bone lesions

It is the criteria described by Morgan M. et al. to characterize the aggressiveness of lytic lesions on radiographs, depending upon the zone of transition. In 2016, modified criteria were described by Schmid J., which categorize lesions into three classes [1, 2].

(1) Well-defined geographic margins: A – sclerotic rim, B – no sclerotic rim.

(2) Ill-defined margins, moth-eaten appearance (**Figure 3**).

(3) Wide zone of transition, permeative lesion.

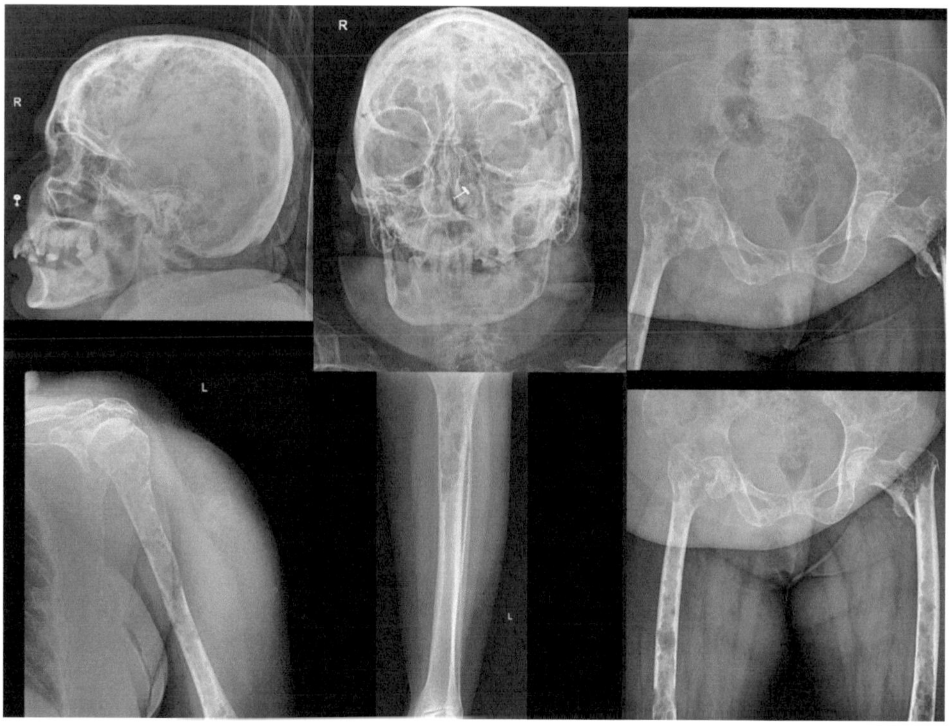

Figure 3.
Skeletal survey – Radiographs of skull lateral and AP view, pelvis, femora, humerus, and left tibia show multiple innumerable lytic lesions in the skull. Differentials include metastasis, leukemia, and multiple myeloma. Pathologic fractures are seen in the left femur per trochanteric region and the right femur neck.

Standard MRI MSK Tumor Protocol comprises Axial T1W, T2W, Coronal STIR, Sagittal PD Fat – saturated, and fat-saturated post-contrast sequences in three planes. MRI of malignant BTs shows cortical/medullary tumors with cortical destruction, neurovascular bundle invasion, joint/growth plate involvement, ± intra lesional hemorrhage/fluid–fluid levels, extent of soft tissue involvement with variable post-contrast enhancement, and loco-regional lymphadenopathy [3–5]. Full-length Coronal T1W MRI of the long bone should be obtained in Ewing's sarcoma and osteosarcoma to detect satellite lesions.

A radiologist creates a roadmap for the operating surgeon and assists the clinician in selecting adequate imaging tests. The ACR Appropriateness Criteria [6], whose objective is to guide clinicians in making appropriate imaging referrals based on clinical signs and symptoms, and divides patients into four scenarios for BT evaluation:

- Persistent clinical symptoms: negative radiograph.
- Definite X-ray benign appearance.
- Suspected malignant appearance.
- Clinically suspected osteoid osteoma.

Apart from routine radiography, MRI is indicated and scores a maximum of up to nine in all cases; radionuclide bone scans and CT scans are performed in atypical scenarios, when an MRI facility is not available or for radiographically occult lesions.

There has been a transition from the WHO classification of Bone Tumors 2013 (4th edition) to 2020 (5th edition). Based on the famous "Know your Pathology – Make your Radiology" dictum, Rad-Path correlation is essential to reach a definitive diagnosis, and histopathology is the diagnostic gold standard. Few tumors are "leave me alone lesions," that is, do not require treatment, while some tumors need surveillance or symptomatic management [7, 8]. As per UK practice guidelines, all malignant BTs are referred to the BT treatment center for biopsy and management. Comprehensive details of advanced BT imaging, including dual-energy CT, MR spectroscopy, dynamic contrast-enhanced MRI, ADC value estimation, and whole-body MRI, are beyond the scope of this chapter [9].

The treatment plan for malignant BTs requires a combined multidisciplinary surgical and oncological (chemo/radio therapeutic) approach, depending upon immune-histochemistry and molecular markers. From the management perspective, for primary bone sarcoma, neo adjuvant chemotherapy is indicated to reduce the size of the localized tumor, followed by wide margin resection surgery for limb salvage procedures. Adjuvant chemotherapy usage can also help to eradicate micro metastasis, with radiation therapy for margin-positive tumors as an adjunct to surgery. Wide margin excision followed by chemotherapy is recommended in high-grade dedifferentiated chondrosarcoma. Prophylactic nailing is advised for tumors that have destroyed more than 50% of the cortex. Decompression spinal surgery and stabilization procedures are performed for unstable malignant vertebral compression fractures with a risk of cord compression. Chemotherapy is the mainstay of treatment for bony metastasis, lymphoma, leukemia, and multiple myeloma; stem cell transplantation can be an option for the last two neoplasms.

Over the last few decades, extensive literature has been published on BT. This chapter aims to provide a review of BT, along with insights from recent literature. Lastly, leukemia and multiple myeloma are presented because of their bone marrow involvement, although they do not belong to the WHO BT classification but rather to hematopoietic and lymphoid tissues [10]. Syndromes associated with BT are also mentioned. The description of rare tumors that are rarely encountered in clinical practice, as well as an extensive management description, is beyond the scope of this chapter.

3. Bone – RADS (reporting and data system)

The Society of Skeletal Radiology has published guidelines for the management of solitary bone lesions on CT (lytic, sclerotic/mixed density lesion) and MRI (low/high signal intensity) in adults. It excludes multiple bone lesions. Few validation studies have been published, but they have yet to be clinically applied across the globe [11, 12].

Recently, the ACR released a white paper on the management of potentially neoplastic bone lesions on radiographs. Like BIRADS (Breast Imaging Reporting and Data System), it grades bone lesions from 0 to IV, with a numerical score of 1–7, depending on the presence of aggressive features.

- Bone-RADS 1: likely benign; leave alone lesion.
- Bone-RADS 2: incompletely assessed on imaging; additional imaging modality required.
- Bone-RADS 3: indeterminate entity; follow-up imaging (at 6, 12, and 24 months after initial detection).
- Bone-RADS 4: suspicious for malignancy – aggressive; biopsy ± oncologic referral.

3.1 Bone tumor staging

The AJCC system for primary bone sarcoma has replaced the Enneking classification, published in 1980, which stages tumors according to their extent, i.e., intra- or extra-compartmental. The AJCC, published in 2003, emphasizes T staging based on size <8 cm (T1) or >8 cm for (T2) and skip metastasis (T3), as well as the presence or absence of nodal disease and metastasis, along with histological grade -G1 (well differentiated), G2 (moderately), G3 (poorly differentiated). The revised AJCC 8_{th} Edition, published after 2017, added the Anatomic site specific staging i.e. (1) Appendicular skeleton, trunk, skull, and facial bones, (2) Spine, and (3) Pelvis as well as M1b stage, that is, metastasis to sites other than the lungs (M1a). An AJCC classification for pelvic and spinal tumors defines the tumor as localized to 1, 3, or 4 vertebral segments, with stage T4 indicating spinal canal invasion, vascular encasement, or tumor thrombus. Additional points to consider include involvement of the growth plate, intra-articular involvement (tumor extending to other articular surfaces and involving tendons or ligaments), and vessel encasement (<180 degrees) [13].

4. WHO classification of bone tumors

4.1 Chondrogenic

4.1.1 Osteochondroma

Osteochondroma is the most common benign tumor of young age and arises from the metaphysis. It is a bony outgrowth with cortical and medullary continuity with the host bone. It can be sessile or pedunculated (**Figures 4** and 5); the latter is directed away from the joint. The former usually resolves spontaneously after puberty.

As per the guidelines of the Musculoskeletal Tumor Society (MSTS) and the Radiological Society of North America (RSNA), cartilage cap thickness on MRI should be <2 cm, with peripheral or without enhancement; an intensely enhancing cap and continued growth after skeletal maturity indicate suspicion for malignant transformation to chondrosarcoma (CS), which requires follow-up radiographs. Other complications include fractures, mechanical osteoarthritic sequelae, synovitis, bursitis, and soft tissue, neurologic, and vascular complications [14, 15].

Pathogenesis: It grows slowly and arises in the bones formed by endochondral ossification, typically originating from the osteochondral junction.

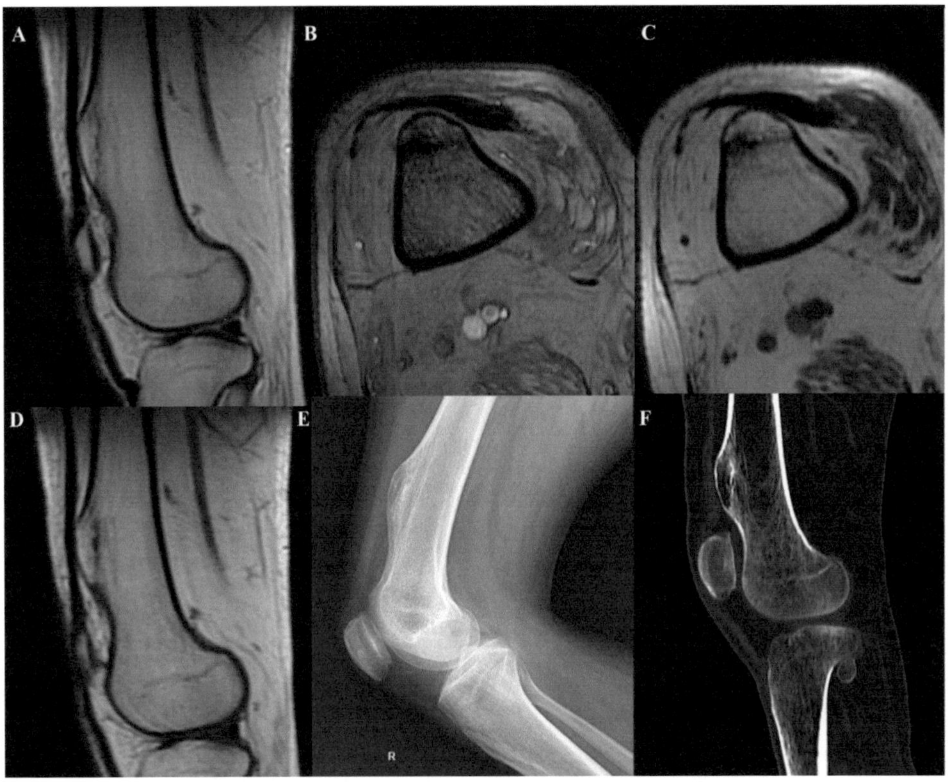

Figure 4.
Sessile osteochondroma of the left femur. MRI, Xray, and CT bone window sagittal images show a broad-based bony outgrowth seen in the region, with cortico-medullary continuity. On axial MRI images (B and C), no discernible cartilage cap seen.

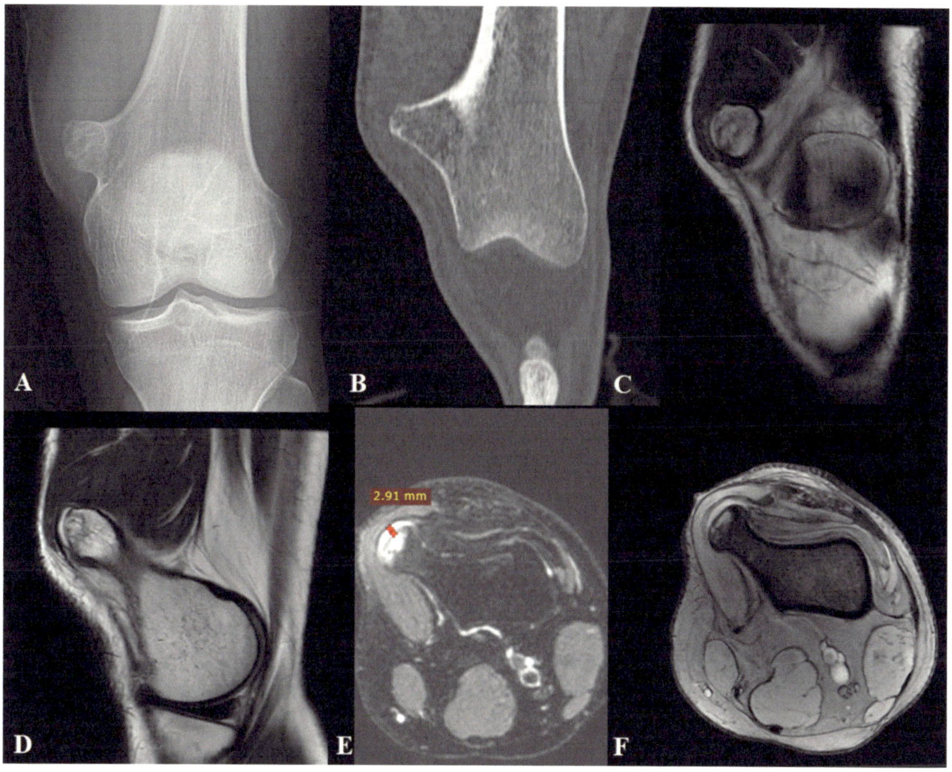

Figure 5.
Sessile osteochondroma of the left femur. Xray, CT bone window, and MRI images show a pedunculated bony outgrowth seen in the metaphyseal region anteriorly with cortico-medullary continuity. On axial MRI images (E and F), a small width cartilage cap is seen that represents benign etiology.

Molecular: Characteristic bi allelic inactivation of EXE1 and EXE2 genes. IDH1 and IDH2 mutations are not present. In multiple hereditary exostosis (MHE), germ line mutations of EXE1/EXE2 are reported.

Gross: An irregular, stalk-like bony outgrowth capped by cartilage.

Microscopy: Osteochondroma has the microscopic appearance of an epiphyseal plate. It has a cartilaginous cap, covered by periosteum, with underlying trabecular bone. The junction between the cartilage and trabecular bone displays enchondral ossification, where the cartilage is being ossified into bone. The trabecular bone is contiguous with the native medullary bone, a key diagnostic feature. Secondary chondrosarcomas may arise from long-standing osteochondromas, particularly in MHE.

Differential diagnosis: Features suggestive of chondrosarcoma are an increased thickness of the cartilage cap (>2 cm in adults), cytologic atypia of the chondrocytes, invasion of the underlying bone, with the cartilage extending into the native bone trabeculae.

Management: Mostly conservative in asymptomatic cases, with surgical resection recommended if there is pain, swelling, deformity, or suspicion of malignancy.

4.1.2 Subungual exostosis

Pathogenesis: By definition, subungual exostosis affects the distal phalanx, most commonly of the big toe, where it lifts the nail bed and may ulcerate and deform the nail plate. It occurs in young individuals; more than 50% are less than 18 years old.

Gross: Small cartilage and bone fragments are usually received.

Molecular: Translocation t(X;6) causing collagen gene *COL12A1* (at chromosome 6) to fuse with insulin substrate receptor gene *IRS4,* leading to increased expression of IRS4 at the protein level.

Microscopy: It has a fibro-cartilaginous cap and bone trabeculae forming the stalk; enchondral ossification is present, or bone may be directly formed from the spindle cells. Chondrocytes may show increased cellularity and nuclear atypia. The inter-trabecular area is fibrous and vascular.

Differential diagnosis: Osteochondroma, which is uncommon in the bones of the hands and feet, does not have chondrocyte atypia, lacks the high cellularity and vascularity of the subungual exostosis, and is continuous with the host medullary bone [16].

4.1.3 Bizarre parosteal osteochondromatous proliferation

Pathogenesis: Bizarre parosteal osteochondromatous proliferation (BPOP) most frequently involves the short tubular bones of the hands and feet, particularly the phalanges or metacarpals/metatarsals. Less often, it may develop in the long bones of the upper limb or leg. The lesion is parosteal, arising on the outer cortical aspect of the bone (juxtacortical), but it lacks connection to the host medullary bone, a feature that distinguishes it from osteochondroma.

Molecular: Translocation t(1;17), inv(7), and inv(6).

Gross: Exophytic bone lesion with a cartilage cap.

Microscopy: An admixture of cartilage, fibrous tissue, and bone. The cartilage has an increased number of chondrocytes and may show atypia and mitosis, enchondral ossification, and spindle cell proliferation in the inter trabecular spaces. The bone formed has a bluish tinge, therefore called "blue bone."

Differential diagnosis:

- Osteochondroma: It maintains structural continuity with the medullary cavity, lacks the blue bone and cartilage atypia, and shows fatty inter trabecular spaces.

- Subungual exostosis lacks the blue bone and is located in the distal phalanx.

4.1.4 Chondroblastoma NOS

It is a rare benign lytic epiphyseal lesion of cartilage origin in long bones, with slight bony expansion and a thin sclerotic rim, occurring around 10–20 years of age. Benign BTs typically arise in the epiphyseal area of long bones, with a predilection for the knee joint. Its characteristic feature is adjacent bone marrow edema. It is considered a giant cell tumor variant (**Figure 6**).

Pathogenesis

Molecular: These tumors are characterized by the substitution of H3.3 P.Lys36Met in the *H3F3B* gene on chromosome 17.

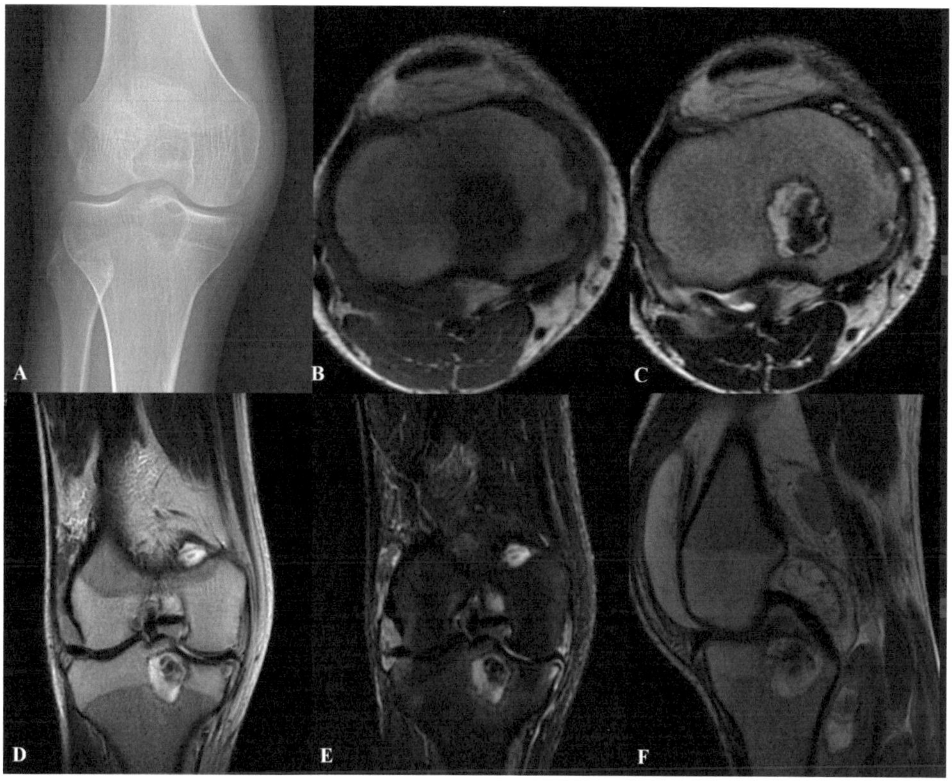

Figure 6.
Chondroblastoma of the right tibia. Right knee radiograph (a) shows a well-defined lytic lesion with a sclerotic rim in the tibial plateau epiphysis in the sub region. MRI axial and sagittal images (b–f) show a T1 hypo intense, T2, STIR hyper intense mass with hypo-intense foci – chondroid matrix, adjacent bone marrow, and reactive joint effusion.

Gross: The lesion has gray-blue chondroid areas, with a rim of sclerotic bone, often containing hemorrhagic spaces resembling an aneurysmal bone cyst.

Microscopy: The tumor displays sheets of plump, polyhedral chondroblasts with interspersed multinucleated giant cells. Chondroblasts have central nuclei with longitudinal grooves (coffee bean). Fine calcifications, often referred to as chicken wire calcifications, encircle each chondroblast.

Differential diagnosis: Giant cell tumor of bone, which arises from the epiphysis of skeletally mature adults, shows numerous evenly distributed giant cells with many nuclei and lacks chicken-wire calcifications. Chondroblastoma occurs in younger patients, is blue on low power, and has grooved chondrocytes and fewer giant cells.

Management: Curettage and bone grafting with adjuvants like phenol and cryotherapy will cure the disease. There is a 10–35% recurrence rate.

4.1.5 Enchondroma and atypical cartilaginous tumor (ACT)

It is a common benign intra medullary bone neoplasm, predominantly found in the tubular bones, around the knee, and in the proximal humerus. It has a thin sclerotic rim, a chondroid matrix with rings and arcs/popcorn-type calcification, and a narrow zone of transition (**Figures 7a**, **7b**, **8**). It should be differentiated from

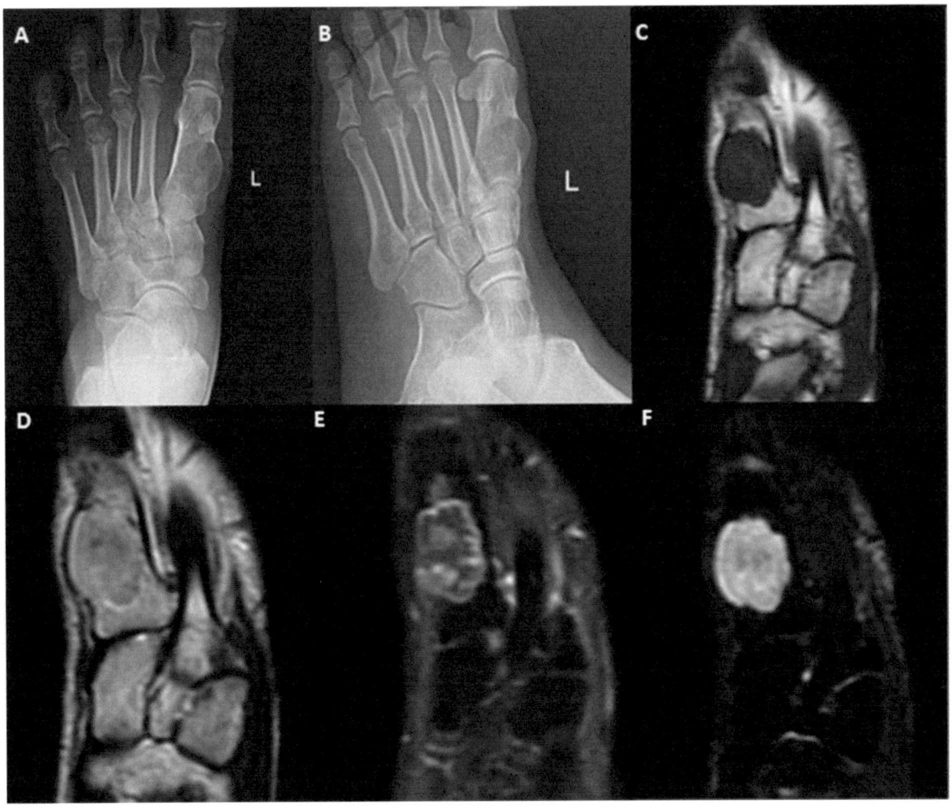

Figure 7a.
Enchondroma of the left 1st metatarsal. (a) Radiograph AP and oblique views show expansive osteolytic lesion. Multiplanar coronal images of the left foot (b–e) show an expansile osteolytic lesion in the shaft of 1st metatarsal with a markedly hyper intense signal on the STIR sequence (e), representing cartilage content.

a bone infarct on Xray, which has a serpiginous outline with few calcific foci but displays fat content on MRI.

The worrying features for developing ACT/secondary low-grade chondrosarcoma on the background of enchondroma (EC) are: length of lesion >5 cm, endosteal scalloping that extends for greater than two-thirds of the lesion's length, greater than two-thirds of the thickness of the cortex, and a wide zone of transition [17].

Management: Curettage and bone grafting are the mainstays of treatment.

The Birmingham Atypical Cartilaginous Tumor Imaging Protocol (BACTIP) provides guidelines and a flowchart as a practical approach for general radiologists in the management of central cartilaginous tumors (CCT) in the appendicular skeleton, ranging from benign to malignant, that is, when to discharge, follow (MRI-Wait and-scan policy), and when to refer to a BT specialist center.

It categorizes CCT into three grades on MRI: I, II, and III, based on the size of size <, >4 cm or any size with aggressive features (bone expansion and/or cortical thickening, periostitis, cortical destruction, and a soft tissue mass), respectively. It further subcategorizes into types A, B, and C based on focal or generalized endosteal scalloping. MRI change is described as an increase in the cranio-caudal length of the lesion >1 cm [18, 19].

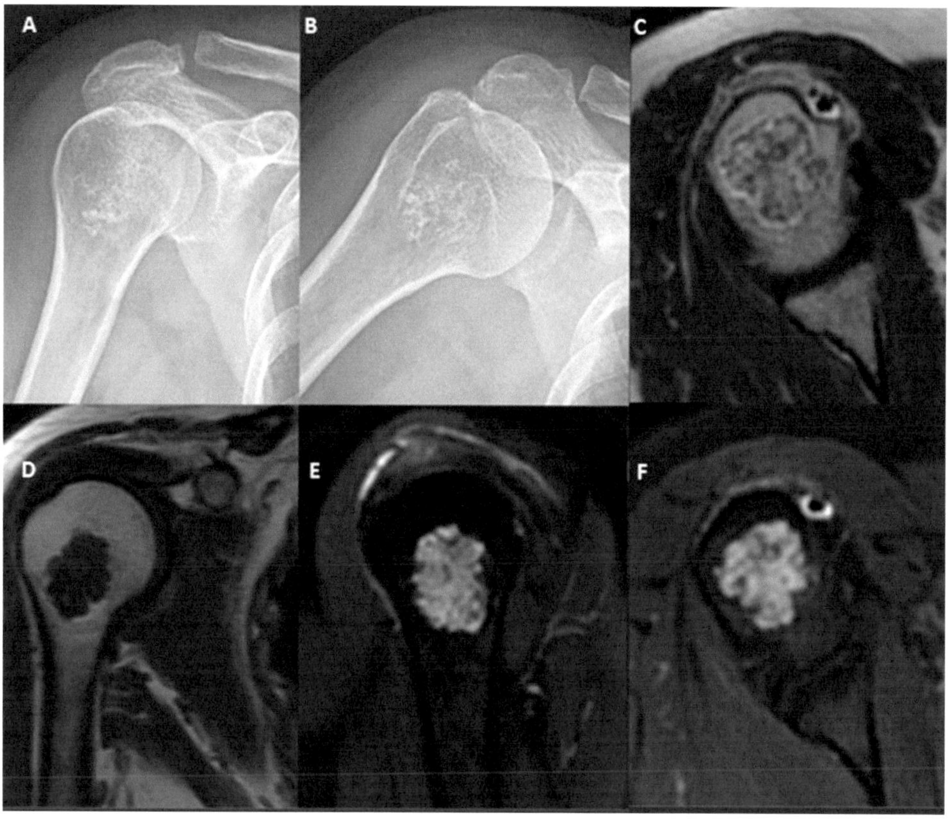

Figure 7b.
Right humeral head enchondroma – radiographs of the right shoulder joint (a, b) show an intra osteolytic lesion with rings and arc pattern calcification (chondroid matrix). MR sequences (c–f) show hypointense foci – calcification.

Pathogenesis: Enchondromas are benign cartilage forming tumors that they arise in the small tubular bones of the hands and feet. They are usually present in as single lesions, but multiple enchondromas may be seen in Enchondromatosis.

Molecular: Mutations in IDH1 and IDH2 genes.

Microscopy: The lesion shows chondroid and focally myxoid matrix with uniformly dispersed chondrocytes situated within the lacunae (**Figures** 5). Chondrocytes lack nuclear hyperchromasia, atypia, and mitosis. In the short tubular bones of the hands, enchondromas tend to be more cellular, and the nuclei show open chromatin, which can mimic an aggressive lesion. Chondrosarcoma may rarely arise within an enchondroma.

4.1.6 Atypical cartilaginous tumor/ Chondrosarcoma, grade 1

Pathogenesis: These low-grade chondroid neoplasms arise from the medullary cavity, and have a potential for cortical erosion and soft tissue extension. Tumors in the long bones are referred to as atypical cartilaginous tumors (ACT), due to their resectable nature. Tumors in the axial skeleton are referred to as Chondrosarcomas Grade 1 due to their aggressive behavior and limited surgical access.

Molecular: IDH1/ IDH2 mutations.

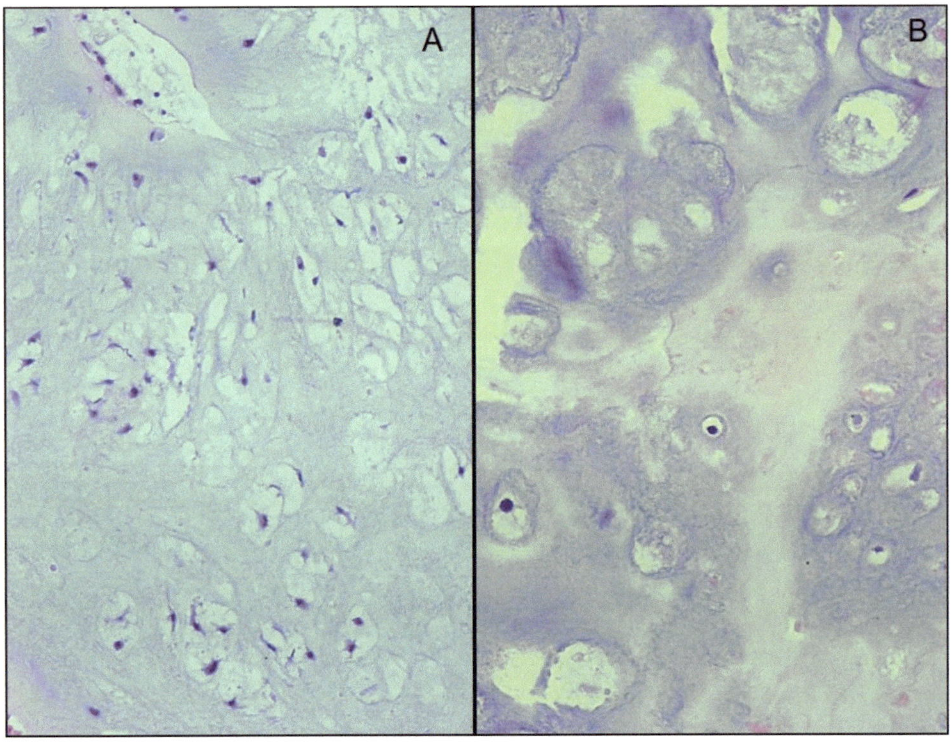

Figure 8.
Enchondroma: A chondroid matrix and chondrocytes within the lacunae.

Microscopy: These tumors are composed of hyaline cartilage lobules with low-mild cellularity and the chondrocytes show slight nuclear atypia. Tumor lobules entrap the medullary trabeculae, breach the bone cortex, and extend into the surrounding soft tissues. The World Health Organization has recently defined this entity in the latest classification.

4.1.7 Chondrosarcoma

Chondrosarcoma (CS) is the 3rd most common type of malignant BT, characterized by a chondroid matrix, following OS and MM. It most commonly appears after 40 years of age, in the axial skeleton, including the ribs, spine, pelvis, and also in long bones (**Figures 9** and **10**) [20]. Based on its location, it can be:

- Central: depending on the intramedullary location.
- Peripheral: appearance over osteochondroma.

Depending on its origin, it can be:

- Primary, when it develops de novo.
- Secondary, when it develops over a benign cartilaginous lesion.

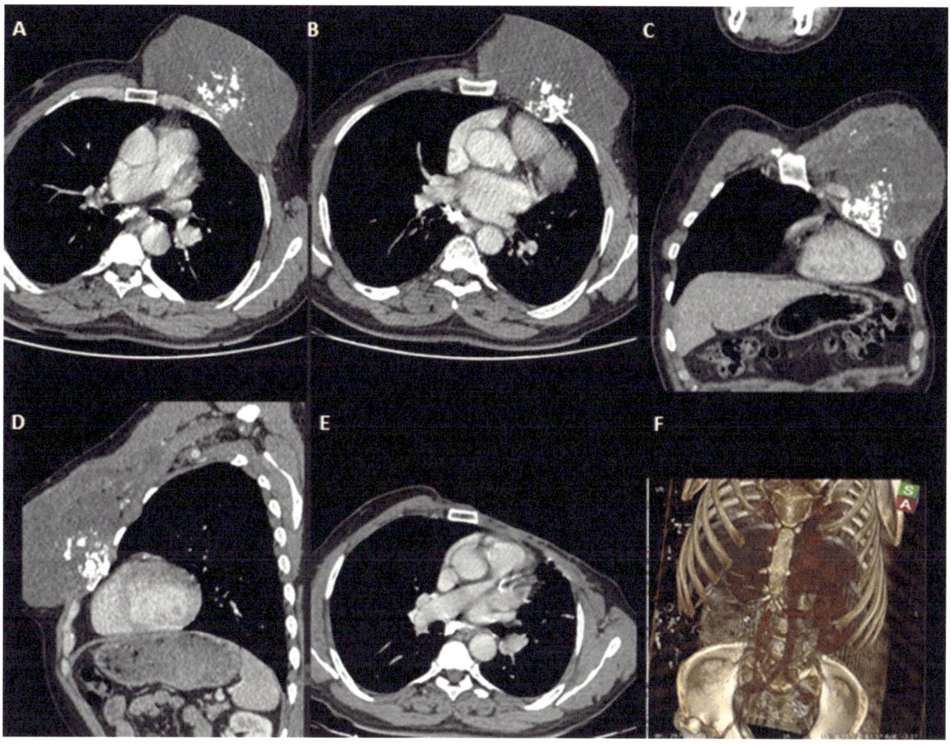

Figure 9.
Chondrosarcoma of the rib. CT scan axial and sagittal sections show peri-osseous soft tissue mass with chondroid matrix calcification in the chest wall. Post-operative CT scan (E, F) shows no recurrent or residual mass. Resected ribs on volume-rendered image (f).

Other types of CS are:

- Periosteal chondrosarcoma (juxtacortical) that arises from the bone surface.
- Dedifferentiated chondrosarcoma – histologically has a biphasic pattern of chondroid sarcoma.
- Clear cell chondrosarcoma – epiphyseal in location and composed of clear-cell chondrocytes.
- Mesenchymal chondrosarcoma – biphasic morphology of a primitive mesenchymal tumor and a well-differentiated cartilaginous component (**Figure 11**).

4.1.8 Grade 1 chondrosarcoma/atypical cartilaginous tumor

Pathogenesis: These are low-grade chondroid neoplasms arising from the medullary cavity, showing potential for cortical erosion and soft tissue extension. Tumors in the long bones are referred to as ACT due to their resectable nature. Tumors in the axial skeleton are referred to as chondrosarcoma Grade 1 due to their aggressive behavior and limited surgical access.

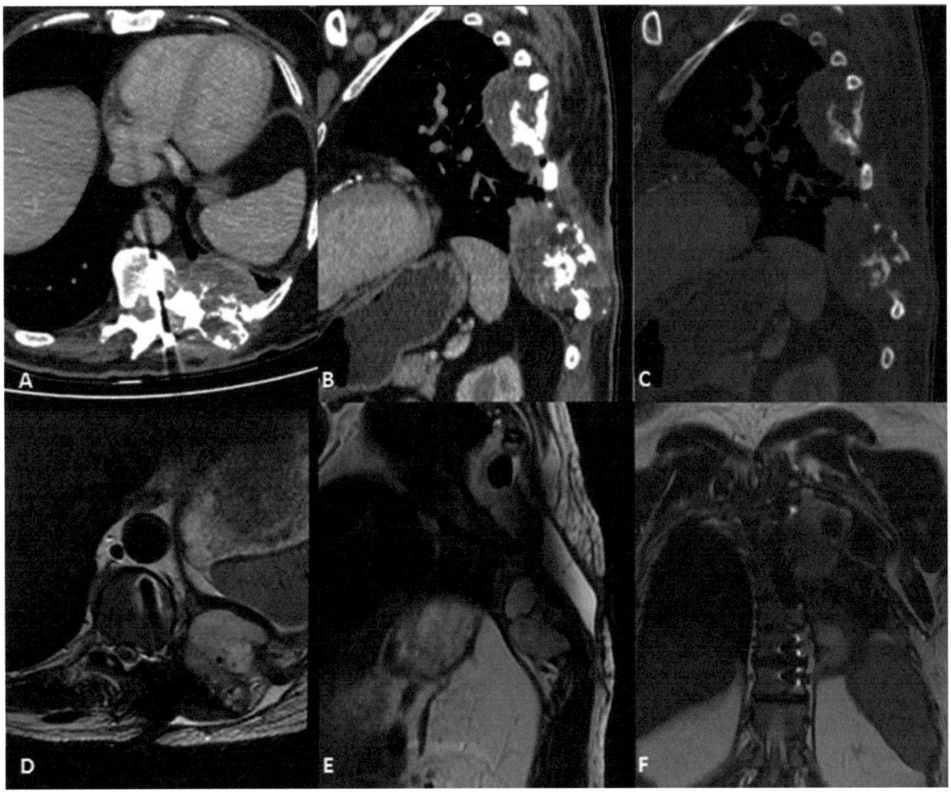

Figure 10.
WHO grade III chondrosarcoma of the rib. CT and MRI images show soft tissue masses along the chest wall protruding into lung with chondroid matrix calcification. Spinal fixator seen in place.

Molecular: IDH1/IDH2 mutations. Multiple enchondromatosis with somatic gain-of-function IDH1/IDH2 mutations predisposes patients to the development of chondrosarcoma.

Gross: The tumor appears as gray-blue lobules of cartilage within the medullary cavity. It may show cortical erosion and infiltration into the soft tissue.

Microscopy: The tumor is composed of hyaline cartilage lobules with low-to-mild cellularity. The chondrocytes are located within the lacunae, show slight nuclear enlargement compared to normal chondrocytes, and exhibit rare mitosis. Tumor lobules may entrap the medullary trabeculae, breach the bone cortex, and extend into the surrounding soft tissues. Myxoid alteration of the cartilaginous matrix may be observed.

Differential diagnosis: Enchondromas are frequently located in the tubular bones of the hands and feet and lack the myxoid matrix and entrapment of host bone. The WHO classification has recently defined this entity in its latest classification.

4.1.9 Central chondrosarcoma (Grade 2 and Grade 3)

Pathogenesis: Malignant cartilage-forming tumors arising from the medulla and characterized by progressive cytologic atypia and invasive growth. Mutations in

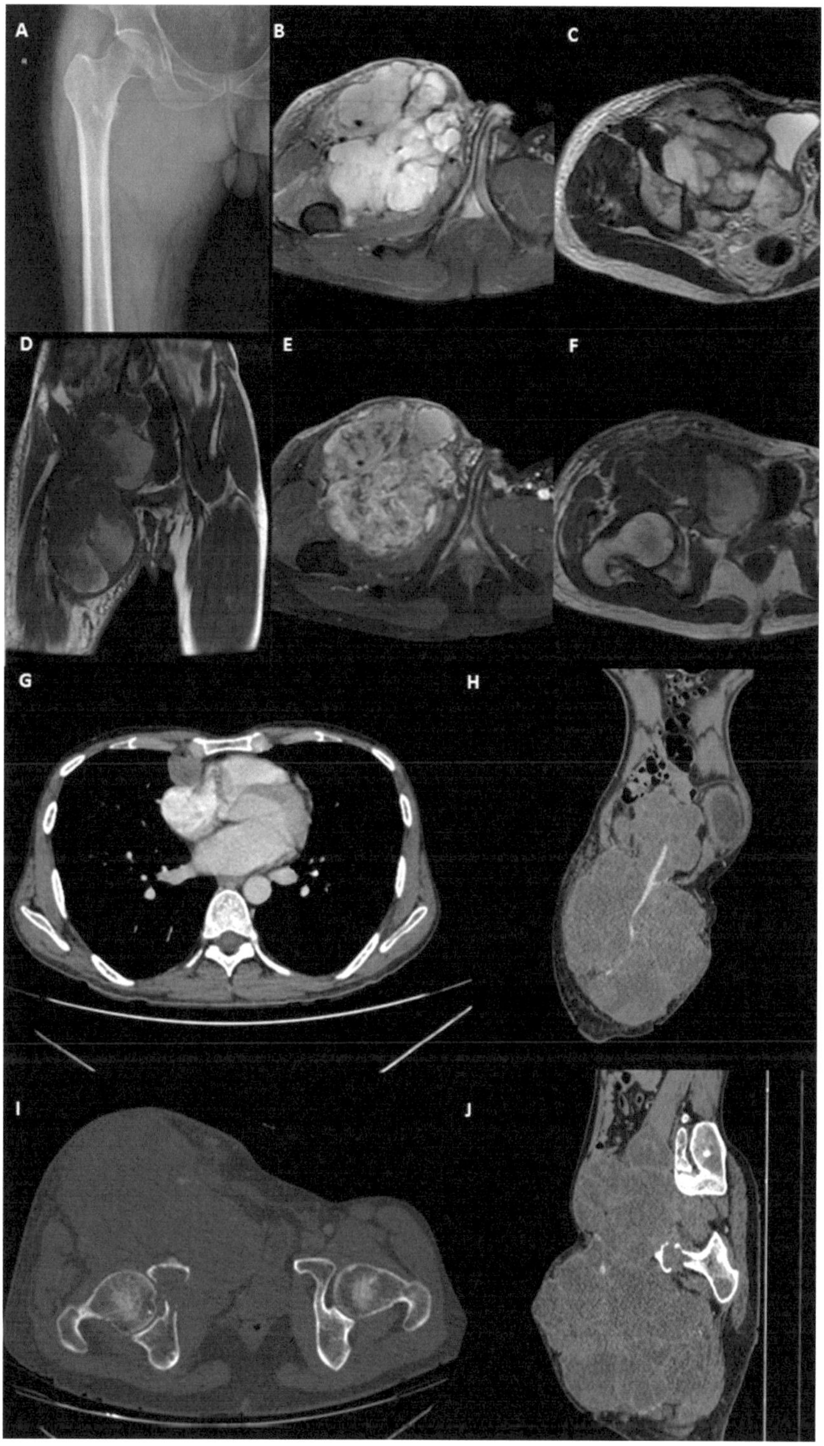

Figure 11.
Extra skeletal mesenchymal chondrosarcoma. Radiograph shows a soft tissue mass in the thigh with blurred fat planes. MRI shows a lobulated mass in the and adductor thigh s with myxoid content and acetabular invasion. CT shows soft tissue mass with vascular encasement of right superficial femoral artery and pulmonary metastasis.

IDH1 and IDH2, CLOA2A1, TP53, and RB1 pathway genes (loss of p16 and CDKN2A, amplification of CDK4). High-grade tumors often exhibit complex karyotypes and chromosomal instability [21].

Gross: Lobulated blue-gray cartilaginous tumors with myxoid areas and foci of calcification.

Microscopy: Blue-gray cartilage lobules invade the marrow trabeculae and may erode the cortical bone to infiltrate the surrounding adipose or muscle tissues. Tumor cells do not produce osteoid. The degree of cellularity, chondrocyte nuclear atypia, and myxoid change in the matrix increases with tumor grade. However, the grading is subject to inter observer variability.

Grade 2: Moderate cellularity, with small, condensed nuclei and inconspicuous mitotic activity.

Grade 3: Highly cellular, with spindled chondrocytes, enlarged nuclei showing an open chromatin pattern, frequent mitoses, and a more myxoid matrix. Foci of necrosis may be present.

IHC: positive for S100, negative for cytokeratin.

Differential diagnosis: Chondroblastic osteosarcoma is diagnosed in a younger age group and demonstrates direct osteoid production by the tumor cells.

4.1.10 Secondary peripheral chondrosarcoma

Pathogenesis: This tumor arises from preexisting osteochondroma, particularly in patients with multiple osteochondromas.

Molecular: Chromosomal instability and complex karyotypes; TP53 and RB1 pathway gene mutations in high-grade tumors.

Gross: The tumor shows a preexisting stalk.

Microscopy: Areas of osteochondroma may be recognized alongside the chondrosarcoma. Grading and molecular genetics are similar to those of central chondrosarcoma. Differential diagnosis: Periosteal osteosarcoma.

4.1.11 Clear cell chondrosarcoma

Pathogenesis: These are low-grade chondrosarcomas of the epiphysis, and two-thirds are located in the head of the femur and the humerus.

Molecular: The tumor displays characteristic loss of chromosome 9 and gain of chromosome 20. IDH1 and IDH2 mutations are absent.

IHC: S100 +, collagen II, and collagen X. Pancytokeratin may be positive, and P53 overexpression may be present.

Microscopy: Round or polyhedral cells, possessing ample clear cytoplasm and centrally placed prominent nuclei, are arranged in lobules with intermixed trabeculae of woven bone and giant cells.

Dedifferentiated chondrosarcoma:

Pathogenesis: The tumor shows a characteristic juxtaposition of a high-grade chondrosarcoma and a high-grade non-cartilaginous sarcoma, with a distinct and sharp interface between the two components.

Molecular: IDH1/2 and p53 gene mutations are commonly present, and the IDH mutation is shared by both components, confirming a clonal relationship.

Gross: The tumor displays gray-blue cartilage lobules alongside yellow-tan areas representing dedifferentiation.

Microscopy: The well-differentiated areas typically correspond to chondrosarcoma grades 1–2. The dedifferentiated component of the tumor is most often fibrosarcoma-like, with spindled tumor cells, but it may resemble an osteosarcoma, pleomorphic undifferentiated sarcoma, angiosarcoma, leiomyosarcoma, or epithelial elements like squamous adamantinoma.

IHC: The IDH1 antibody detects only a minor amount of positive tumor cells. Cytokeratin may be positive in dedifferentiated tumors.

Periosteal chondrosarcoma

Pathogenesis: The tumor originates along the metaphyseal surface of long bones and is usually larger than 5 cm. The tumor may erode the cortex, with medullary invasion occurring only rarely.

Molecular: IDH1 and IDH2 gene mutations are present.

Differential diagnosis: periosteal osteosarcoma and periosteal chondroma.

4.1.12 Mesenchymal chondrosarcoma

Pathogenesis: This rare, aggressive tumor presents in the second or third decade and involves bones, soft tissue, intracranial sites, craniofacial bones, ribs, chest, femur, ileum, and vertebrae, with these being the favored sites, commonly arising in the medullary cavity.

Molecular: Characteristic fusion of the HEY1 and NOCA2 genes.

Gross: Gray-white, soft, circumscribed masses with areas of calcification and necrosis.

Microscopy: Histologically, the lesion shows a biphasic pattern consisting of sheets of small, round cells and nodules of mature cartilage. The small cells possess scant cytoplasm with large nuclei and often surround irregular, staghorn-shaped blood vessels.

Immunohistochemistry: The small cell component is positive for CD99, S100, NKX2.2, and SOX9, whereas the chondroid areas express S100 and SOX9. FLI1 negativity helps differentiate the tumor from Ewing sarcoma.

Management: Wide margin excision followed by chemotherapy in high-grade dedifferentiated tumors. Radiation and chemotherapy are not as effective in low-grade chondrosarcoma.

4.2 Osteogenic

4.2.1 Bony island/enostosis

A well-defined intramedullary benign lesion, composed of compact lamellar bone with smooth margins or marginal bony spicules. It is an incidental finding on imaging that requires no follow-up (**Figure 12**).

Diagnostic dilemma

It should be differentiated from osteoblastic metastasis (described later) and osteopoikilosis, a rare hereditary benign condition that presents with multiple para-articular radio-opaque spots and skin nodules.

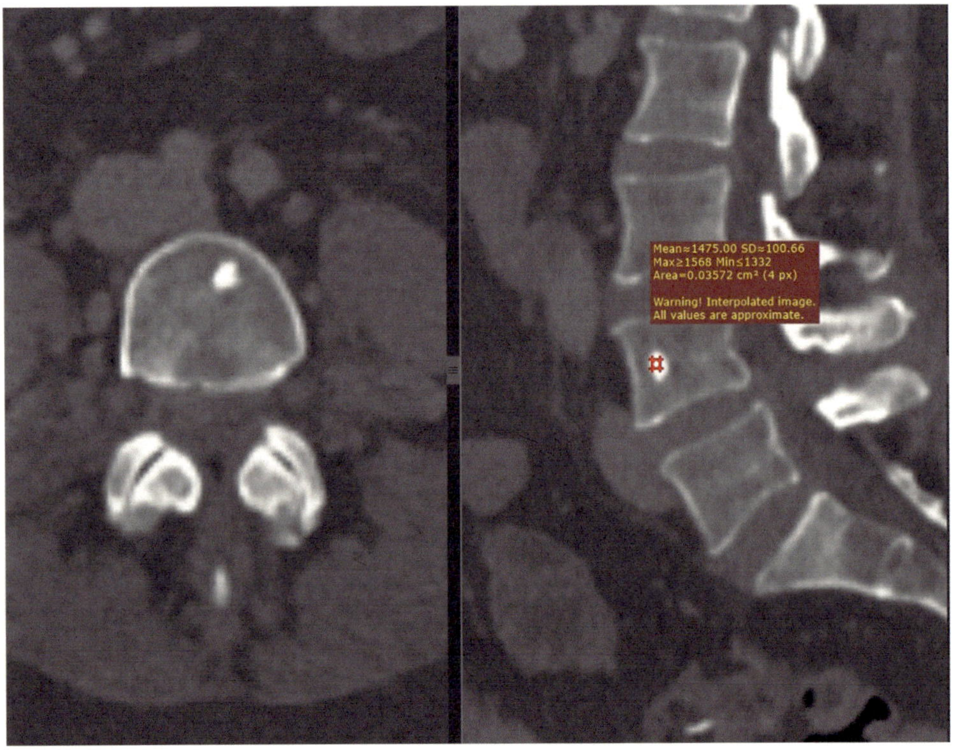

Figure 12.
Enostosis. CT axial and sagittal lumbar spine sections- bone window show a bony island seen in the L4 vertebra with an HU attenuation value of 1,475 units.

4.2.2 Osteoma

A well-differentiated, broad-based bony outgrowth from the cortex, found in the skull and para-nasal sinuses, with a size less than 2.5 cm. It shows no medullary continuity. It has two types:

- Dense variety: ivory osteoma (**Figure 13a–c**).
- Spongy variety that occurs in the cranial vault (**Figure 13d–f**).

Pathogenesis: A benign, slow-growing BT usually seen in the elderly that affects the bones formed by membranous ossification, such as craniofacial and jaw bones. These tumors arise from the surface of bones without cortex invasion. Osteoma-like lesions present in the medullary cavity are termed bone islands. Intramedullary lesions arise from the epiphysis or metaphysis of long bones. Most osteomas are asymptomatic, and when symptoms are present, they are related to the affected site.

Molecular: Multiple osteomas suggest Gardner syndrome, an autosomal dominant disorder with an APC mutation. Osteopoikilosis (spotted bone disease) is associated with multiple bone islands linked to LEMD3 gene mutation.

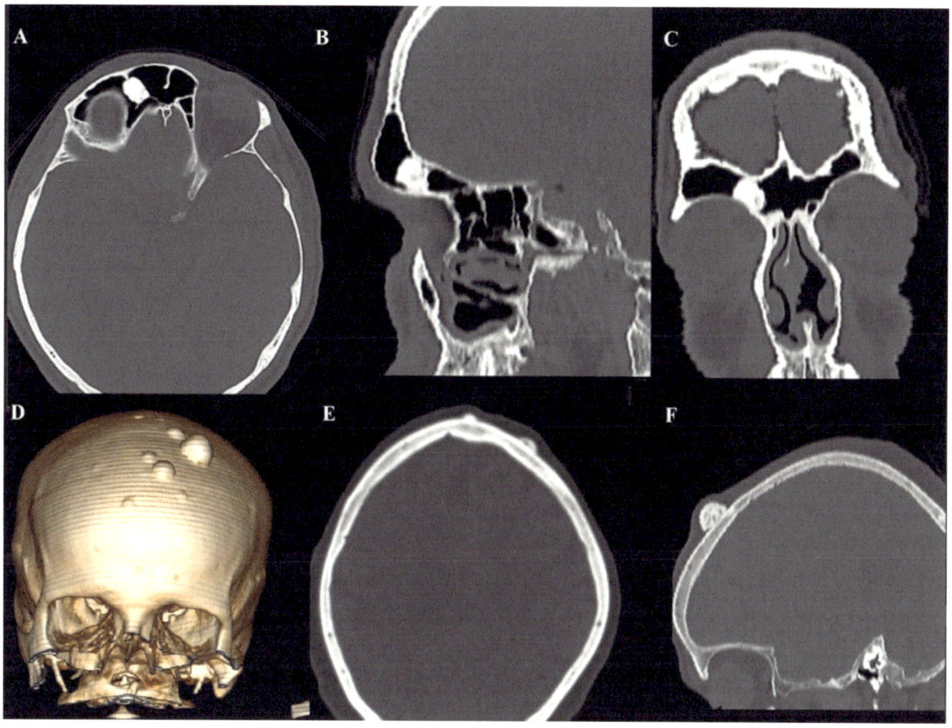

Figure 13.
*CT scan of the skull in bone windows sections (A-C, E, F) and volume-rendered image (D). Osteoma spongy variety (**Figure a–c**) in the right frontal sinus and Ivory osteomas (**Figure d–f**). show multiple osteomas seen along the table of the skull and.*

Gross: Typically single, small, sessile, hard, and bony, with a broad base. Microscopy: Composed of cortical (more commonly) or lamellar bone, with an admixture of woven and mature bone patterns. Bone trabeculae are thick and may show osteoblastic rimming in active lesions; inter trabecular contain fibrous stroma.

Management: Osteoma that is causing obstruction or compression, such as nasal sinus blockage, will be treated by surgical excision.

4.2.3 Osteoid osteoma

Radiological features: Osteoid osteoma (OO) is a cortical-based osteolytic lesion (composed of an intensely enhancing nidus, seen on MRI) with a size of <2 cm, surrounded by a zone of sclerosis and periosteal new bone formation. It may have a central linear sclerotic focus on Xray imaging and CT. MRI may show adjacent marrow edema. Intra capsular proximal femoral OO can present with joint effusion (**Figure 14**).

On radionuclide imaging, it shows central severe uptake surrounded by ill-defined, less intense uptake.

Diagnostic dilemma: OO needs to be differentiated from:

- Osteoblastoma: nidus greater than 2 cm.
- Chronic sclerosing osteomyelitis.

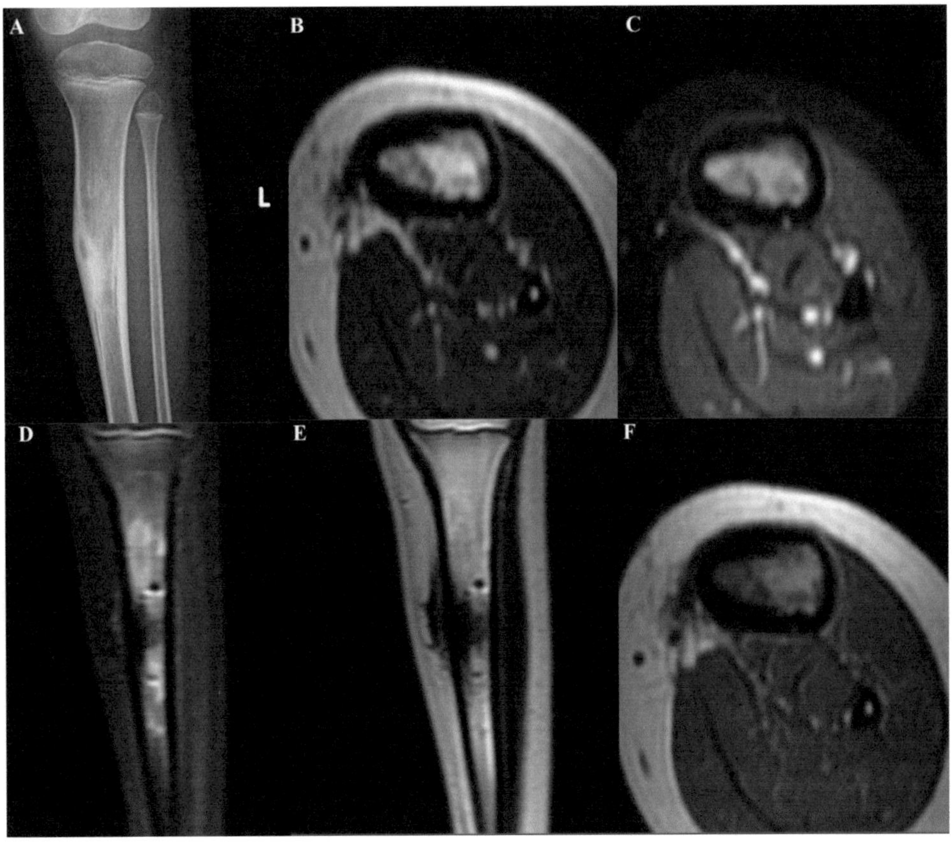

Figure 14.
Radiograph of the left leg shows an eccentric sclerotic lesion along the medial cortex of the tibia with a central lucent nidus. MRI images show an enhancing intra medullary nidus with adjacent bone marrow edema.

- Stress fracture.

Pathogenesis: A benign bone-forming tumor originates within the cortical region of long bones (tibia and femur are the most common), though it may also occur in the tubular bones of the hands, feet, and posterior spine. In about 75% of cases, the lesion is cortical, and in 25%, it is medullary. It usually manifests in the second decade, with localized nocturnal pain that responds to non-steroidal anti-inflammatory drugs (NSAIDs), attributed to prostaglandin production by the nidus.

Molecular: FOS gene rearrangement.

Gross: A round to oval small mass of gritty tan tissue, showing an outer rim of sclerotic bone and a central nidus. The size of the nidus differentiates osteoid osteoma from osteoblastoma, which is smaller than 2 cm in osteoid osteoma and larger in osteoblastoma.

Microscopy: The central nidus is composed of irregular osteoid seams lined by plump osteoblasts, set in a highly vascular and fibrous stroma. A sharp demarcation exists between the nidus and the surrounding zone of reactive, sclerotic bone, which may have a cortical or lamellar pattern.

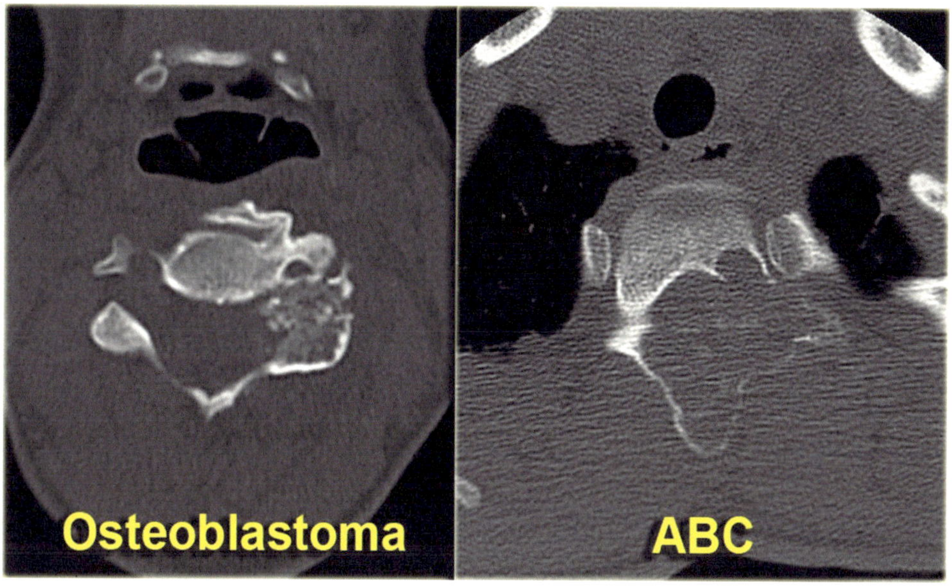

Figure 15.
CT spine bone window axial sections show the of osteoblastoma and aneurysmal bone cyst (ABC) (Reproduced with kind permission from the Dr. Robin Smithuis, Radiology Assistant – educational site of the Radiological Society of the Netherlands).

Management: Pain is responsive to NSAIDs like ibuprofen, and surgical excision if it is ineffective. The nidus of the tumor causing pain can be treated by CT-guided radiofrequency ablation.

4.2.4 Osteoblastoma

Radiological features: It has a nidus greater than 2 cm, and the posterior neural elements of the spine and flat bones are the sites of predilection. It can show multiple fluid–hemorrhagic levels that represent secondary aneurysmal bone cysts (ABC) (**Figure 15**).

Diagnostic dilemma: Aggressive osteoblastoma with an adjacent soft tissue component can be difficult to differentiate from OS. Osteosarcoma shows permeation of the host bone, lack of zonation pattern, nuclear atypia, and atypical mitoses.

Pathogenesis: Osteoblastoma is a benign but aggressive osteogenic tumor that predominantly affects the vertebral bodies and long bones in adolescents, most often during the second decade of life. It presents with localized pain that exacerbates at night and fails to respond to NSAIDs.

Molecular: FOS gene rearrangement.

Gross: Gritty, tan, irregular mass with a hard and sclerotic rim and a softer, vascular central nidus. The lesion is usually larger than 2 cm, distinguishing it from osteoid osteoma.

Microscopy: It shows a central core of immature trabeculae of woven bone and osteoid, lined by active osteoblasts, in a vascular connective tissue stroma. At the periphery, the nidus transitions to sclerotic cortical or lamellar bone. The lesion has well-defined margins.

Management: surgical excision is the mainstay of treatment; bone grafting can be done for lesions that are well-contained. Radiotherapy is used for lesions that are at risk of malignant transformation.

4.2.5 Osteosarcoma

Radiological features: Osteosarcoma, the most frequent primary bone sarcoma, arises in the long bones of skeletally immature individuals. It occurs in the age range of 10–25 years and presents with local clinical symptoms. Radiographs demonstrate aggressive/malignant features with an eccentric, ill-defined metaphyseal osteolytic lesion containing an osteoid matrix, multiple sclerotic foci with bony trabeculae, calcification, and Codman's type/sunray/laminated (multi-layered) periosteal reaction. Chest Xray/CT scan may show ossified pulmonary metastases with a propensity for pneumothorax [22–24] (**Figures 16–22**).

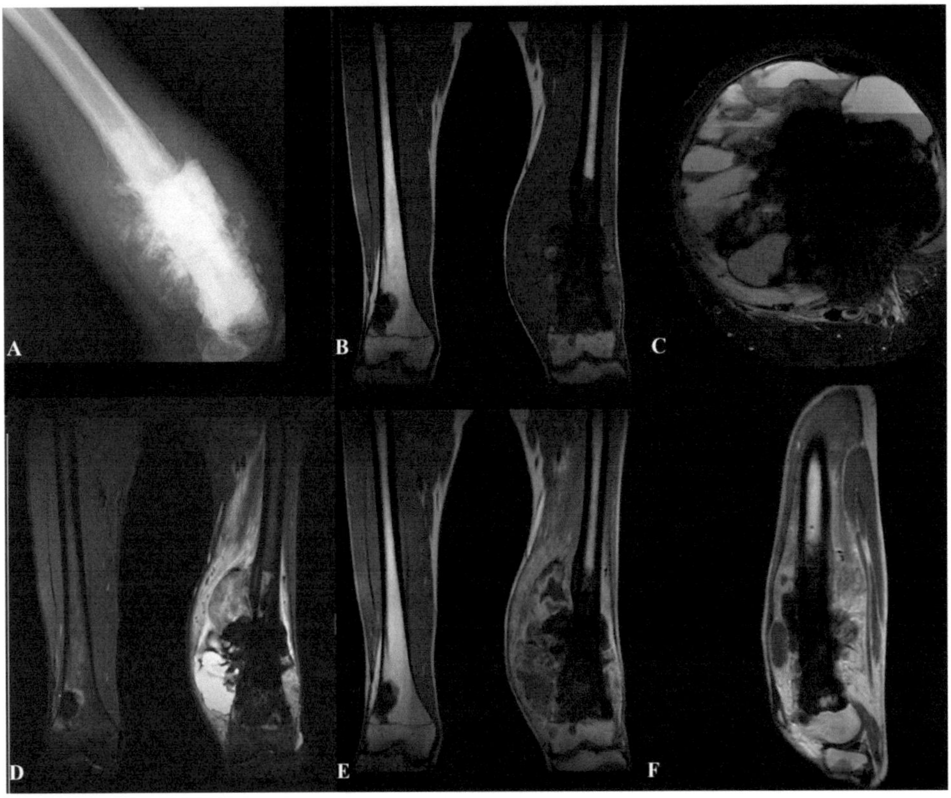

Figure 16.
Chondroblastic osteosarcoma in a 17-year-old male who presented with thigh pain and swelling. Radiograph lateral view (a) Shows an aggressive metadiaphyseal sclerotic lesion of the left femur with osteoid matrix, wide zone of transition with sunburst type and Codman's periosteal reaction and adjacent soft tissue swelling with blurred fat planes. MRI T1W coronal (b), Axial STIR (c) and coronal STIR (d), coronal and sagittal post-contrast sections (e–f) show markedly hypo intense mass with invasion, cortical destruction, growth plate and soft tissue invasion with fluid–fluid levels and metastatic deposit in the right femur metaphysis.

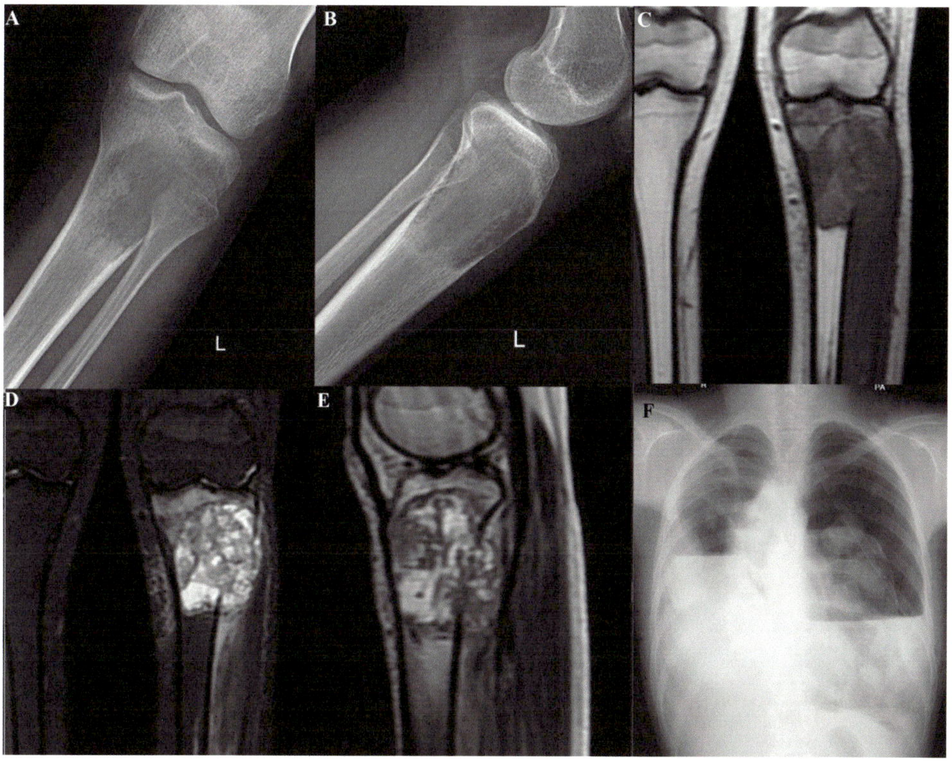

Figure 17.
Telangiectatic osteosarcoma. Radiograph AP view and lateral view (a–b) show an ill-defined lytic lesion in the left proximal tibial metaphysis with periosteal reaction along the posterior cortex. MRI images (c–e) show a T1 intermediate signal, T2 and STIR hyper intense mass with fluid–fluid levels, growth plate and soft tissue invasion, and marrow edema. CXR shows pulmonary metastasis with left-sided hydro pneumothorax.

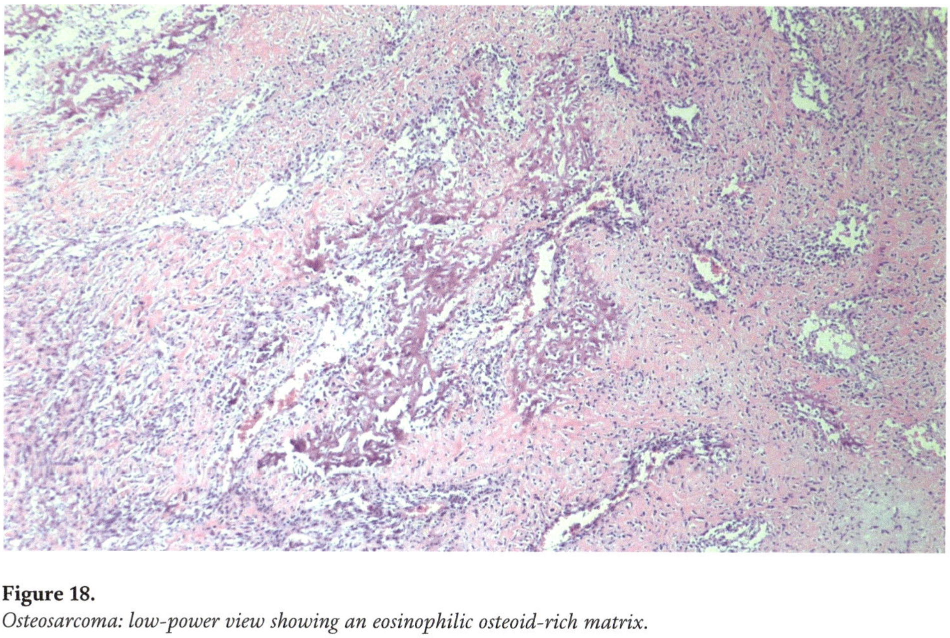

Figure 18.
Osteosarcoma: low-power view showing an eosinophilic osteoid-rich matrix.

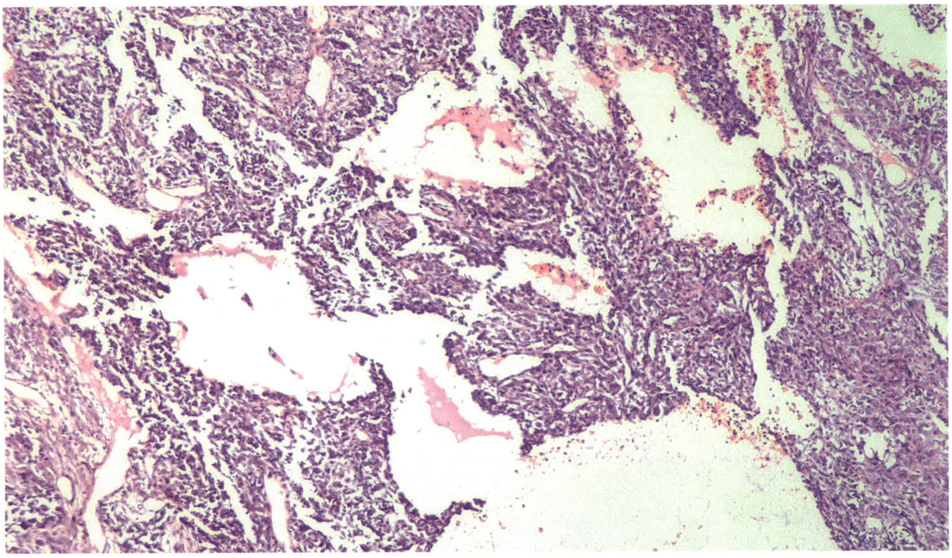

Figure 19.
Telangiectatic osteosarcoma showing blood-filled vascular spaces and surrounding malignant tumor cells.

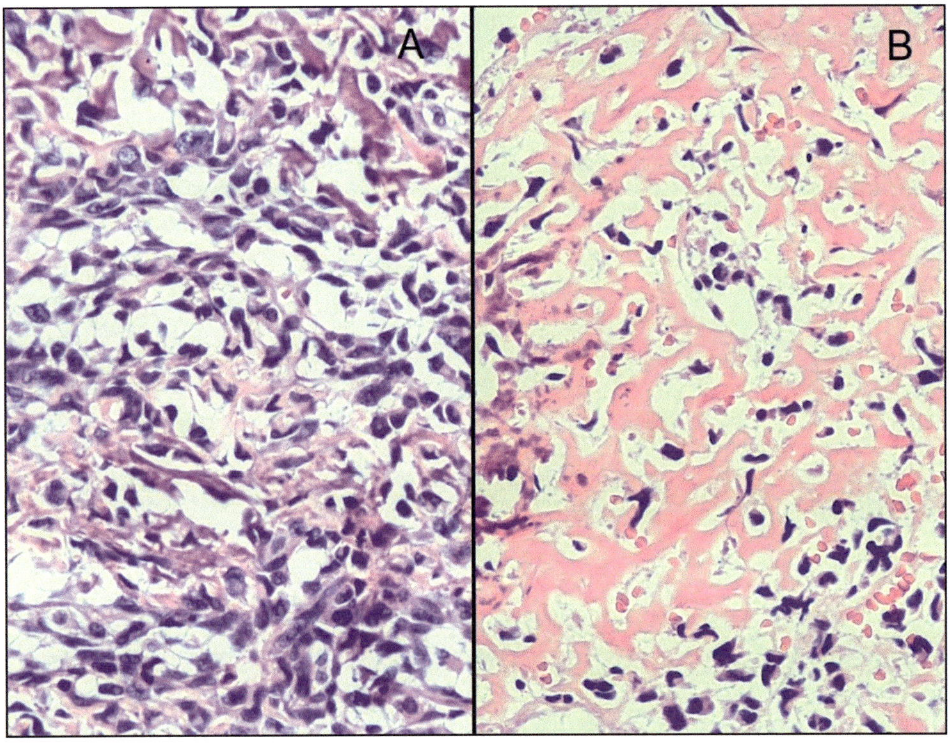

Figure 20.
Osteosarcoma: Thin lace-like osteoid production by the tumor cells, which may appear basophilic (a) or eosinophilic (b).

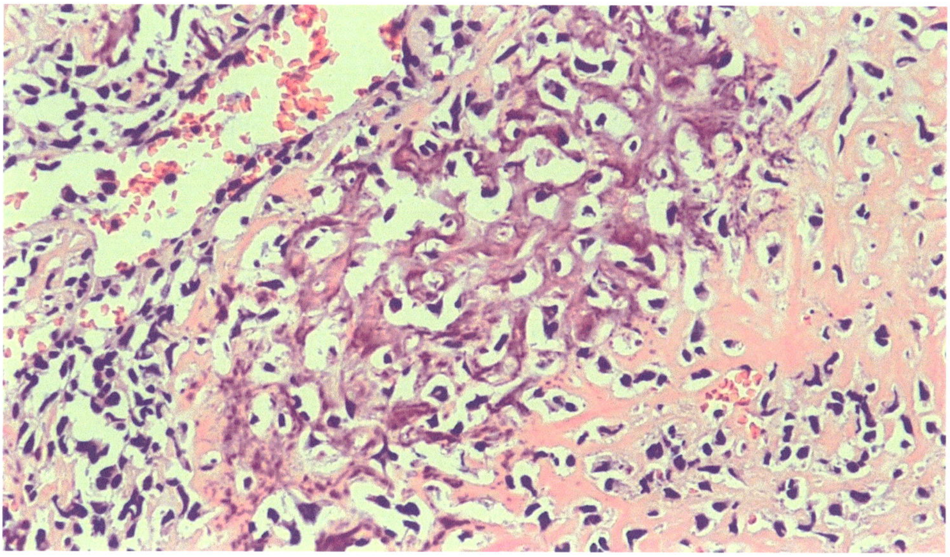

Figure 21.
Osteosarcoma: osteoid with mineralization.

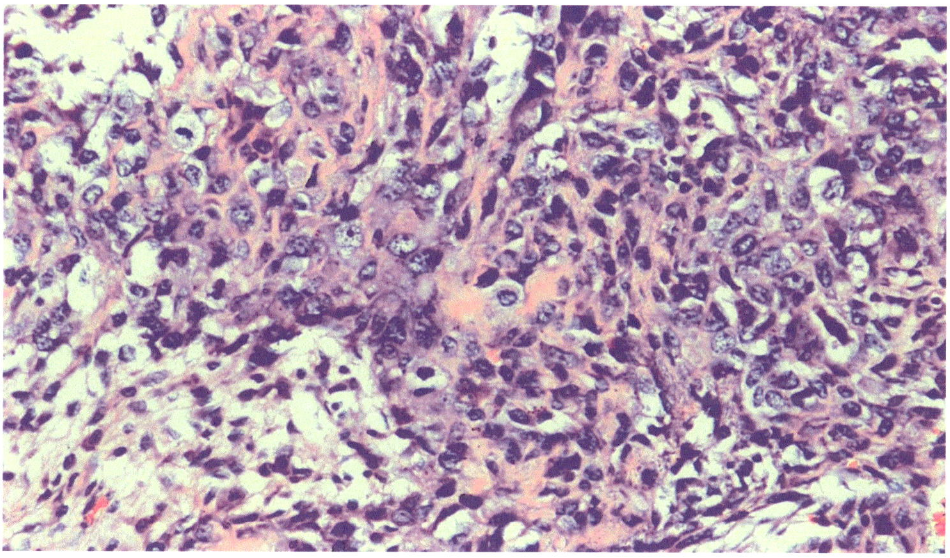

Figure 22.
Osteosarcoma: tumor cells with vesicular nuclei, mitosis, and minimal eosinophilic osteoid.

Its subtypes include:

- Classic intramedullary OS.
- Telangiectatic type (**Figure 17**). It shows multiple fluid-hemorrhagic levels that represent a secondary aneurysmal bone cyst.
- Juxtacortical (surface periosteal) OS.

- Parosteal OS.
- Extra skeletal OS.
- Secondary OS occurs in chronic bone injury, Paget's disease, or after radiotherapy.

Diagnostic dilemma

1. OS and osteomyelitis both have an aggressive radiographic appearance. MRI is the gold standard non-invasive test to differentiate the two.

2. Parosteal OS needs to be differentiated from post-traumatic myositis ossificans (MO), as both present as an ossified mass on imaging, with a thin sliver of normal tissue between the tumor and the mass. MO changes on sequential imaging and has peripheral ossification, compared with OS, which has central ossification.

3. Telangiectatic type OS and aneurysmal bone cyst both have fluid levels; the former has an enhancing soft tissue component.

4. If the chondroid/fibrous matrix predominates, OS mimics chondro/fibrosarcoma on imaging.

Pathogenesis: Osteosarcoma is defined by malignant cells that directly synthesize osteoid.

Molecular: Most osteosarcomas present with complex genomic rearrangements, resulting in highly unstable chromosomes and significant intratumoral diversity. This phenomenon has been named "chromothripsis" (which literally means shattering of chromosomes) [25].

Inactivation of the TP53 gene occurs in the majority (about 90%) of OS cases, including patients with Li-Fraumeni syndrome.

Mutation of RB1 gene (in 56%) and those with hereditary RB gene mutation, MDM2 and CDK4 amplification in low-grade central OS.

Gross: Osteosarcoma typically manifests as a bulky intramedullary lesion with cortex and soft tissue invasion. The cut section is variable, often displaying gray-white and gritty foci of osteoid, yellow necrosis, and red-brown hemorrhage.

Microscopy: The key diagnostic feature of osteosarcoma is the direct osteoid production by tumor cells without an intervening chondroid. Tumor cells may be markedly pleomorphic or small and plasmacytoid. Mitosis and necrosis are frequent. Osteoid is a thin, lace-like eosinophilic matrix between the tumor cells, which may undergo mineralization and ossification. Cartilage may be present and is usually of high grade.

Major histological patterns of OS are as follows:

- **Osteoblastic OS**: Rich in osteoid matrix with bone formation.
- **Chondroblastic OS:** Dominated by malignant cartilage. It must be distinguished from chondrosarcoma. Osteosarcoma is a disease of young adults. The

cartilage in osteosarcoma is high-grade; the peripheries of the chondroid lobules are more cellular, showing spindled cells, and osteoid is usually present. Chondrosarcoma usually occurs in the axial skeleton of adults and is rare in the jaw. It displays low-grade cartilage without osteoid.

- **Telangiectatic OS**: It comprises large blood-filled cystic spaces, mimicking an aneurysmal bone cyst, but lined by pleomorphic tumor cells with mitosis and osteoid production.

- **Fibroblastic OS**: The tumor contains spindle cells arranged in fascicles, resembling fibrosarcoma, with scattered osteoid deposition.

- **Small cell OS**: Tumor cells are mainly small, round, blue cells forming osteoid, resembling Ewing sarcoma.

  Immunohistochemistry: Osteosarcoma is positive for osteoblastic differentiation markers: SAT-B2 (highly specific), osteonectin, osteopontin, and RUNX. The tumor may also be variably positive for S100, actin, CD99, and keratins.

- **Low-grade central OS:**

  A rare intramedullary low-grade tumor that typically arises in the metaphyseal region of long bones in young adults.

  Microscopy: The tumor shows a fibroblastic spindle cell stroma arranged in fascicles. The intervening bone trabeculae are broad, parallel, and lamellar. The spindly tumor cells exhibit low atypia and minimal mitosis.

  Differential diagnosis: Fibrous dysplasia, which shows curvilinear woven bone trabeculae without osteoblastic rimming.

  Molecular: MDM2 and CDK4 amplifications detected by immunohistochemistry or FISH.

- **Periosteal OS:**

  An intermediate-grade OS developing on the diaphyseal surface of the bone, below the periosteum. It occurs in long bones in young adults and shows prominent chondroid formation.

  Molecular: TP53 mutations; the tumor lacks MDM2 and CDK4 mutations, differentiating it from parosteal and central osteosarcomas.

  Gross: Broad-based, lobulated, and fusiform mass on the outer bone cortex, beneath the periosteum, elevating and sometimes infiltrating into the cortex.

  Microscopy: The tumor comprises lobules of atypical cartilage, with intervening areas of typical osteosarcoma showing immature osteoid production by tumor cells. The tumor is located above the cortical bone, with a layer of periosteum on the surface. Spindle cells may be present beneath the periosteum.

  Differential diagnosis

  1. Periosteal OS: It occurs in middle aged adults and is characterized by well-differentiated cartilage without osteoid.

  2. Parosteal OS: It contains mature bony trabeculae, low-grade spindle stroma, and MDM2 positivity.

- **Parosteal OS:**
  A low-grade osteosarcoma arising from the outer surface of the bone cortex, typically at the posterior distal femur, although it may involve other long bones. It represents the most common surface osteosarcoma.
  Molecular: Supernumerary ring chromosomes, leading to MDM2 and CDK4 amplification, are detected by immunohistochemistry or fluorescence in situ hybridization.
  Gross: The tumor is attached to the cortex of the bone as a lobulated soft tissue mass and may be invading the cortex and medullary cavity.
  Microscopy: Parallel, curvilinear, or anastomosing trabeculae of woven bone with intervening spindle stromal cells. Trabeculae may show osteoblastic rimming. In a series, 24% of cases dedifferentiate to a high-grade OS [26].
  Immunohistochemistry: MDM2 and CDK4-positive. MDM2 amplification detected by FISH.

- **High-grade surface OS:** It is a high-grade sarcoma originating on the external cortical bone surface. The diaphysis of the humerus, tibia, and femur are the favored sites. Although primarily periosteal, it may invade the endosteum and cortex. Microscopy is similar to conventional osteosarcoma.

4.3 Fibrogenic

4.3.1 Desmoplastic fibroma

Radiology: It presents as a locally aggressive, solitary, large destructive tumor in young adults, with an ill-defined area of osteolysis in the metaphysis of long bones and a sclerotic rim. It mimics the desmoid tumor of the anterior abdominal wall. Fibrous dysplasia is its differential.

It is the bony counterpart of desmoid-type fibromatosis, slow-growing and locally aggressive.

Gross: White, firm specimen with a whorled cut surface and rounded margins.

Microscopy: Bland spindle cells in an abundant collagenous matrix, without significant nuclear atypia or mitosis. The margins are infiltrative.

Immunohistochemistry: Cells express variable reactivity to actin and β-catenin. Differential diagnosis: Low-grade central osteosarcoma and fibrous dysplasia.

Management: Wide local excision can be performed, as recurrence is high – up to 30–40% – if not removed completely.

4.3.2 Fibrosarcoma NOS

Radiology: This tumor shows a malignant appearance on imaging, with an ill-defined area of osteolysis in the metaphysis of long bones. It occurs in the 3rd to 6th decade and is devoid of osteoid or cartilaginous matrix. The most common location is around the knee. It can invoke a little sclerotic reaction. Rarely, it arises in the fibrous wall of a medullary infarct.

Consider a diagnosis of exclusion after the advent of immunohistochemistry and molecular genetics. The femur is the most commonly reported site.

Microscopy: A fish-flesh or fascicular pattern of cellular arrangement; spindle cells show mild to moderate nuclear atypia. Severe pleomorphism is unusual in fibrosarcoma. The presence of osteoid or cartilage, or expression of immunohistochemical stains, excludes a diagnosis of fibrosarcoma.

Differential diagnosis

Chondrosarcoma: Cartilage, S100 positive.

Osteosarcoma: Osteoid and positive for SATB2. Synovial sarcoma: Epithelial marker and SS18 expression are present in synovial sarcoma. Solitary fibrous tumor: STAT6 positive. Leiomyosarcoma: ASMA, Caldesmon.

Management: Treatment depends on the stage, with surgical removal followed by chemoradiotherapy, especially for high-grade or metastatic tumors.

4.4 Vascular

4.4.1 Intra-osseous hemangioma

Radiology: A well-defined intra medullary lytic lesion with thickened trabeculae, that is, polka dot, corduroy appearance (**Figures 23** and **24**).

Pathogenesis: It is a common benign vascular tumor of young age, which most commonly occurs in the vertebral bodies; craniofacial bones are the next most frequent site.

Gross: Dark-red, soft, with sclerotic bone and spongy, blood-filled spaces.

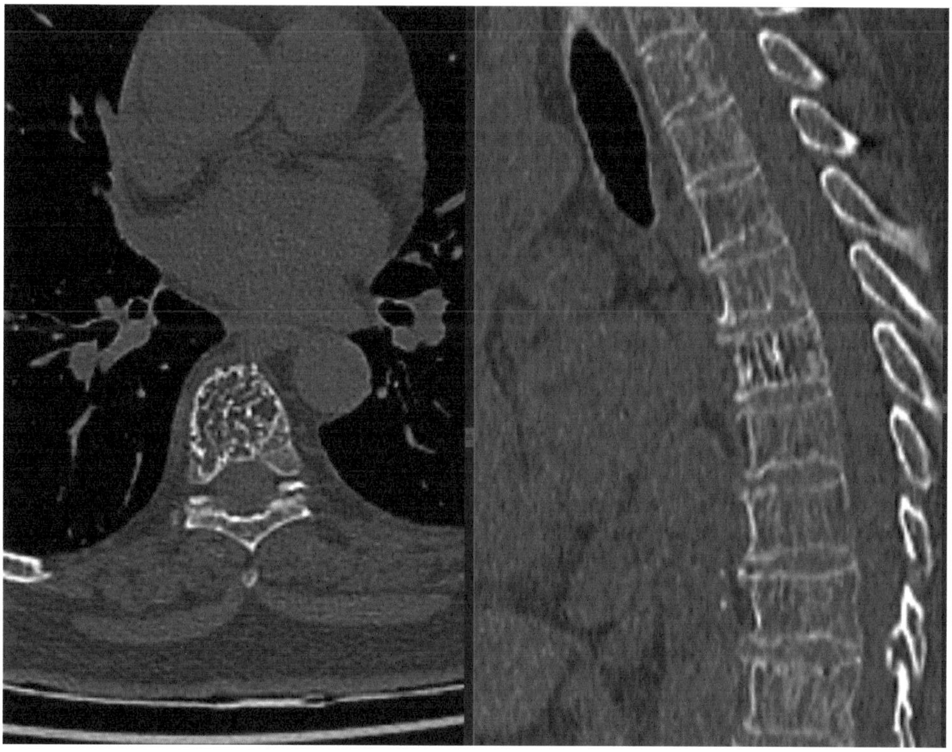

Figure 23.
Vertebral hemangioma. CT of the dorsal spine bone windows [axial and sagittal] sections shows a mid-dorsal vertebral body lesion with polka-dot appearance with intervening thickened vertical trabecula.

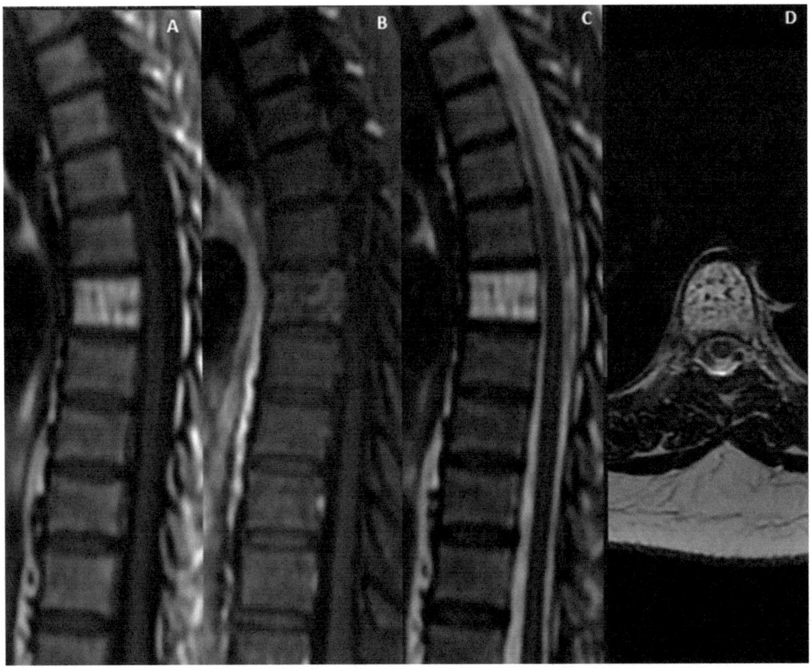

Figure 24.
Vertebral hemangioma. MRI sagittal T1W pre-contrast (a) and fat-saturated post-contrast (b), sagittal and axial T2W (c, d) show a mid-dorsal vertebral body fatty signal intensity lesion with hypointense foci, that is, E. serpiginous vessels.

Microscopy: Hemangiomas are usually present in the inter trabecular areas of the bone and may expand and erode the cortex. Hemangiomas show vessels lined by endothelial cells that lack nuclear atypia. Hemangiomas may contain variable amounts of fat, smooth muscle, hemosiderin, and reactive bone [27].

Its four types are:

- Capillary hemangiomas: lobules of capillaries.
- Cavernous hemangiomas: larger vascular channels
- Venous: Thin-walled vessels, which are of mixed cavernous and capillary types.
- Arteriovenous: interconnected arteries and veins.

Immunohistochemistry: CD31, CD34, ERG, FLI-1, and Factor VIII positive.

Management: Most commonly, they regress spontaneously in infantile cases. Sometimes, beta-blockers are used for problematic ones. Surgery or embolization is reserved for deep and symptomatic hemangiomas.

4.4.2 Angiosarcoma

Radiology: Aggressive lytic lesion on radiograph with intense vascularity on MRI.

Pathogenesis: A highly malignant tumor with vessel formation.

Molecular: Amplification of 2q and 17q. RB1 pathway is involved, with p16 loss and cyclin D1 overexpression.

Gross: Red-brown, hemorrhagic tan masses involving mostly tubular bones; may be multifocal, with bone cortex, medulla, and soft tissue invasion.

Microscopy: It may be well-differentiated with readily identifiable vessels, but mostly it is highly atypical and requires a large panel of immunohistochemistry to identify the vascular differentiation in tumor cells. The endothelial cells can be spindle-shaped or epithelioid, exhibiting pleomorphic nuclei and mitotic figures. The formation of vascular spaces, tumor cells with small cytoplasmic lumina containing red blood cells (RBCs), and tumor stroma containing extravasated neutrophils, eosinophils, RBCs, and hemosiderin give some clues to the diagnosis of angiosarcoma.

Immunohistochemistry: CD31, CD34, ERG, Factor VIII, and FLI-1 stains are positive. ASMA, D2-240, and keratins may also be positive.

Differential diagnosis: Metastatic carcinoma, particularly, and any other high-grade sarcoma.

4.5 Osteoclastic (giant-rich cell containing)

4.5.1 Non-ossifying fibroma

Radiology: It is a benign, non-neoplastic osteolytic lesion with a lobulated, well-defined outline and a thin sclerotic rim. With time, the lesion undergoes sclerosis and ossification and has a natural tendency to regress. Simple bone cyst, fibrous dysplasia, and aneurysmal bone cyst are its differentials (**Figures 25** and **26**).

Pathogenesis: Also referred to as fibrous histiocytoma of bone, it is the most commonly encountered bone lesion in children and young adults. It typically arises in the metaphysis of long bones in the extremities, around the knee and ankle joints.

The lesion, when confined to the cortex, is termed a fibrous cortical defect, whereas lesions extending into the medulla were historically called metaphyseal fibrous defects, a term currently not recommended by the WHO.

Gross: Circumscribed red-brown lesions.

Microscopy: Bland, fibrous, spindle-shaped cells in a storiform pattern, admixed with osteoclast-like multinucleated cells and reactive bone formation.

Management: They usually resolve spontaneously in younger children and need surgical intervention for larger lesions, with a risk of fracture or pathological fracture.

4.5.2 Aneurysmal bone cyst

Radiology: It is a benign, non-neoplastic, blood-filled, expansile osteolytic tumor with a lobulated, well-defined outline, a soap bubble appearance with fluid–fluid levels, and a thin sclerotic rim. The most common location is at the metaphysis of the long bones in individuals under 20 years of age. In the spine, it most commonly involves the neural arch (**Figures 27** and **28**).

Pathogenesis

Molecular: Cytogenetic rearrangements of USP6 at chromosome 17p13.2.

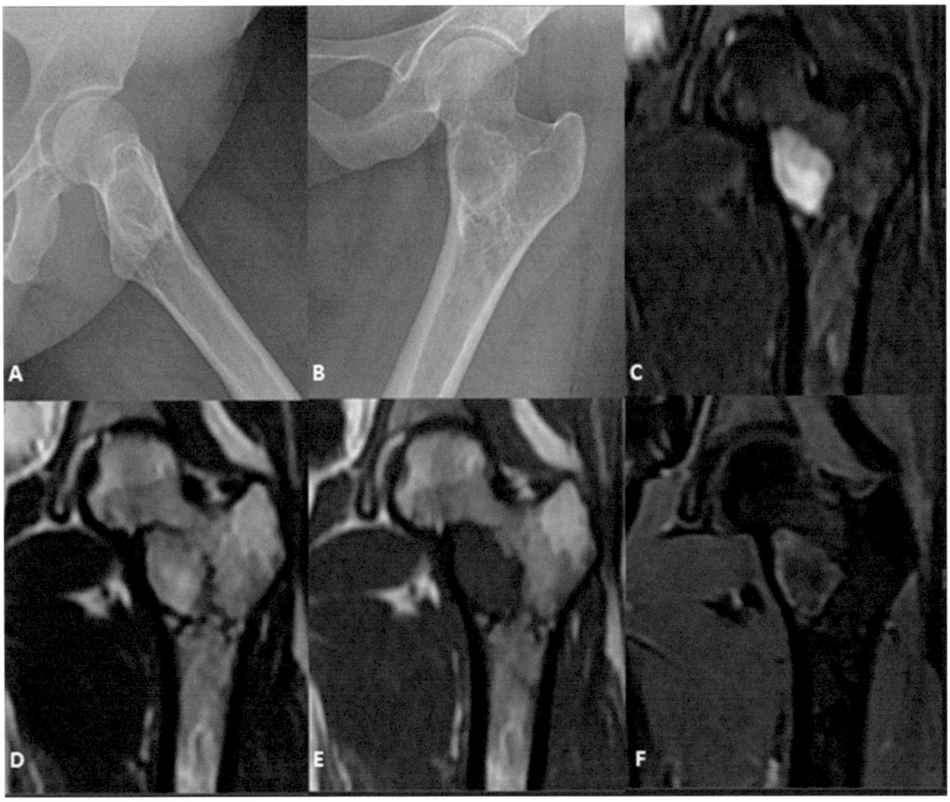

Figure 25.
Simple bone cyst/non-ossifying fibroma. Radiograph (a, b) shows a well-defined eccentric lytic lesion with a thin rim in the neck of the left femur medially accompanied by mild bony expansion and remodeling deformity. On coronal MRI STIR (c), T2W (d), T1W (e), GRE (f) sequences, it shows fluid content – a benign "leave me alone" lesion.

Gross: Multiloculated, blood-filled cystic cavities bordered by gritty septa and an outer shell of thin reactive bone.

Microscopy: Large, blood-filled cavernous spaces delineated by fibrous septa containing osteoclast-like multinucleated cells. Reactive bone lined by osteoblasts, hemosiderin-containing macrophages, and mild amounts of lymphocytes may be present in a fibrous stroma, seen in young age groups. ABC-like changes may be seen in other benign lesions, such as chondroblastoma and fibrous dysplasia.

Immunohistochemistry: Negative for H3.3 p.Gly34Trp.

USP6 rearrangement detected by FISH.

Management: Various treatment plans can be opted for, for example: curettage and bone grafting, en bloc resection for recurrent lesions, and selective arterial embolization for spinal and pelvic lesions. Recently, minimally invasive percutaneous sclerotherapy or agents like bisphosphonate and denosumab have been used in selective cases.

4.5.3 Giant cell tumor (NOS and malignant type)

Radiology: Giant cell tumor (GCT), also known as osteoclastoma, is a sub-articular eccentric expansile osteolytic lesion occurring in individuals aged 20–40

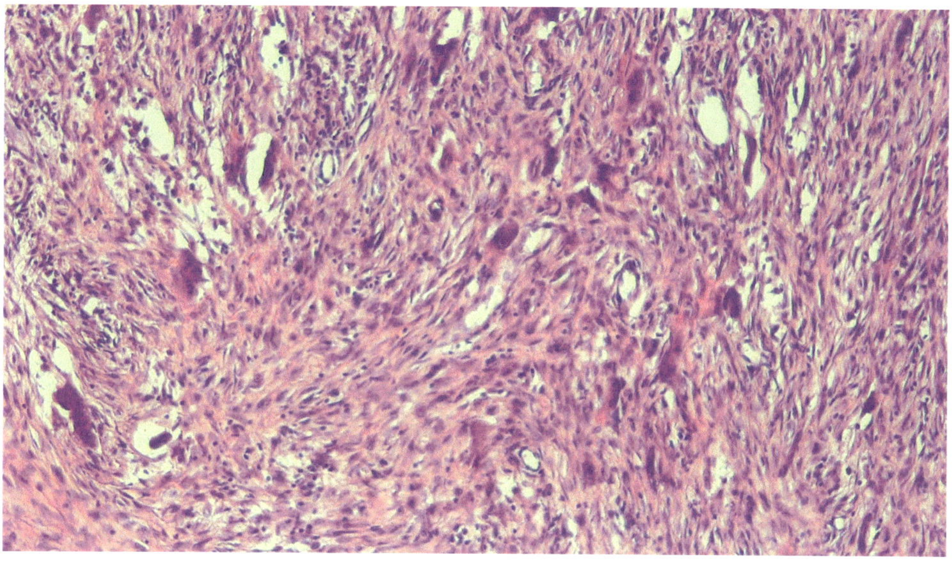

Figure 26.
Non-ossifying fibroma: Bland fibrous stromal cells in a storiform pattern and interspersed giant cells.

years. It is an intermediate-grade BT, mostly affecting the epiphysis of long bones. Bones adjacent to knee joint are the favored site (**Figures 29–32**). In the axial skeleton, the sacrum and vertebral bodies may be involved. In an immature skeleton, the metaphysis may be involved. It may rarely involve the pelvis and the bones of the hands and feet. It has no sclerotic rim and is primarily a solid tumor with possible hemorrhage and secondary aneurysmal bone cystic components. It can rarely undergo malignant transformation. Brown tumor of hyperparathyroidism, chondroblastoma, and sub-articular geode are its differentials. These can be differentiated from GCT by bony texture, age, and adjacent osteoarthritic changes, respectively.

Pathogenesis

Molecular: H3-3A (H3F3A) mutation occurs in 95% of GCT, 90% of which have H3.3 p.Gly34Trp. Malignant GCT has TP53 and HRAS mutations. Telomeric association with the ring chromosome is the most common chromosomal abnormality. A crucial role of the RANK/RANKL pathway in the pathogenesis of GCT has been demonstrated. The mononuclear stromal cells in GCT are of osteoblastic lineage, most likely represent the neoplastic component, and express (pre)osteoblastic stem cell markers SATB2, SP7, RUNX, and ALP. The mononuclear stromal cells express RANKL and recruit mononuclear cells to form giant cells [28].

Gross: GCT expands the epiphysis, may cause cortical thinning and breach, and possibly extend into the surrounding tissues; GCT usually does not involve the joint spaces. It is predominantly red-brown, friable, and hemorrhagic, with pale white fibrous areas.

Microscopy: GCT exhibits neoplastic proliferation of mononuclear stromal cells and interspersed multinucleated giant cells. The stromal cells are usually plump, with vesicular nuclei and indistinct nucleoli, or they can appear fibroblast-like, set against a collagen-rich matrix. The giant cells have abundant cytoplasm,

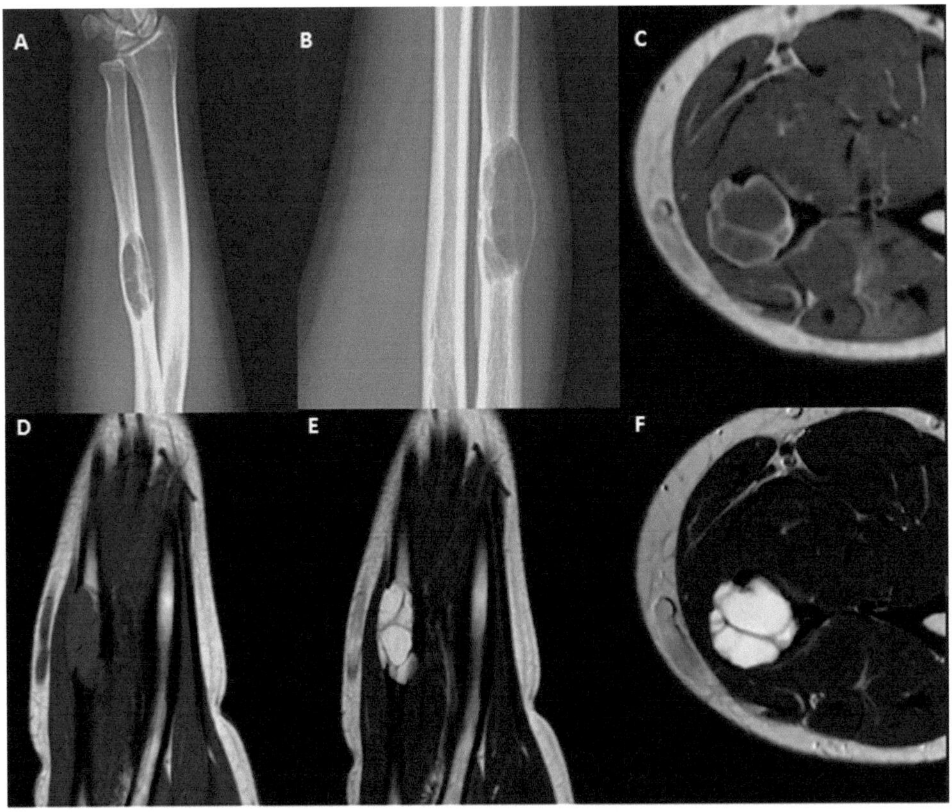

Figure 27.
Aneurysmal bone cyst in the ulna (a, b). Knee radiograph AP view and oblique view (a, b) show a soap bubble-type lesion in the diaphysis with thin septa and thinned out cortex. Post-contrast T1W axial MRI (c), T1W (d), T2W coronal (e) and axial (f) images, shows fluid content in the lesion with thin hypointense enhancing septa.

numerous vesicular nuclei, and small nucleoli, resembling those of mononuclear cells. Mitotic figures are frequent. GCT may display variable areas of fibrosis, hemorrhage, necrosis secondary to fracture, foamy macrophages, reactive bone formation, and secondary ABC-like areas. Vascular invasion may also be observed.

Immunohistochemistry: Positive for H3.3 p.Gly34Trp. Stromal cells express SATB2.

Differential diagnosis: Giant cell-rich osteosarcoma shows osteoid production. Undifferentiated pleomorphic sarcoma with marked cellular pleomorphism and mitosis requires immuno-histochemical and radiological correlation.

Management: Curettage and bone grafting are indicated for small lesions, and cement packing is recommended for large lesions. Adjuvants like phenol or liquid nitrogen are also used in selective cases. For aggressive or recurrent cases, Denosumab, an osteoclast RANKL inhibitor, is used first to shrink the lesion, forming a capsule around the tumor margin, thereby making wide resection an easier task.

Malignant GCT: Primary malignant GCT occurs when a high-grade sarcomatous component arises de novo in GCT. Secondary malignant GCT develops after treatment with denosumab, curettage, bone graft, or radiotherapy. The malignant transformation may result in pleomorphic undifferentiated sarcoma or

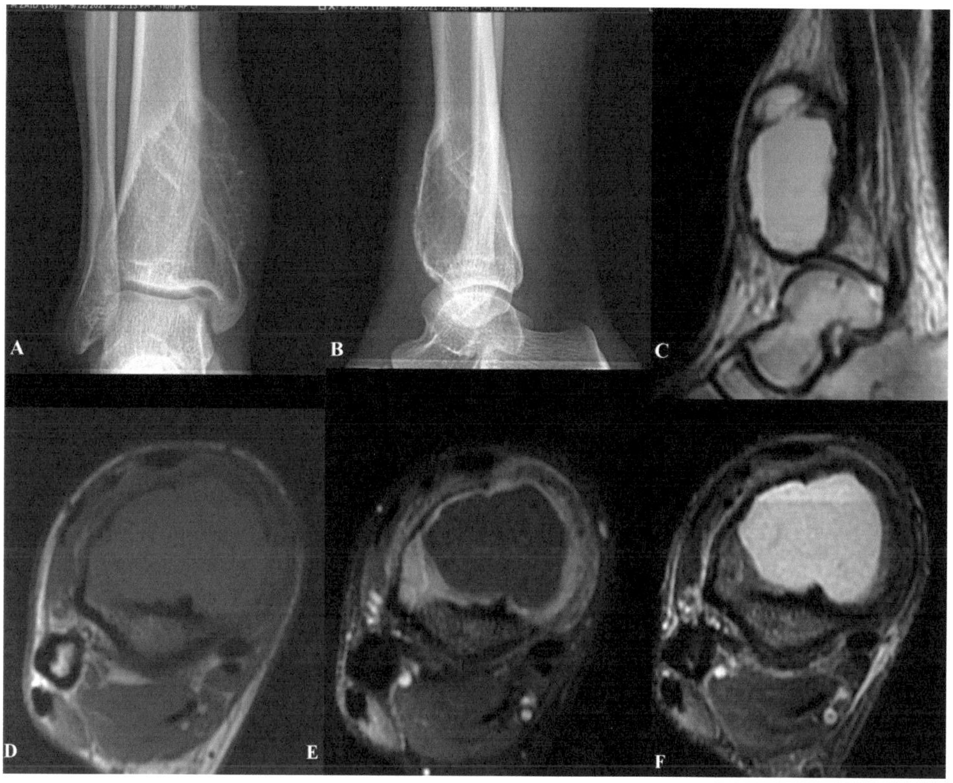

Figure 28.
Aneurysmal bone cyst of the tibia. Knee radiograph AP view and lateral view (a, b) of the right leg show a soap bubble-type lesion with thin septa and an out cortex, multi-sequential MRI images (c–e) show a lobulated metaphyseal lesion with fluid–fluid levels and sclerotic enhancing rim and enhancing septa that reaches up to the articular surface.

osteosarcoma. Secondary malignant GCT after radiotherapy is more common. Tumors have two components: one typical of GCT and the other of sarcoma. Malignant cells may be positive for H3.3 p.Gly34Trp and may exhibit higher expression of TP53 and Ki67.

Denosumab-treated tumors may show complete disappearance of giant cells; instead, stromal cells acquire a bland fibrous look, with immature osteoid. However, these cells do maintain their reactivity for H3.3 p.Gly34Trp. Treatment has been linked to increased recurrence, and malignant transformation to osteosarcoma or malignant GCT has been reported [29, 30].

4.6 Notochordal

4.6.1 Chordoma

Radiology: It is a midline expansile osteolytic tumor of adult age (30–70 years), most commonly involving the base of the skull or spine, the spheno-occipital region, and the sacrococcygeal region, in the midline. It arises from remnants of the notochordal cell rests. Its characteristic feature is a marked T2 hyper intense signal

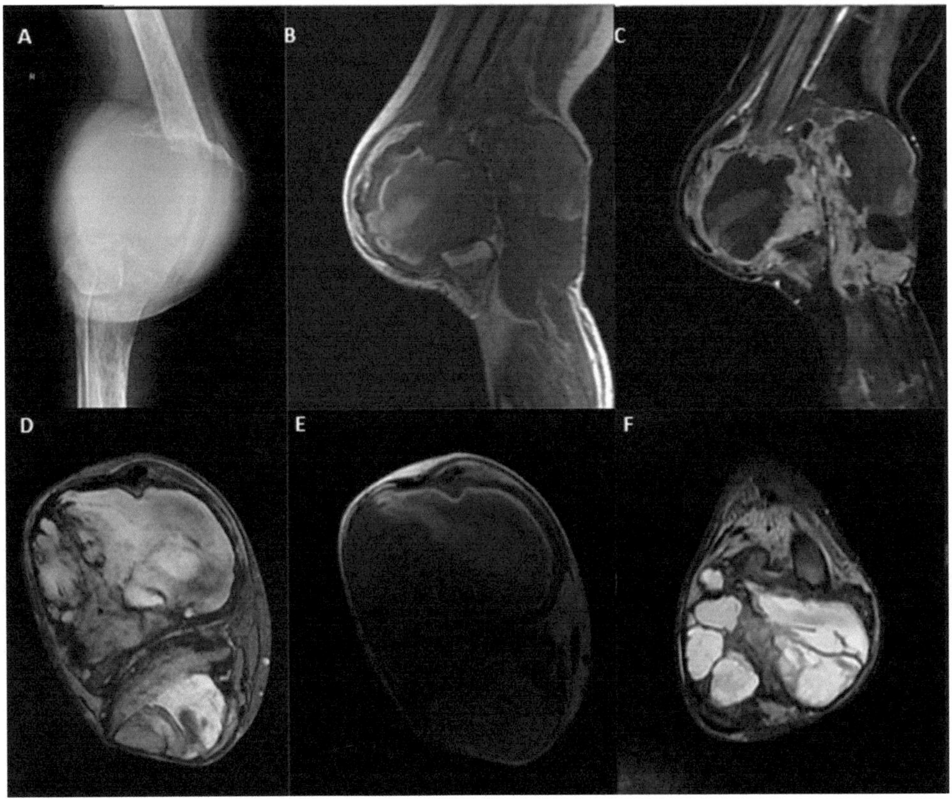

Figure 29.
Giant cell tumor of the right femur. Radiograph oblique view shows an osteolytic sub articular lesion with a soft tissue component and cortical thinning. On T1W image (b), it shows hemorrhagic content with post-contrast enhancement (c), and fluid content on (d, f). Popliteal fossa and Hoffa fat pad invasion are evident.

on MRI, due to fluid, mucoid, or gelatinous material, with a honeycomb pattern of enhancement (**Figure 33**). At the base of the skull, it should be differentiated from petro-clival chondrosarcoma, which has a chondroid matrix and occurs at synchondrosis (eccentric location).

Pathogenesis:

Molecular: TBXT gene mutation causes Brachyury protein overexpression.

Gross: Lobulated, gelatinous, expanding the bone and extending into the soft tissue.

Microscopy: Lobulated tumor with an abundant myxoid matrix, blue background, and interspersed large bubbly cells that have been traditionally called "physaliphorous cells." Tumor cells may show nuclei with marked pleomorphism or may have bland nuclei; mitoses are not abundant.

Differential diagnosis chondrosarcoma, metastatic carcinoma, and chordoid meningioma. All of these tumors are Brachyury-negative.

Immunohistochemistry: Brachyury, cytokeratins, S100, and EMA positive.

Poorly differentiated chordoma: This rare tumor displays sheets of epithelioid cells with pronounced nuclear atypia, necrosis, mitosis, and occasional rhabdoid differentiation. Physaliphorous cells are absent. *SMARCB1* gene mutation is detected

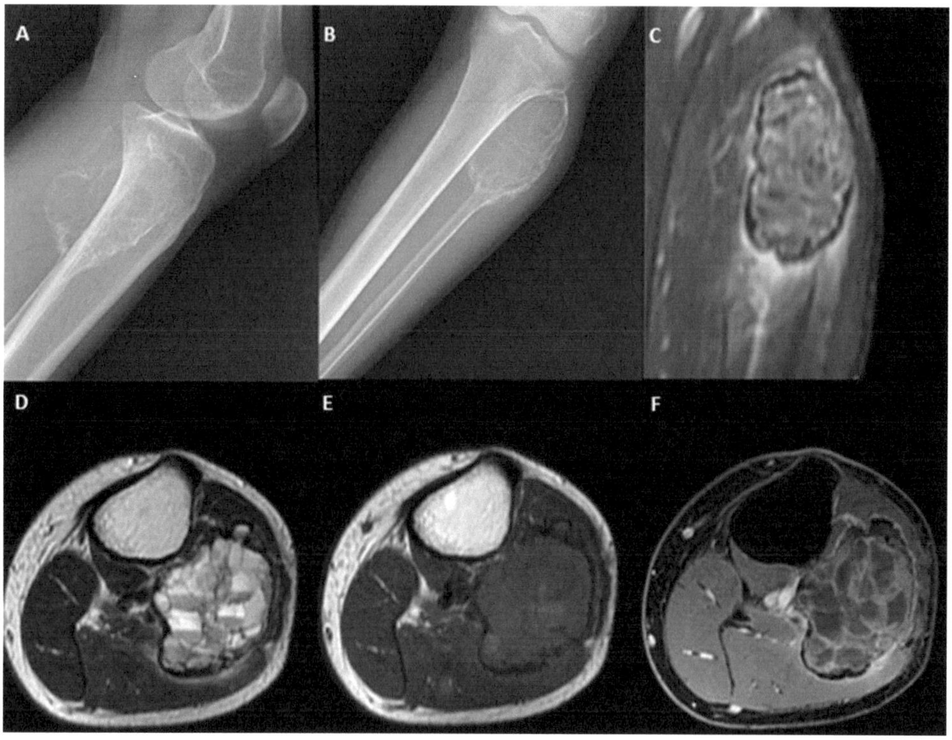

Figure 30.
Giant cell tumor with secondary aneurysmal bone cyst in the head of the fibula. Knee radiograph AP view and lateral view show a soap bubble-type lesion with thin septa and thinned-out cortex. Axial MRI T2W, T1W show fluid–fluid levels, and fat-saturated post-contrast image shows cortical erosions, enhancing septa and eccentric intra osseous soft tissue. Sagittal STIR image shows adjacent soft tissue edema.

by the loss of SMARCB1 (INI1) immunostaining in the tumor. The tumor is positive for keratins, brachyury, and S100 stains.

Dedifferentiated chordoma: This variant exhibits typical chordomatous areas and an abrupt transition to a high-grade sarcoma, typically osteosarcoma or pleomorphic undifferentiated sarcoma. The dedifferentiated sarcomatous areas are negative for brachyury.

4.7 Mesenchymal tumors of the bone

4.7.1 Simple bone cyst

It usually arises in the proximal humerus and femur, less commonly in the tibia and other long bones.

Radiology: It is a benign bony osteolytic metaphyseal/diaphyseal lesion in growing age, without a discernible matrix and with a narrow zone of transition. When it undergoes fracture, it shows a fallen fragment sign because of the fluid content (**Figure 36**). The term “unicameral” is omitted from the WHO classification, 5th edition, because it can be uni- or multi-locular in appearance (**Figure 21**).

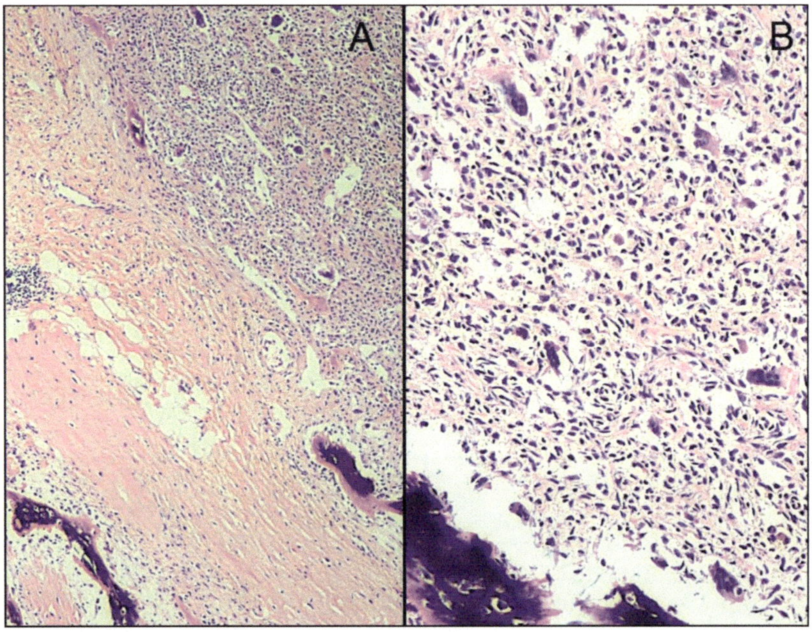

Figure 31.
Giant cell tumor: The tumor eroded the bone cortex and is extending into the fibroadipose tissue (A). A rim of host bone is visible around the tumor (B).

Gross: The cyst is typically received in multiple fragments, usually unilocular, lined by fibrous tissue, and may contain blood after a pathological fracture.

Microscopy: There is no epithelium or endothelium, and the cyst has a fibrous wall with degenerating eosinophilic fibrin cloud-like material in the lumen and wall, which may calcify. The cyst wall may also contain foam cells, hemosiderin, and reactive bone, particularly after fracture, when it becomes difficult to differentiate it from aneurysmal bone cyst and cystic fibrous dysplasia.

Management: Mostly left as such unless causing symptoms like pain, discomfort, or fracture. However, the prognosis is good, with little chance of recurrence. Bone grafting and bone mineral substitutes are used to fill the defect.

4.7.2 Fibrous dysplasia

Radiology: It is a benign, non-neoplastic, bony metaphyseal/diaphyseal osteolytic lesion in the growing age, with a ground-glass appearance matrix, a thick sclerotic rim, and remodeling bone, that is, shepherd's crook deformity. It has both monostotic and polyostotic forms. The femur, tibia, and craniofacial bones are the most common sites. It can be monostotic, involving a single bone, or polyostotic, involving multiple bones. Monostotic forms present in childhood or adolescence, while polyostotic forms present in adulthood. Fibrous dysplasia may be associated with McCune–Albright syndrome. Pain, deformity, and fracture may be the presenting symptoms (**Figure 34**). Depending on its appearance, it has to be differentiated from Paget's disease, which has a similar appearance but occurs in old age, and the lesion extends up to the articular surface.

Pathogenesis

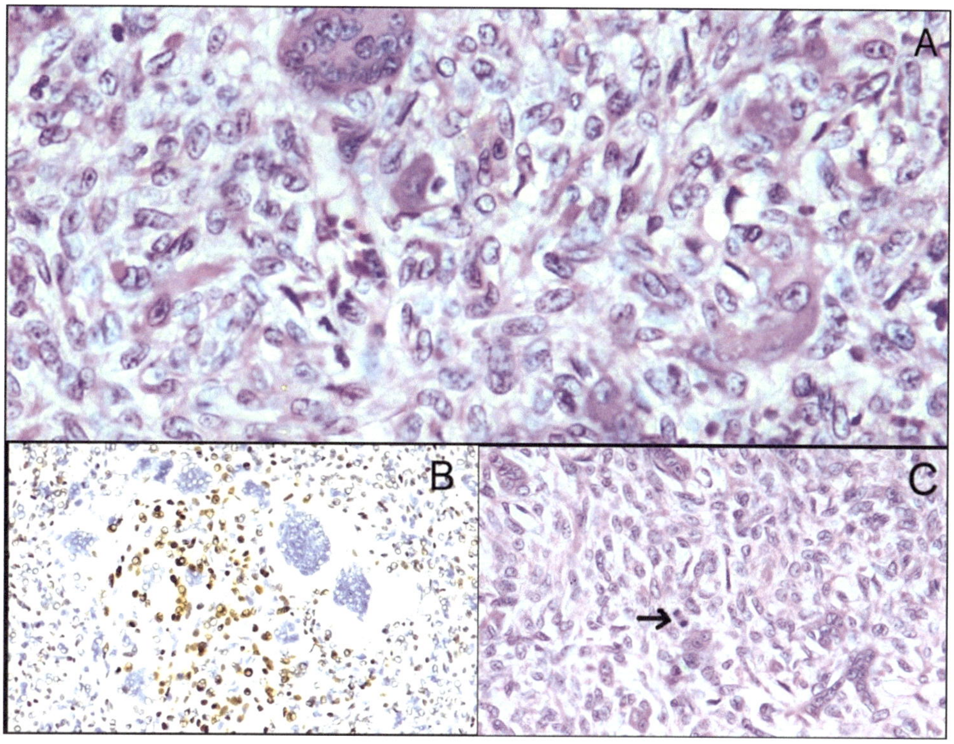

Figure 32.
Giant cell tumor: Mononuclear stromal cells and giant cells having similar vesicular nuclei (A). Stromal cells are positive for the immunohistochemical stain p63 (B). Mitosis in the stromal cells (arrow, C).

Molecular: The GNAS gene codes for the α-subunit of the G stimulatory protein and exhibits a missense mutation, activating the WNT/β-Catenin signaling in the osteoprogenitor cells.

Gross: There is expansion of the medulla of the bone by gray-white gritty bone, cartilage, and cystic changes, which may be present.

Microscopy: Fibrous dysplasia is a biphasic tumor. It consists of a bland fibrous stroma and interspersed curvilinear, Chinese-letter-shaped woven bone trabeculae. Osteoblasts are present but inconspicuous, and focally, secondary aneurysmal bone cystic areas can be present.

Management: Pain killers and bisphosphonates are used for symptomatic relief. Pathological fractures are treated by surgery and corrective osteotomy for deformities of the bones. A definitive cure is still not possible.

4.7.3 Adamantinoma

Radiology: It is a biphasic tumor of epithelial and osteofibrous components, that is, a malignant, indolent, cortical-based, multi-loculated cystic lesion with a sclerotic rim that occurs at ages between 15 and 55 years. It has a predilection for the tibial diaphysis. MRI can show the soft tissue component, periosteal reaction, and skip lesions.

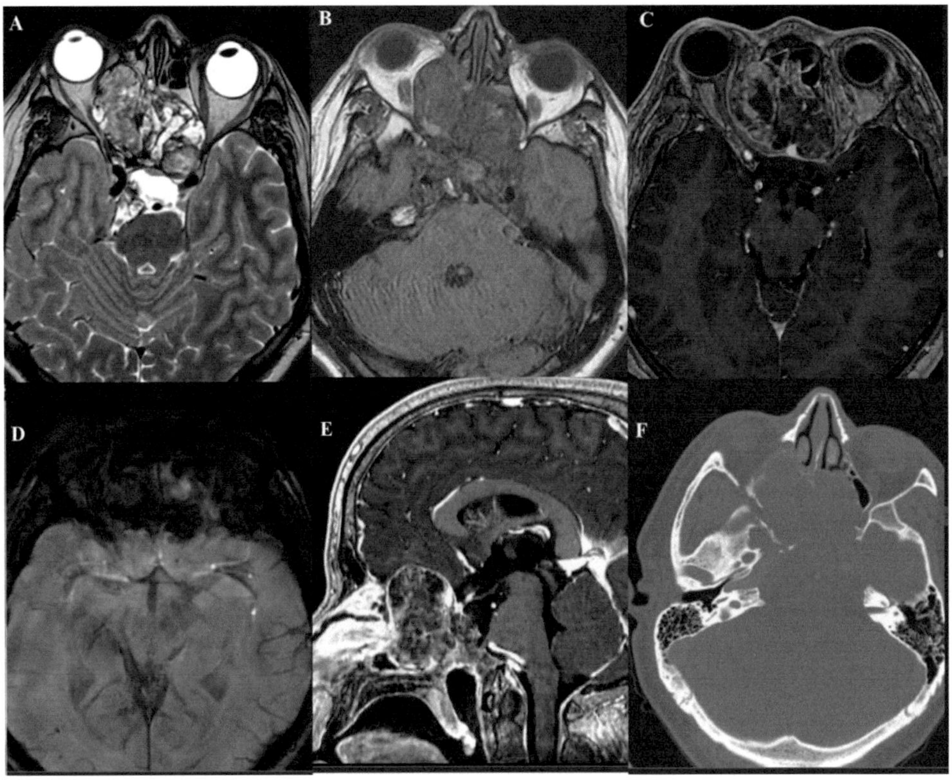

Figure 33.
Chordoma of the basi sphenoid. MRI shows a heterogeneously enhancing lesion in the of the with a honeycomb pattern of enhancement and hemorrhagic foci. Expansile osteolytic lesion involving the wing of sphenoids, jugum sphenoidale, clivus and bilateral petrous apices with bony spicules. It extends anteriorly into nasopharynx and nasal cavities.

Pathogenesis:

Gross: Classic adamantinoma presents as a white, lobulated cortical tumor, which may extend into the medullary cavity and invade the cortical bone with a soft tissue component.

Microscopy: Classic adamantinoma shows a prominent epithelial component of basaloid, squamous, or tubular cells embedded in a fibrous stroma. The bone trabeculae are rimmed by osteoblasts. In the OFD-like adamantinoma, the osteofibrous areas predominate, with clusters of epithelial cells. The differentiation between OFD and OFD-like adamantinoma depends on the amount of these epithelial cells; OFD has only single clusters of epithelial cells in the stroma. Dedifferentiated adamantinoma has classic areas with dedifferentiated areas, where the tumor may show sarcomatous or giant cell morphology with a high mitotic count.

Immunohistochemistry: The epithelial components were positive for basal and broad-spectrum keratins, and the stroma was positive for vimentin.

Management: Wide margin excision to amputation is the treatment option; however, the tumor is resistant to radiotherapy and chemotherapy.

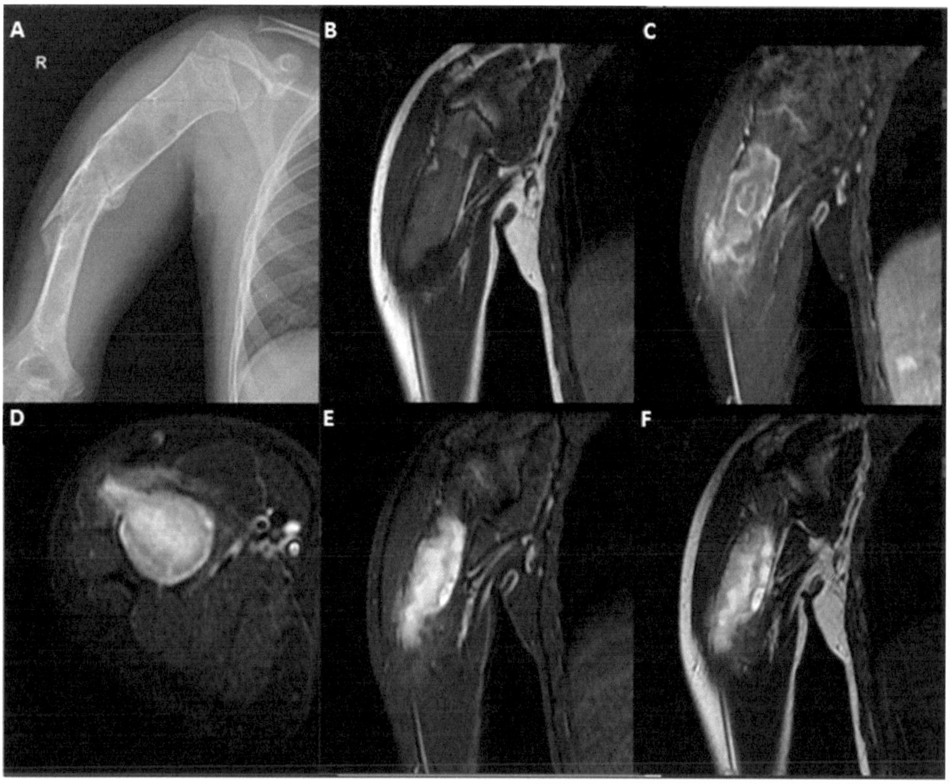

Figure 34.
Fibrous dysplasia of the right humerus. Radiograph AP view of the arm shows an expansile osteolytic lesion of the right humerus with a ground glass matrix, remodeling deformity and pathologic fracture. Coronal and axial MRI images (B-F) show an intramedullary fluid signal intensity lesion with heterogeneous post-contrast enhancement.

4.7.4 Osteofibrous dysplasia

Radiology: A benign, non-neoplastic, fibro-osseous cortical-based lesion with a similar radiologic appearance that mimics Adamantinoma, but it has a relatively well-defined outline and smaller size (that is, 6–7 cm versus 10–17 cm for the latter). Its age of presentation is around 10 years and it exclusively involves the tibia and fibula.

Pathogenesis

Gross: Solid, white, and gritty; usually confined to the cortex.

Microscopy: A fibro-osseous lesion with a close differential diagnosis of fibrous dysplasia. The lesion consists of irregular trabecular woven bone in a background of fibrous connective tissue. The bone trabeculae have prominent osteoblastic rimming and tend to show a zonal pattern, with the bone trabeculae becoming more prominent toward and merging with the peripheral host bone. The center of the lesion is fibrous, showing bland spindle cells without any significant mitotic activity.

Immunohistochemistry: stromal cells may show occasional cells with keratin positivity.

Diagnostic dilemma:

- Typical cortical location and an early age differentiate osteofibrous dysplasia from fibrous dysplasia, with less osteoblastic rimming of bone trabeculae.
- Adamantinoma is also located in the cortex of the tibia in the young age group; however, it shows prominent epithelial cells, which can be easily identified on keratin stains.

Management: wide margin excision to amputation is the treatment option; however, it is resistant to radio- and chemotherapy.

4.7.5 Intra osseous lipoma

Radiology: It is a relatively rare, benign intra medullary tumor, with fatty signal intensity on MRI. It may show bony septa and central calcification, that is, the Cockade sign [31]. It most commonly occurs in the calcaneum and the metaphysis of the femur, tibia, humerus, and fibula. The axial skeleton is less commonly involved. In 2016, Hafeez et al. documented a rare case of bilateral intraosseous lipomas of the sphenoid body on CT and MRI [32]. Lipoma should be differentiated from lipo-sclerosing fibro-osseous tumor (LSMFT), which has fat, myxoid, and fibrous content.

Pathogenesis:

Gross: Yellow, lobulated, soft, circumscribed; the cut surface may be gritty due to the presence of bone trabeculae.

Microscopy: Adipocytes in lobules, separated by thin fibrous septa; trabecular bone may be present within or surrounding the lipoma.

Management: No treatment is required.

4.7.6 Ewing's sarcoma

Radiology: Ewing sarcoma (ES), also known as malignant round cell tumors of bone, is the second most common primary malignant BT in children; it is predominantly diaphyseal in location, with a predilection for long bones, femora, pelvis, and ribs, and typically occurs between 15–30 years of age. Apart from its aggressive features, it exhibits a multilayered onion skin periosteal reaction, a soft tissue component, cortical erosion, and a saucerization defect [25] (**Figures 35** and **36**).

Diagnostic dilemma:

- It closely mimics eosinophilic granuloma (aggressive form – Lodwick type III), osteosarcoma, and lymphoma on radiographs and MRI, and can be differentiated on histo-pathological grounds.
- It also mimics osteomyelitis on Xray imaging; later on, MRI shows sequestra, cloaca, sinus tract, intra medullary abscess, and soft tissue inflammatory changes.

Pathogenesis

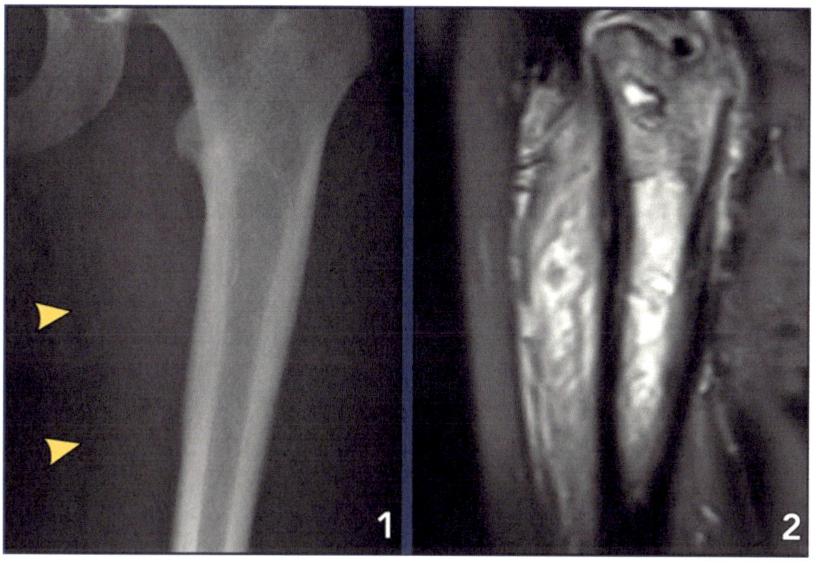

Figure 35.
Ewing's sarcoma of the left proximal femur. Radiograph shows an ill-defined medullary lytic lesion with a soft tissue mass and blurred fat planes (arrows). MRI shows intra and extra-osseous bony tumor (Reproduced with kind permission from author Dr. Robin Smithuis, Radiology Assistant – educational site of the Radiological Society of the Netherlands).

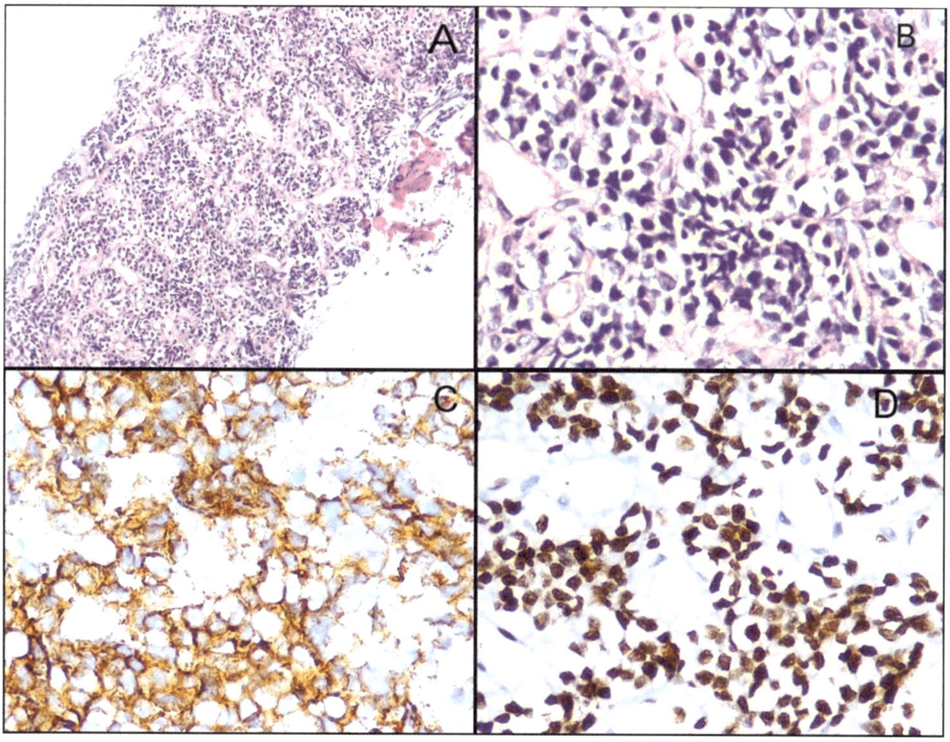

Figure 36.
Ewing sarcoma: small round blue cells (A), having small round basophilic nuclei and indistinct cytoplasm (B). CD99 stain: tumor cells have membranous positivity (C). NKX2.2: tumor cells are nuclear positive (D).

Gross: gray-white friable tumor involving the diaphysis of long bones; any bones or soft tissue may be involved.

Molecular: Genetically, FET-ETS fusion genes – the most common being the t (11:22) translocation with EWSR1:FLI1 gene fusion – result in over-expression of the protein in 80% of cases.

Microscopy: Ewing sarcoma has a monotonous population of small, round, blue cells with some spindling and formation of pseudorosettes around the blood vessels. Tumor cells have scant cytoplasm; round, basophilic, and uniform nuclei with indistinct nucleoli; usually, brisk mitosis and tumor necrosis are present. Immunohistochemical staining for CD99 showed strong membranous positivity in tumor cells. NKX2.2 has higher specificity and shows a nuclear staining pattern. Additionally, FLI-1 and ERG exhibit nuclear positivity, reflecting over-expression of the respective proteins. It is potentially curable by chemotherapy.

4.7.7 Bone metastasis

It can be lytic (due to destruction of bony trabeculae) or sclerotic in appearance (because of the osteoblastic response). Osteoblastic metastases are from prostate, breast, bladder, and mucinous GI tract carcinoma, while the lytic metastases are from the lungs, liver, renal, and thyroid in adults (**Figures 37–39**). In children,

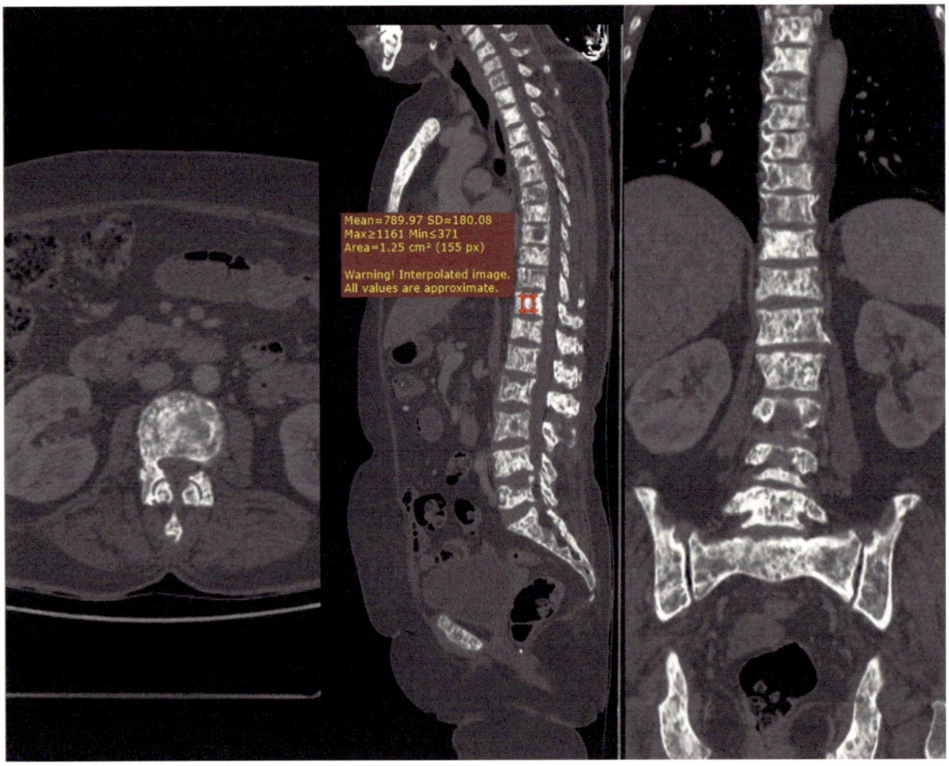

Figure 37.
Sclerotic bony metastases throughout the axial skeleton in a patient with prostate carcinoma with raised serum PSA of 1,099 mg/dl. Multiple sclerotic lesions are seen in the spine and pelvic bones. HU is less than 1,000.

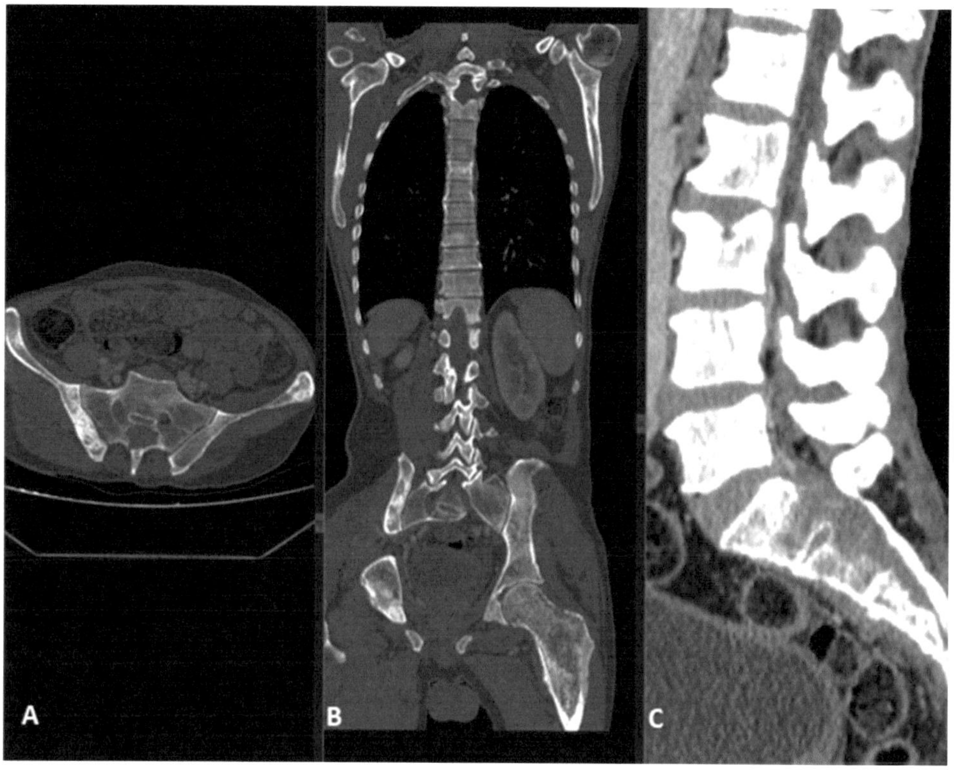

Figure 38.
Sclerotic bony metastases throughout the axial skeleton with a sacral intra spinal soft tissue component.

metastases from neuroblastoma, osteosarcoma, rhabdomyosarcoma, and Ewing sarcoma are seen.

Common sites for metastasis include the femoral and humeral metaphysis, as well as the vertebral bodies. CT scans and radioisotope bone scans are recommended for diagnosis, monitoring, and assessing response to treatment. Bone metastasis can occur from rarer malignancies and sarcomas. Immunohistochemistry is usually required, along with a radiological workup, in cases with an unknown primary site. In 2019, Hafeez M. reported a rare case of leiomyosarcoma (LMS) of the renal vein with bone metastasis. Histopathology of the specimen showed spindled to oval-shaped, medium-sized cells with eosinophilic cytoplasm and markedly pleomorphic nuclei. Mitotic figures and foci of necrosis were noted. Immunohistochemical stains were performed, which showed ASMA positivity, favoring LMS [33, 34].

4.7.8 Metastasis reporting and data system for prostate cancer

In clinical trials, MET-RADS-P is a standardized tool for the interpretation and reporting of whole-body MRI (WB-MRI) in advanced prostatic cancer. WB-MRI combines anatomical and functional (diffusion-weighted MRI) imaging. It comprises T1W, in-phase, opposed-phase, T2W, STIR, DWI, and ADC maps. It classifies patients into subgroups: nodal, bone, visceral, primary disease, and assesses

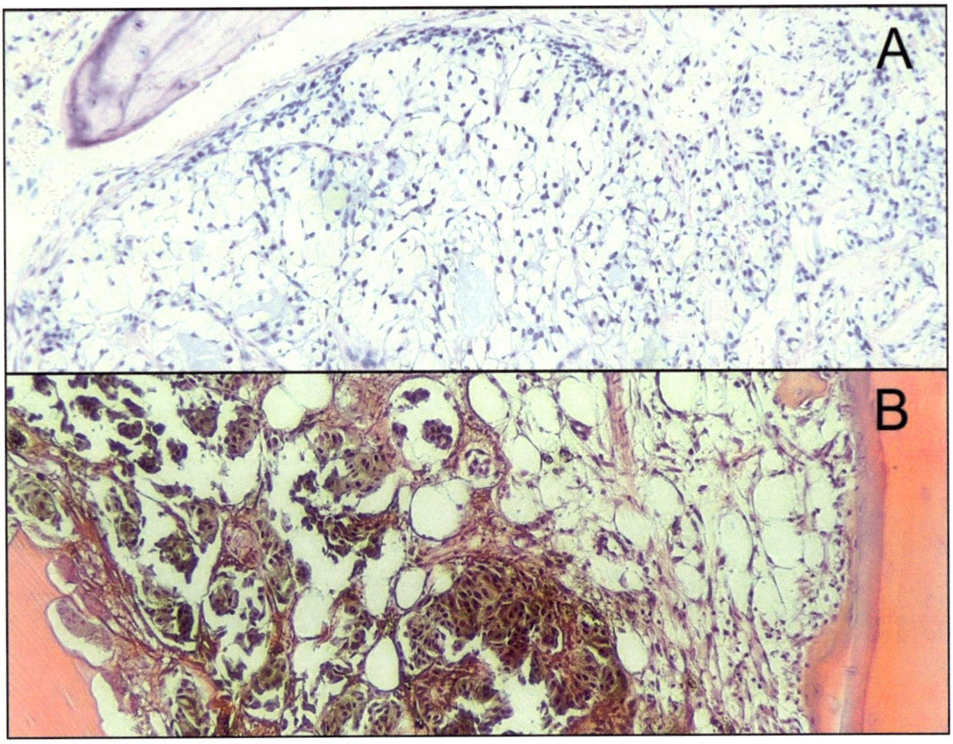

Figure 39.
Bone metastasis: mucoepidermoid carcinoma showing mucous cells with clear cytoplasm (A). Malignant melanoma: tumor cell nests having pigmented brown cytoplasm (B).

overall disease burden (oligo/poly metastatic) and location (axial versus peripheral skeleton) [35].

Diagnostic dilemma:

- Differentiating the bony island (also known as enostosis) from sclerotic bone metastasis remains a challenge in cancer patients. In one recent study, the Hounsfield unit (HU) attenuation measurements ranging from 885–1,060 on the CT scan for a bone lesion favor metastasis, whereas a density >1060 favors a bony island because of its compact texture [29]. Another differentiating feature is that, on a bone scan, enostosis doesn't show uptake, while metastasis does!

- Diffuse bony sclerosis is seen in OB and needs to be differentiated from myelofibrosis, mastocytosis, fluorosis, Paget's disease, and osteopetrosis.

- On skeletal surveys, when multiple lytic lesions are encountered, the differentials are metastases, multiple myeloma, lymphoma, and leukemia; appropriate imaging tests can differentiate.

- Blow-out metastasis (soap bubble, i.e., expansile osteolytic multiloculated appearance on radiograph) is seen in renal carcinoma, thyroid carcinoma, and melanoma. GCT, ABC, plasmacytoma, and chordoma are the differentials.

- In the case of a known malignancy undergoing therapy, a new sclerotic bone lesion can represent pseudo-progression, which is a sclerotic response to occult bony metastasis. It can be distinguished from true progression through a positive response to therapy at other sites [30].

- Malignant vertebral compression fracture is differentiated from osteoporotic fracture by the presence of pre-/para-vertebral and epidural soft tissue components, absence of a linear horizontal fracture line, and multiplicity of lesions.

- On planar bone scintigraphy, diffuse skeletal radionuclide uptake with loss of renal uptake results in a super scan appearance; this could be due to metastatic or metabolic causes; the former is confined to the axial skeleton, while the latter has diffuse axial and appendicular skeletal uptake [36, 37].

4.8 Hematopoietic neoplasms

4.8.1 Langerhans cell histiocytosis NOS/eosinophilic granuloma (EG)

Radiology

Langerhans cell histiocytosis (LCH) represents the neoplastic proliferation of myeloid-derived dendritic (i.e., histiocyte) cells. It is a disease of childhood; the later the age, the more the lesions are confined to the skeleton only. The milder form, "EG," is seen in young adults or the pediatric group and involves the long bones, ribs, pelvis, skull, and spine (**Figure 40**). When it involves a solitary vertebra, it reduces height, that is, vertebra plana appearance. When it is present in the skull, a button sequestra appearance, that is, a lytic lesion with central devascularized bone and beveled edge, is seen due to disproportionate involvement of the inner and outer tables of the skull. When it is located in the jaw, it causes a lytic lesion in the alveolus with loss of the lamina dura, that is, floating tooth appearance. On radiograph, its aggressive form should always be considered as a differential diagnosis of bizarre bone lesions and has to be differentiated from Ewing's sarcoma, lymphoma, and osteomyelitis.

Pathogenesis

Molecular: MAPK pathway activation, including BRAF or MAP2K1 mutations.

Microscopy: Langerhans cells are present in a background of mixed inflammatory cells, such as eosinophils, neutrophils, lymphocytes, and plasma cells. Langerhans cells are intermediate in size, having pale, ample cytoplasm and irregular, grooved (coffee bean) nuclei.

Immunohistochemistry: LCH cells are S100, CD68, CD1a, CD207 (Langerin), Cyclin D1, and BRAF p.Val600Glu positive. Birbeck granules are observed by electron microscopy.

4.8.2 Langerhans cell histiocytosis – disseminated

The rare multisystem LCH disease is seen in infants when two or more organs/systems, such as bone marrow, lymph nodes, lungs, liver, spleen, and skin, are involved. The two associated disease forms are:

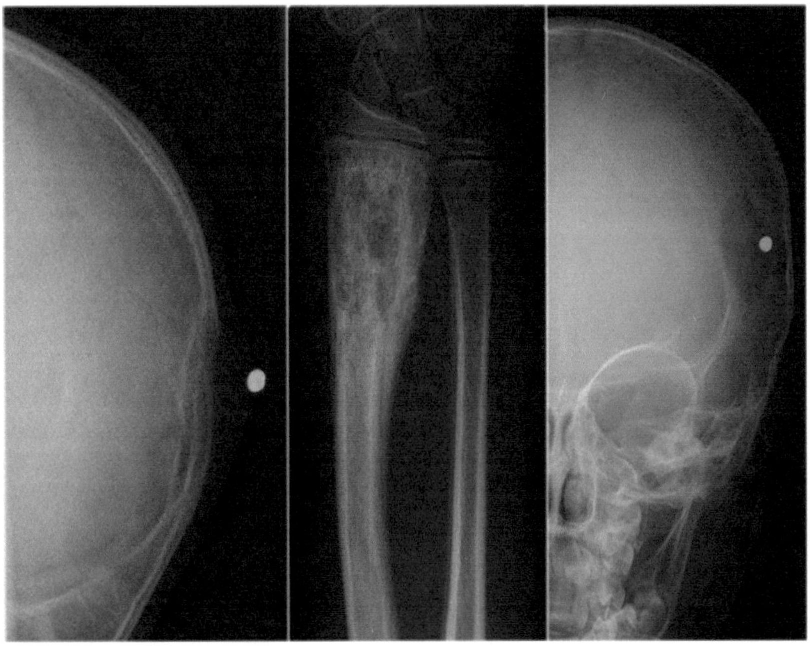

Figure 40.
Eosinophilic granuloma. Skull radiograph shows a lytic lesion with beveled edges. Radial distal metaphyseal aggressive lesion mimicking osteomyelitis and Ewing's sarcoma (reproduced with kind permission from author Dr. Robin Smithuis, Radiology Assistant – educational site of the Radiological Society of the Netherlands).

Letterer–Siwe disease: It is a syndrome characterized by rash, bleeding gums, and respiratory symptoms. The lytic lesions have a predilection for the flat bones and meta-diaphyseal regions. Pulmonary involvement closely mimics miliary tuberculosis.

Hand–Schüller–Christian disease: It is a triad of exophthalmos, diabetes insipidus, and lytic bone lesions due to histiocytosis; the former two conditions are due to lesions around the orbit and hypophysis.

4.8.3 Lymphoma

It involves the proliferation of malignant lymphoid cells primarily in lymph nodal organs in Hodgkin's type and in any organ of the body in non-Hodgkin's type; the latter is also known as extranodal lymphoma, which can be of B-cell or T-cell type. It can be primary (when arising in non-lymphoid tissue) or secondary (hematogenous spread to organs). The thymus, Waldeyer's lymphatic ring, spleen, liver, lungs, brain, lymph nodes, and bones can be involved. It can involve the bone marrow focally or diffusely (**Figures 41** and **42**). Diffuse large B-cell lymphoma (DLBCL) is the most common type of primary bone lymphoma that involves the marrow. The most common site is the metadiaphysis of the femur, followed by the pelvis.

Burkitt lymphoma involves the jaw bones, that is, the maxilla and mandible. Various classification systems have been used in clinical practice over the decades, including the Ann Arbor, Lugano, and Lymphoma Response to Immuno-modulatory Therapy Criteria (LYRIC), which are beyond the scope of this chapter [38, 39].

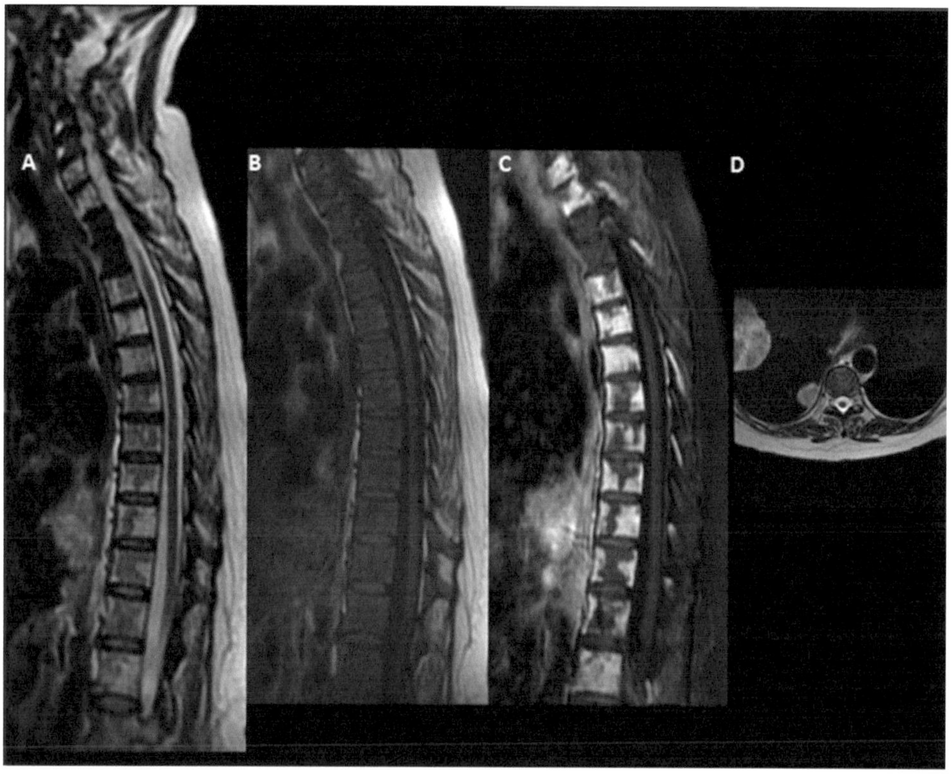

Figure 41.
Diffuse large B-cell lymphoma. Sagittal T2W, T1W pre (a, b) and fat-saturated post-contrast (c), sagittal and axial T2W MRI (c, d) show diffuse patchy involvement of the marrow. Upper two dorsal vertebrae return hypo-intense marrow signals on all the sequences due to post-radiotherapy changes. The axial T2W MRI (d) shows pulmonary metastasis.

5. Miscellaneous

5.1 Leukemia

It is primarily a malignancy of white blood cells. It can be of the myeloproliferative or lymphoproliferative type. Apart from the blood, the spleen, liver, lungs, brain, lymph nodes, and bones can be involved. It can affect the bone marrow either focally or diffusely. Distribution and age vary according to the type of leukemia. Common types of leukemia are acute/chronic myeloid leukemia and acute/chronic lymphoblastic leukemia. The diagnosis is made via blood smear or bone marrow biopsy.

5.2 Solitary plasmacytoma

On imaging, it shows an expansile osteolytic "soap bubble" lesion.

Pathology

Single localized intraosseous neoplasm, composed of a clonal population of plasma cells, with the absence of features of multiple myeloma, such as bone involvement or end-organ damage.

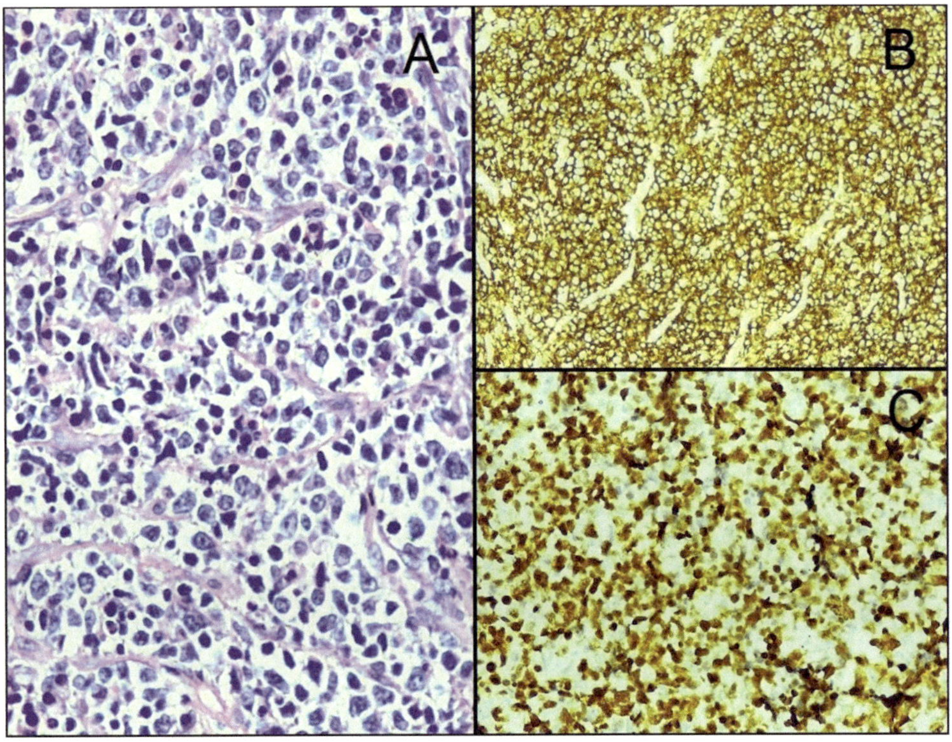

Figure 42.
Diffuse large B-cell lymphoma: tumor cells with large vesicular nuclei (A) that are strongly positive for CD20 IHC stain (B) and have a very high proliferation index on Ki-67(C).

Microscopy: Plasma cell sheets may be mature, with some nuclear enlargement, or may be immature, with marked nuclear atypia (**Figure 43**).

Immunohistochemistry: Positive for CD138, CD38, Mum-1, CD56, and negative for CD20, CD19, CD3, and CD56.

5.3 Multiple myeloma

It is the most common primary malignant BT in adults and one of the most common hematologic neoplasms. It is due to the infiltration of plasma cells in the bone marrow.

The British Society of Hematology and the National Institute for Clinical Excellence recommend MRI as the baseline imaging test for bone marrow infiltration. On imaging, it can be diffuse (with multiple lytic lesions or osteopenia), focal on diffuse, micronodular, solitary extra or para-medullary forms (**Figures 44–47**).

Apart from routine basic hematologic tests and biochemical tests, specific serologic tests include Bence-Jones proteins and serum protein electrophoresis, monoclonal paraproteins, and immunoglobulin estimation.

The International Myeloma Working Group (IMWG) has published the "CRAB" criteria for the diagnosis of MM, that is:

C – Hypercalcemia (>1 mg/dL) higher than the upper limit of normal.

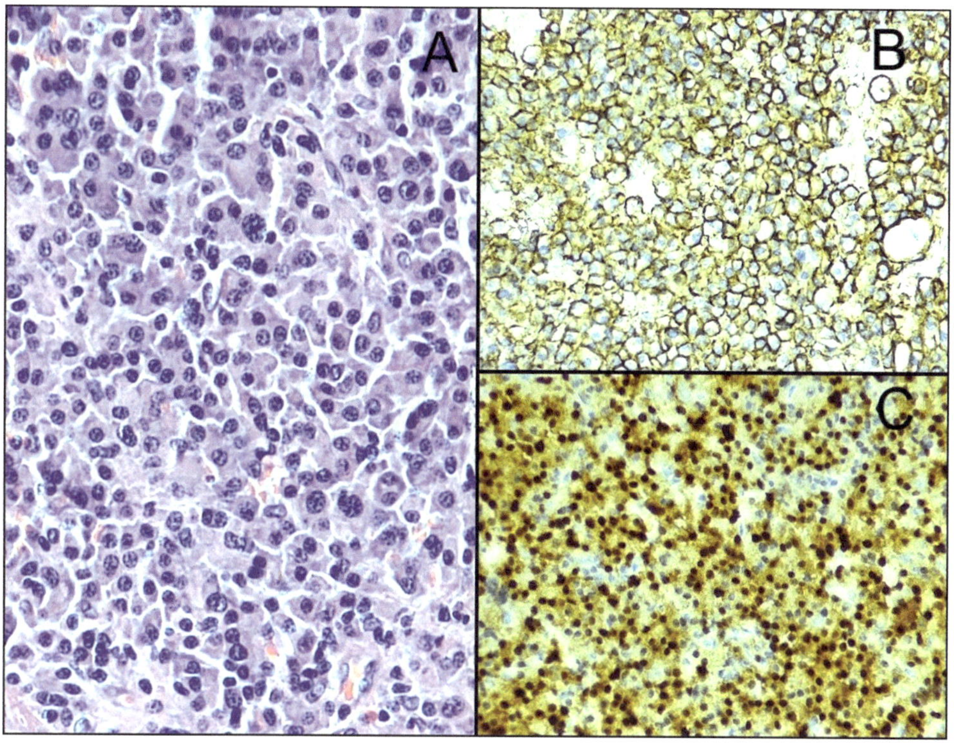

Figure 43.
Plasmacytoma: sheets of plasma cells having abundant cytoplasm and "cart-wheel" or "clock-face" nuclei (A). Plasma cells are positive for CD138 in a membranous pattern (B) and for MUM-1 in a nuclear pattern (C).

R – Renal failure: serum creatinine >2 mg/dL.

A-anemia hemoglobin value <100glt.

B – Bone osteolytic lesions identified in the skeletal survey, CT, or MRI.

Myeloma-defining events (MDE) indicate active MM: CRAB plus abnormal free light chain ratio, MRI bone marrow lesion of at least 5 mm, and 60% clonal plasma cells on bone marrow trephine exam (histologic diagnosis).

The IMWG has recommended guidelines for the imaging standardization, acquisition, and interpretation of Whole body MRI [40–42]. Multiple myeloma (RADS), like RECIST criteria, has Response Assessment Criteria (RAC) based on ADC values:

I: highly likely to be responding.

II: likely to be responding.

III: no change.

IV: likely to be responding.

V: highly likely to be progressing.

Diagnostic dilemma

1. The moth-eaten (multiple innumerable lytic lesions, that is, rain drop appearance) pattern of MM in the calvaria needs to be differentiated from lytic lesions, that is, the salt-and-pepper skull of hyperparathyroidism; the latter would have an abnormal bony texture [43].

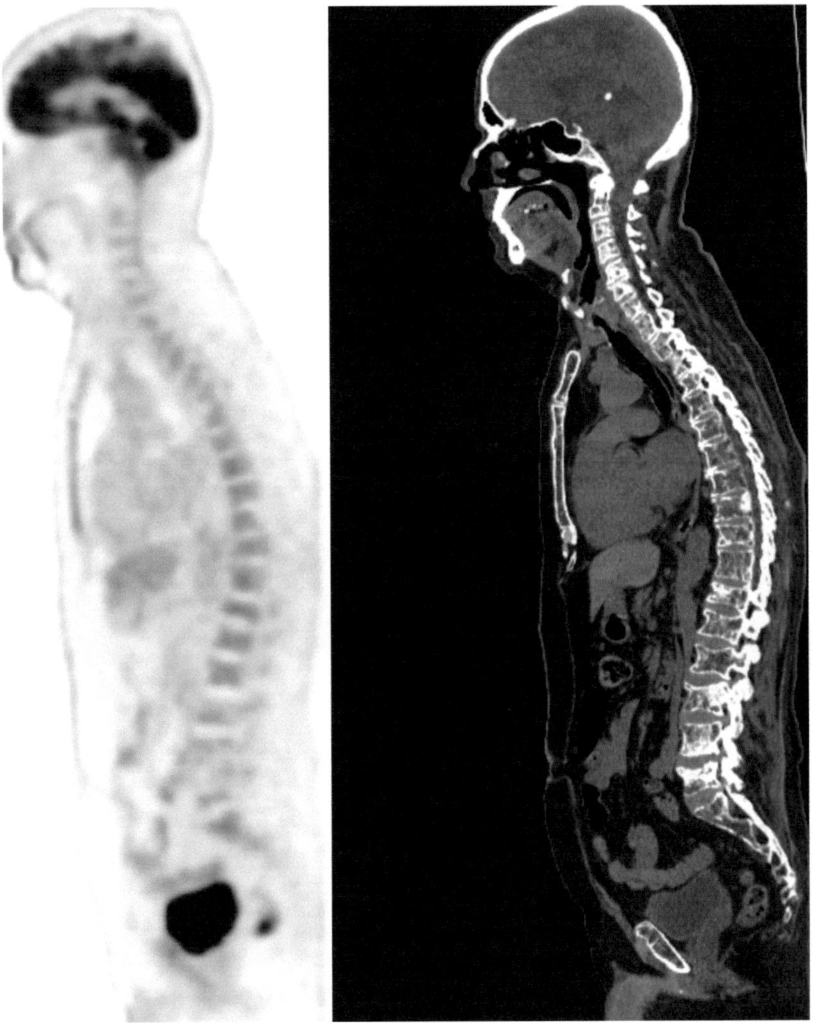

Figure 44.
Multiple myeloma. PET CT and CT scan sagittal sections show radiotracer uptake dorsolumbar vertebral bodies and marked osteopenia, respectively.

2. MM mimics osteoporosis on imaging, as both present with reduced bone density and compression fractures. OP has residual foci of normal marrow.

3. MM appears the same as lytic bony metastasis on radiographs. A negative bone scan and pertinent serologic tests for MM can help differentiate.

6. Syndromes associated with Bone Tumors

Paget's disease: A bone metabolic disorder with bony remodeling deformity and altered osteoclastic and osteoblastic activity. Pain, focal areas of osteolysis, and raised alkaline phosphatase levels indicate possible malignant sarcomatous transformation.

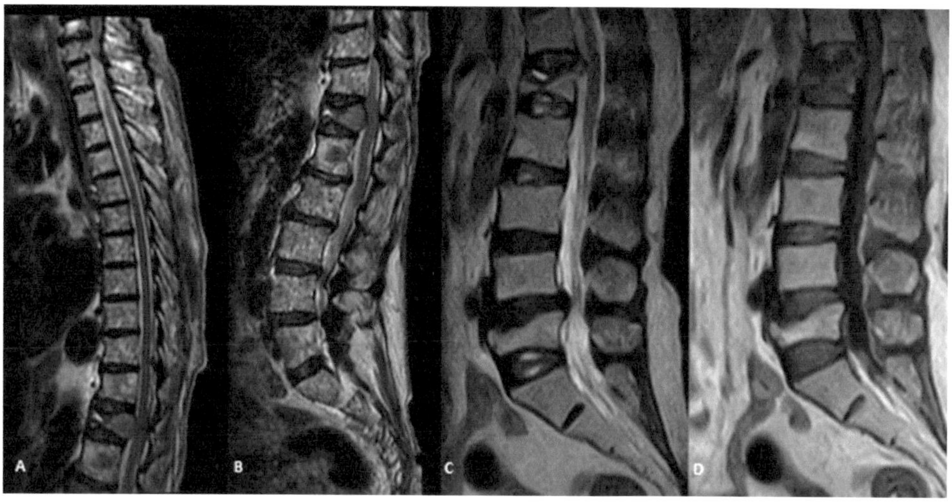

Figure 45.
Variegated pattern of dorsolumbar spine bone marrow involvement in multiple myeloma (a, b). Coexistent malignant D2 vertebral compression fracture with bowing of the posterior cortex. L1 and L5 post-traumatic compression fractures (c, d) in the figure with a L1 hypointense fracture line.

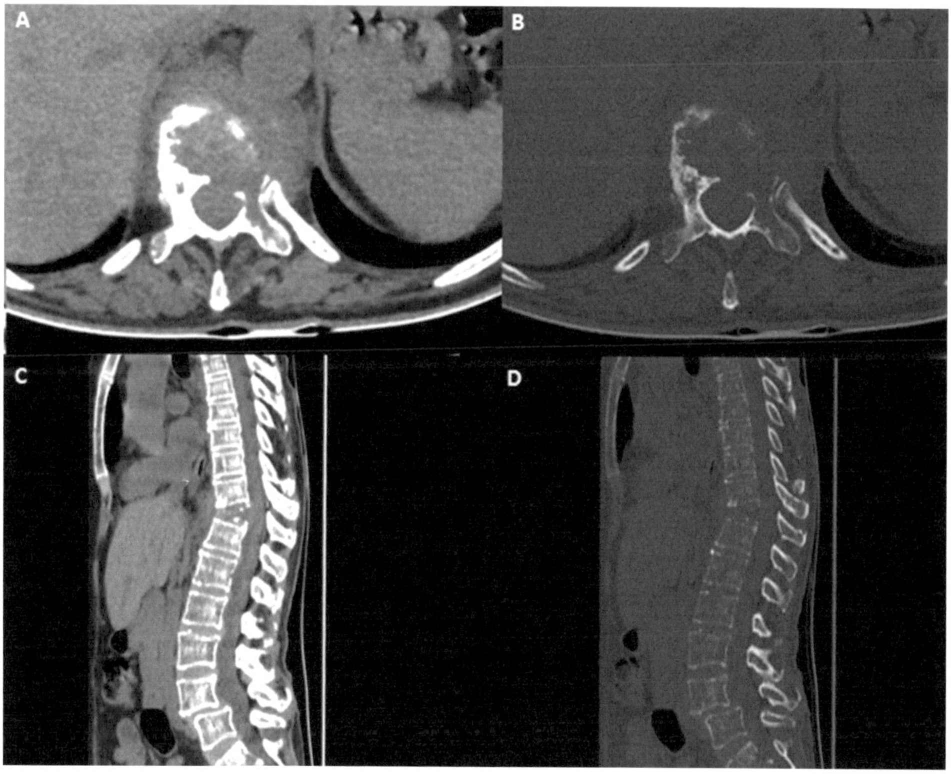

Figure 46.
Multiple myeloma. CT shows marked osteopenia in the dorsolumbar vertebral bodies. D11 vertebral body deposit with a compression fracture.

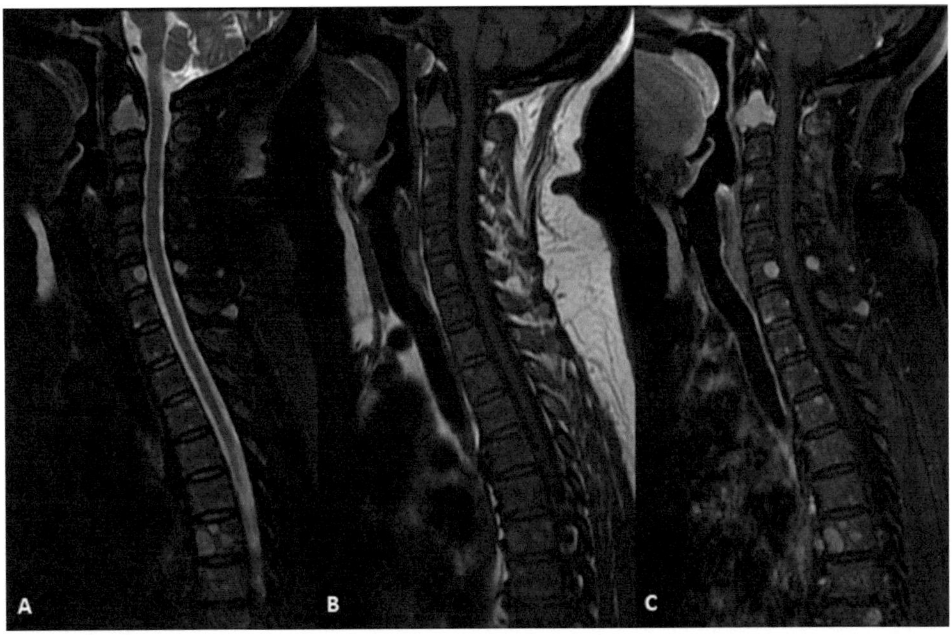

Figure 47.
Nodular lesion on the background of diffuse multiple myeloma. Cervico-dorsal spine sagittal T2W (a), T1W post-contrast (b), and saturated T1W images (c) show multiple deposits in the bodies and spinous processes. Diffuse hypo intensity on T1W image represents diffuse marrow involvement.

Gardener's syndrome: A syndrome comprising multiple osteomas and familial adenomatous polyposis.

Ollier syndrome: A syndrome comprising multiple enchondromas.

Maffucci syndrome: A syndrome comprising multiple enchondromas with soft tissue hemangiomas.

Hereditary multiple exostosis: Multiple osteochondromas indicate hereditary multiple exostosis with an increased risk of CS, up to 3–5%, and require a skeletal survey and genetic testing.

POEMS syndrome: It is an acronym associated with multiple myeloma and stands for polyneuropathy, organomegaly, endocrinopathy and monoclonal gammopathy and skin changes.

McCune–Albright disease: A triad of polyostotic fibrous dysplasia, precocious puberty, and cutaneous pigmentation.

Hutchinson syndrome: It comprises clinical symptoms, that is, anemia, limping gait, and irritability, associated with bone metastasis in neuroblastoma. Its characteristic feature is sutural diastasis associated with calvarial bony deposits.

Acknowledgment

The authors are grateful to Dr. Robin Smithuis, Radiology Assistant – Educational site of the Radiological Society of the Netherlands, for granting permission to reproduce **Figures 1, 2, 15** and **31**.

Conflict of Interest

The authors declare no conflict of interest.

Authors' contribution

Mahnoor Hafeez contributed to correspondence, the clinical and radiological parts, diagnosis, and the designing of the manuscript; Ruqaiya Shahid and Malik Osama Tanweer contributed to the pathogenesis and management parts of the chapter, respectively. All three authors were involved in the preparation of the manuscript, conducted the literature search, and approved the final manuscript.

Author details

Mahnoor Hafeez[1]*, Ruqaiya Shahid[2] and Malik Osama Tanweer[3]

1 Dow Institute of Radiology, Dow University of Health Sciences, Ojha campus, Karachi, Pakistan

2 Department of Pathogenesis, Dow University of Health Sciences, Ojha Campus, Karachi, Pakistan

3 AO Hospital (Trauma, Orthopaedics, Spinal and Sports Surgery), Karachi, Pakistan

*Address all correspondence to: mahnoor.hafeez@yahoo.com

References

[1] Morgan M, Schmid J, Bell D, et al. Lodwick classification of lytic bone lesions. In: Radiopaedia.org. 2025. DOI: 10.53347/rID-33206. Available from: https://radiopaedia.org/articles/lodwick-classification-of-lytic-bone-lesions

[2] Schmid J, Knipe H. Modified Lodwick-Madewell classification of lytic bone lesions. Radiopaedia.org. DOI: 10.53347/rID-74090. [Accessed: 2025-October-01]

[3] Sutton D. A textbook of radiology and imaging

[4] The radiology assistant : Bone tumors. The Radiological Society of the Netherlands. (n.d.). Available from: https://radiologyassistant.nl/musculoskeletal/bone-tumors

[5] Rafiee, Hameed SGC, editor. Bones. Chapman & Nakielny's aids to radiological differential diagnosis. Elsevier Health Sciences, 2019. 5th Edition. Elsevier Health Sciences; 2013:3–36

[6] Stacy GS, Mahal RS, Peabody TD. Staging of bone tumors: A review with illustrative examples. American Journal of Roentgenology. 2006;**186**(4):967–976

[7] Choi JH, Ro JY. The 2020 WHO Classification of Tumors of Bone: An updated review. Advances in Anatomic Pathology. 2021;**28**(3):119–138. DOI: 10.1097/PAP.0000000000000293

[8] Kumar V, Abbas AK, Jon CJ, Aster, editors. Robbins & Kumar Basic Pathology Pathologic Basis of Disease. 8th **II**. United States (Philadelphia): Saunders, Elsevier; 2022. ISBN-10 032353113X

[9] Murthy S, Thakur U, Ghasemi A, Ahlawat S. Advances in musculoskeletal tumor imaging. Seminars in Roentgenology. 2024;**59**(4):477–488. DOI: 10.1053/j.ro.2024.07.002

[10] Bell D, Gaillard F. WHO Classification of Tumors of Haematopoietic and Lymphoid Tissues. Radiopaedia.org; 2010. DOI: 10.53347/rid-9250. Available from: https://radiopaedia.org/articles/who-classification-of-haematolymphoid-tumours

[11] ACR. Bone-Reporting and Data System (Bone-RADSTM). (n.d.). Available from: https://www.acr.org/Clinical-Resources/Clinical-Tools-and-Reference/Reporting-and-Data-Systems/Bone-RADS

[12] Chang CY, Garner HW, Ahlawat S, et al. Society of Skeletal Radiology– White paper. Guidelines for the diagnostic management of incidental solitary bone lesions on CT and MRI in adults: Bone reporting and data system (Bone-RADS). Skeletal Radiology. 2022. DOI: 10.1007/s00256-022-04022-8

[13] Murphey MD, Kransdorf MJ. Staging and classification of primary musculoskeletal bone and soft-tissue tumors according to the 2020 WHO update, from the AJR special series on cancer staging. American Journal of Roentgenology. 2021;**217**(5):1038–1052

[14] Rauf A, Gaillard F. Osteochondroma. Radiopaedia.org. 2008. DOI: 10.53347/rid-1799

[15] Lee KCY, et al. Imaging the Complications of Osteochondromas. Clinical Radiology 2002;**57**:18–28

[16] WHO Classification of Tumors Editorial Board. WHO Classification of Tumours: Soft Tissue and Bone Tumours. 5th ed. **3**. Lyon: International Agency for Research on Cancer; 2020

[17] Roberts D, Gaillard F. Enchondroma vs low grade chondrosarcoma. Radiopaedia.org. 2009. DOI: 10.53347/rid-6245. Available from: https://radiopaedia.org/articles/enchondroma-vs-low-grade-chondrosarcoma-3

[18] Davies AM, Patel A, Azzopardi C, James S, Botchu R. Birmingham atypical cartilaginous tumour imaging protocol (BACTIP) revisited. Clinical Radiology. 2025;**83**:106837

[19] Patel A, Davies AM, Botchu R, James S. A pragmatic approach to the imaging and follow-up of solitary central cartilage tumours of the proximal humerus and knee. Clinical Radiology. 2019;**74** (7):517–526. DOI: 10.1016/j.crad.2019.01.025

[20] Bell D, Datir A. Chondrosarcoma. Radiopaedia.org. 2008. DOI: 10.53347/rid-1121. Available from: https://radiopaedia.org/articles/chondrosarcoma

[21] Amary MF, Damato S, Halai D, et al. IDH1 and IDH2 mutations are frequent events in central chondrosarcoma and central and periosteal chondromas but not in other mesenchymal tumours. The Journal of Pathology. 2011;**224**(3):334–343. DOI: 10.1002/path.2913

[22] Murphey MD, Robbin MR, MCRae GA, Flemming DJ, Temple HT, Kransdorf MJ. The many faces of osteosarcoma. Radiographics. 1997;**17** (5):1205–1231

[23] Bogotá/CO, U.S.C.B.S.a.L.B.H.D.P. O.R.R.G.. Radiological approach to the diagnosis of primary osteosarcomas. ECR 2018 EPOS. Available from: https://epos.myesr.org/poster/esr/ecr2018/C-1231 [Accessed: 2018-January-08]

[24] Armstrong P, Wastie M, Rockall AG Bones. Diagnostic Imaging 6th . Hoboken, New Jersey, USA: John Wiley & Sons; 2010. ISBN-10 1405170395

[25] J EV-I, De Noon S, Trevers K, Elrick H, van Belzen IAEM, Zumalave S, et al. Ongoing chromothripsis underpins osteosarcoma genome complexity and clonal evolution. Cell. 2025;**188**(2): 352–370.e22. DOI: 10.1016/j.cell.2024.12.005

[26] Bertoni F, Bacchini P, Staals EL, Davidovitz P. Dedifferentiated parosteal osteosarcoma: The experience of the Rizzoli Institute. Cancer. 2005;**103**(11):2373–2382. DOI: 10.1002/cncr.21039

[27] Kato K, Teferi N, Challa M, et al. Vertebral hemangiomas: A review on diagnosis and management. Journal of Orthopaedic Surgery and Research. 2024;**19**:310

[28] Noh B-J, Park Y-K. Giant cell tumor of bone: Updated molecular pathogenesis and tumor biology. Human Pathology. 2018;**81**:1–8. DOI: 10.1016/j.humpath.2018.06.017

[29] Nakata E, Kawai H, Fujiwara T, Kunisada T, Inoue H, Futagawa M,

Katayama H, Itano T, Ozaki T. Clinicopathological and histological analysis of secondary malignant giant cell tumors of bone without radiotherapy. Oncology Letters. 2022;**24**(3):319. DOI: 10.3892/ol.2022.13439

[30] Li H, Gao J, Gao Y, Lin N, Zheng M, Ye Z. Denosumab in giant cell tumor of bone. Frontiers in Oncology. 2020;**10**:580605. DOI: 10.3389/fonc.2020.580605

[31] Berlin L. Aunt Minnie's atlas and imaging-specific diagnosis. Radiology. 1997;**204**(1):278

[32] Hafeez M. MRI and CT of bilateral intraosseous lipomas of the Sphenoid Body-A case report. Pakistan Journal of Radiology. 2017;**27**(1):52–55. Available from: https://www.pakjr.com/index.php/PJR/article/view/532

[33] Hafeez M. Insight at Medical Imaging: A Radiologist Experience from Pakistan. Chișinău, Republic of Moldova: Eliva Press; 2023. ISBN-10: 9994988565

[34] Hafeez M, Khan A. Leiomyosarcoma of renal vein with bone metastasis: The radiological findings. Journal of the College of Physicians and Surgeons Pakistan. 2019;**29**(9):902–904

[35] Padhani AR, Lecouvet FE, Tunariu N, Koh DM, De Keyzer F, Collins DJ, et al. Metastasis reporting and data system for prostate cancer: Practical guidelines for acquisition, interpretation, and reporting of whole-body magnetic resonance imaging-based evaluations of multiorgan involvement in advanced prostate cancer. European Urology. 2017;**71**(1):81–92. DOI: 10.1016/j.eururo.2016.05.033

[36] Ulano A, Bredella M, Burke P, et al. Distinguishing untreated osteoblastic metastases from enostoses using CT attenuation measurements. American Journal of Roentgenology. 2016;**207**(2):362–368. DOI: 10.2214/AJR.15.15559

[37] Coakley FV. Pseudoprogression due to healing of bone metastases by sclerosis. In: Pearls and Pitfalls in Abdominal Imaging: Pseudotumors, Variants and Other Difficult Diagnoses. UK: Cambridge University Press; 2010. p. 352–355

[38] Reiser M, Baur-Melnyk A, Glaser C Musculoskeletal Imaging (Direct Diagnosis in Radiology)

[39] Ahmad W, Zaheer I, Waheed KB. Intriguing lymphoma patterns: A radiologist's challenge. Pakistan Journal of Radiology. 2024;**34**(1):26–36

[40] Bell D, Yap K (2010). Multiple myeloma. Radiopaedia.org. 10.53347/rid-9555

[41] K N, Niknejad M. Salt and Pepper Sign (Skull). Radiopaedia.org. 2013. DOI: 10.53347/rid-21561. Available from: https://radiopaedia.org/articles/salt-and-pepper-sign-skull-1

[42] Love C, Din AS, Tomas MB, Kalapparambath TP, Palestro CJ. Radionuclide bone imaging: An illustrative review. Radiographics. 2003;**23**(2):341–358. RSNA. Available from: https://pubs.rsna.org/doi/abs/10.1148/rg.232025103

[43] Messiou C, Hillengass J, Delorme S, Lecouvet FE, Moulopoulos LA, Collins DJ, Blackledge MD,

Abildgaard N, Østergaard B, Schlemmer HP, Landgren O. Guidelines for acquisition, interpretation, and reporting of whole-body MRI in myeloma: Myeloma response assessment and diagnosis system (MY-RADS). Radiology. 2019;**291**(1):5–13. RSNA. Available from: https://pubs.rsna.org/doi/full/10.1148/radiol.2019181949

Chapter 5

Osteosarcoma - Transmission Electron Microscopy and Molecular Biology and Diagnostics Update

Consolato M. Sergi

Abstract

Pediatric small round blue cell tumors are a vast category of tumors occurring in infancy and childhood. Light microscopy of small round blue cell tumors reveals round cells. They usually have a hyperchromatic nucleus and relatively sparse basophilic cytoplasm. Pediatric small round blue cell tumors encompass various entities, including nephroblastoma (Wilms' tumor), neuroblastoma, rhabdomyosarcoma, Ewing sarcoma, retinoblastoma, and malignant lymphoma. These tumors represent the most prevalent diagnoses of solid malignancies in pediatric and adolescent populations. The differential diagnosis of these neoplasms can be intricate or contentious at the light microscopic level, even with immunohistochemistry. Occasionally, subtle staining or an unclear background may impede pathologists' ability to reach an accurate diagnostic conclusion. Molecular biology can generate large volumes of data that are difficult to distinguish. Consequently, electron microscopy can be beneficial for accurately validating the findings from light microscopy. Moreover, the ultrastructural state can provide insights into findings that may be relevant in cases of unclassifiable tumors, informing treatment and supplying data useful to single-cell scientists. This report highlights the electron microscopy findings of osteosarcoma. In this chapter, transmission electron microscopy is reviewed, and the current advantages and disadvantages of electron microscopy relative to molecular diagnosis are presented. Moreover, the most updated knowledge of the molecular biology and pathology of osteosarcoma is reported.

Keywords: osteosarcoma, electron microscopy, round blue cell tumor, childhood, molecular diagnostics, molecular biology

1. Introduction

The role of a pathologist can be quite demanding in both clinical diagnosis and research domains [1–3]. The advancement of light microscopy during the eighteenth century and, particularly, the nineteenth century was impressive. By the mid-nineteenth century, achieving a resolution above 0.5 microns was unfeasible. This is due to the Abbe's formula. Abbe's equation pertains to an ideal optical system ($d = 0.61\ \lambda/NA$) [1–23].

In this equation, d represents the resolution, λ denotes the wavelength of the imaging radiation, and NA signifies the numerical aperture. Abbe's formula defines the diffraction-limited resolution of an optical system. The resolution will be constrained if all aberrations and distortions are eradicated from the optical system. Aberrations and distortions will establish the practical limit of resolution. The resolution can be enhanced by reducing the wavelength, for instance, by applying filters or increasing the NA. The NA can be improved by augmenting the refractive index (n), such as by introducing oil to the specimen or by increasing the angle of incidence of the light (u) approaching the specimen. The limiting angle of resolution can be significantly reduced by increasing the lens diameter. The efficacy of an electron microscope is fundamentally based on the wavelength of electrons, which is shorter than that of light. The development of the cathode ray tube may have played a pivotal role in the history of transmission electron microscopy (TEM) [24, 25]. This tube was critical for surmounting the resolution challenge. The use of electrons rather than light was essential. In the nineteenth century, Hertz (1857–94) proposed that cathode rays constituted a type of wave motion. In 1899, Weichert discovered that these rays could be precisely focused into a point. To achieve this, the researchers employed an axial magnetic field generated by an elongated solenoid, a specific form of electromagnet. The objective of the solenoid is to produce a regulated magnetic field. Subsequently, Busch built a tiny solenoid to converge a beam of electrons, employing the exact mechanism that glass uses to converge sunlight. TEM was developed by two German physicists, Max Knoll and Ernst Ruska. Approximately eight years before the commencement of the Second World War, German engineers Ernst Ruska and Maximilian Knoll achieved the magnification of an electron picture. The initial prototype of the concept was constructed by Ruska two years later, in 1933, resolving 50 nm. Fifty years later, Ruska received the Nobel Prize [25–36].

The inaugural commercially accessible TEM, designated "EM1," was built in England. Metropolitan Vickers, for Imperial College London, constructed the device. Nonetheless, the initial models did not excite light microscopy users or morphologists due to the inadequate region-of-interest (ROI). Subsequently, the analysis of biological specimens using an electron microscope, following osmium treatment and ultra-thin sectioning, altered the practices and methodologies of light microscopy users and morphologists. The inaugural TEM was constructed in 1938 at the University of Toronto, Ontario, Canada, in North America. Conversely, most of the ensuing steps were suspended. They experienced a delay characteristic of the twentieth century due to the Second World War. Subsequently, conventional and commercial electron microscopes emerged for diagnostic applications, achieving an impressive resolution of 1 nm (10^{-3} microns, 10^{-6} mm).

2. Small, round, blue cell tumors – the pediatric consortium

The collection of malignancies classified as the small round blue cell tumor group has been a challenge for pathologists for several decades [1, 3, 35, 37–49]. The challenges appear to commence during residency, when several interpretations may arise from a basic hematoxylin and eosin stain. In recent years, several novel cancers have been identified and categorized within the pediatric round blue cell tumor group. Nevertheless, a fundamental set of 10 diagnoses must be considered when examining a tissue specimen from the pediatric population. This category encompasses malignancies characterized by cells exhibiting hyperbasophilic or hyperchromatic nuclei with a high nucleus-to-cytoplasm ratio. While specific insights can be gleaned from the accurate analysis of a hematoxylin and eosin-stained tissue slide, additional techniques may be necessary to achieve a definitive diagnosis. Before the introduction of polyclonal and monoclonal antibodies and their application in immunohistochemistry, TEM made a significant contribution to the diagnosis of small round blue cell cancers. Since the 1990s, immunohistochemistry has replaced morphological techniques in diagnosis. Presently, numerous novel polyclonal and monoclonal antibodies target antigens associated with small round blue cell carcinoma. During the final decade of the twentieth century and the initial decade of the twenty-first century, molecular biology, encompassing fluorescence *in situ* hybridization and advances from genomic probes to next-generation sequencing, has eclipsed immunohistochemistry as a prominent application in numerous laboratories. Molecular biology protocols are not consistently approved by the Food and Drug Administration (FDA), the Canadian Food Inspection Agency (CFIA), or analogous regulatory entities in other nations. A substantial amount of information is challenging to incorporate into a pathology report for therapeutic applications [1, 3, 35, 37–49].

Meanwhile, immunohistochemical analysis has revealed several issues: epithelial cancers often express mesenchymal markers, and vice versa. The epithelial–mesenchymal transition has blurred several boundaries within pathology classifications [50–53]. In recent years, a resurgence in electron microscopy has become evident in many laboratories worldwide [1, 3, 35, 37–49]. The turnaround time for tissue specimens has been reduced from weeks to three days or less through various techniques that utilize monoclonal or polyclonal antibodies for staining. Furthermore, using an electronic camera integrated with the electron microscope has enabled pathologists to obtain quick images that are compatible with many operating systems. Ultimately, specific antibodies remain difficult to detect in regions affected by necrosis or by alterations resulting from autophagy and ischemia, even after antigen retrieval. Simultaneously, electron microscopy, when conducted by skilled professionals, can yield exceptional results and insights for the accurate classification of unidentified pathological tumors. The pediatric small round blue cell tumor category encompasses neuroblastoma, Wilms' tumor (nephroblastoma), rhabdomyosarcoma, Hodgkin's lymphoma, Ewing sarcoma, peripheral neuroectodermal tumor, hepatoblastoma, retinoblastoma, synovial sarcoma, and osteosarcoma [1–23].

The molecular biology data for the juvenile cohort of tiny round blue cell tumors may be daunting due to the methodologies used. In neuroblastoma, 5-aza-2-deoxycytidine activates FOXO3/FKHRL1, leading to the induction of silent caspase-8 [54]. Additionally, nuclear FOXO3 forecasts unfavorable clinical outcomes and facilitates tumor angiogenesis in neuroblastoma [54, 55]. While papillary renal cell carcinoma is predominantly characterized by papillae rather than small round blue cell features, it may exhibit patches of round cells that necessitate differentiation from other recognized small round blue cell tumors (e.g., Wilms' tumor) by ancillary procedures [56]. Ultimately, metanephric stromal tumors should also be included in the differential diagnosis [57]. The rhabdoid tumor is an exceptionally aggressive juvenile neoplasm, characterized by its renal and extra-renal subtypes. Osteosarcoma is one of the most prevalent malignant bone tumors. It must be judiciously differentiated from Ewing sarcoma of the bone or primitive neuroectodermal tumor of the bone [58]. Electron microscopy can be a valuable tool for achieving a definitive diagnosis by integrating immunohistochemistry and molecular biology.

3. TEM technique

An electromagnetic field, rather than optical lenses, is used to focus a high-energy electron beam (~200 keV) onto the sample for analysis. TEM uses an electron gun positioned at the top of the microscope that generates electrons capable of traversing the instrument's column. A series of condenser lenses reduces the size of the beam fired by the gun and regulates its diameter upon striking the specimen.
A fundamental prerequisite of TEM is that the specimen must be sufficiently thin to allow the passage of the electron beam, typically 100–150 nm thick, in stark contrast to the 200–400 microns required for light microscopy [59]. The objective lenses produce the intermediate magnified image, which is further enlarged by the successive projector lenses. The resultant image is initially viewed by the operator (e.g., TEM technician or a pathologist specializing in TEM) and subsequently photographed using a camera or captured digitally. TEM operates in two modes: bright-field mode, which produces a two-dimensional image based on the intensity of the transmitted beam, reflecting the sample's density or thickness, and dark-field mode, which captures the electron diffraction pattern. Preparing semi-thin and ultra-thin sections can be somewhat difficult. The specimen's delicacy renders it susceptible to bending and fracturing, necessitating exceptional care and competence. The preparation of TEM specimens entails reducing their thickness to electron transparency, with potential artifacts arising at various stages (as discussed below). The process involves the accurate compilation of an EM-sized sample, typically measuring 0.1 mm × 0.1 mm × 0.1 mm. Tissue fixation provides physical stability to cellular structures during subsequent processes. Despite the potential benefits of cryofixation, chemical fixation remains the preferred method because cytoplasmic structures deteriorate and collapse during subsequent water sublimation. Chemical fixing is occasionally employed alongside cryofixation. Glutaraldehyde is the most commonly utilized fixative for electron microscopy. Nonetheless, glutaraldehyde alone fails to adequately preserve all cellular structures. Consequently, several supplementary treatments have been implemented, with tannic acid combined with heavy-metal treatment being particularly advantageous [60, 61]. The utilization of tannic acid residues in the protective mechanism is an exception, as it binds to both proteins and heavy metals, particularly during shrinkage induced by dehydration and drying. The employed solutions consist of 2% glutaraldehyde (TEM grade) in 0.1 M sodium cacodylate, pH 7.3, along with 0.1% aqueous tannic acid and 0.1%–0.2% uranyl acetate in distilled water. The minimum fixing duration for glutaraldehyde is 30 minutes at ambient temperature. The tissue specimen may be refrigerated at 4°C and stored in sealed cryovials or containers for up to seven days to prevent evaporation. Specimens must be returned to room temperature before further processing. Glutaraldehyde is subsequently removed from the sample without washing, after which a tannic acid solution is added, and the sample is incubated at room temperature for 20 minutes. The specimen is thereafter rinsed in three aliquots of distilled water and incubated for five minutes in

the final aliquot. The next stage involves adding the uranyl acetate solution, followed by a 20-minute incubation at room temperature. The post-fixation phase utilizes 0.2 M cacodylate buffer. Both glutaraldehyde buffer and cacodylate buffer exhibit high toxicity. Glutaraldehyde adheres to the skin upon abrupt contact, and cacodylate buffer includes arsenic [62, 63]. The dehydration process entails a sequential exposure to ethanol: 35% EtOH for 15 minutes, followed by 50% EtOH for 15 minutes, then 70% EtOH for 15 minutes, then 95% EtOH for 15 minutes, and finally 100% EtOH for 15 minutes. The procedure involves a 15-minute treatment with propylene oxide followed by an overnight application of a 1:1 mixture of propylene oxide and Epon resin. The subsequent morning encompasses the embedding operation, which involves embedding with Epon: (1) exchange to fresh Epon 812 for one to three hours; (2) embed in fresh Epon 812; (3) arrange polyethylene capsules in a holder with numbered strips of paper. New Epon 812 is introduced into the capsules, and the specimen is thereafter transported to the designated blocks. The blocks are thereafter maintained in a 60-degree oven for 48 hours. The preparation of semi-thin sections is essential for identifying the area of interest (ROI). Semi-thin sections are stained with 1% Toluidine Blue and 2% borate in distilled water. The next step is to place ultra-thin sections (~70 nm) on grids for the final post-fixation step. Grids are subjected to uranyl acetate staining for a duration of five minutes to two hours, followed by lead citrate staining for five minutes. TEM involves a high-voltage electron beam generated by a cathode and focused by magnetic lenses. The beam partially transmitted through the thin, electron-transparent specimen generates the TEM information. This information exhibits spatial variation, leading to a monochromatic graphical representation. A sequence of magnetic lenses subsequently amplifies this image until it is captured by striking a fluorescent screen, a photographic plate, or a light-sensitive sensor, such as a charge-coupled device (CCD) camera. In the 1980s and 1990s, TEM images were displayed in real time on a monitor; however, in the twenty-first century, these images are increasingly shown on a computer.

4. Osteosarcoma under the transmission electron microscope lens

Tumor cells characterized by aggregates of cytoplasmic processes containing neurosecretory granules may indicate neuroblastoma. In contrast, a significant diversity in size, shape, and cytoplasmic differentiation, with most tumor cells exhibiting extensively dilated cisterns of rough endoplasmic reticulum and bundles of thick and thin filaments with well-defined Z-bands, may suggest a diagnosis of rhabdomyosarcoma. The presence of an intracytoplasmic deposit of glycogen may signify Ewing sarcoma. A tubular cellular architecture with a well-defined basal lamina may support the diagnosis of nephroblastoma (Wilms' tumor). Osteosarcoma is predominantly a malignant tumor of the skeletal system, with rare occurrences of extraskeletal manifestations [35, 58, 64–74]. The diagnosis depends on the confirmed presence of malignant (atypical) cells associated with osteoid development. This circumstance is complex because the pathologist receives only limited tissue from the interventional radiologist. Moreover, various growth patterns confuse the landscape. Insights into the molecular foundations of pathology have validated the examination of disease progression through morphological alterations in organs [75]. The genetic lineage of the molecules enhances comprehension of the origins of the noted morphological alterations. Understanding the molecules implicated in a specific disease process and the associated morphological alterations can illuminate the pathway to a comprehensive understanding of therapeutic alternatives. Currently, it constitutes a significant issue in pediatric oncology [35, 58, 64–74]. The degree of differentiation determines cell morphology at the ultrastructural level, as is typically the case [1, 3, 22, 76–80]. There is a certain consistency in the investigation of osteosarcoma cells. Osteosarcoma cells, characterized by poor differentiation, display minimal cytoplasm and a high nucleus-to-cytoplasm ratio. As differentiation advances, the quantity of cytoplasm rises, resulting in a normalized or reduced nucleus-to-cytoplasm ratio (see **Figure 1**).

Within the nucleus, a conspicuous nucleolus is frequently discernible. The nucleolus/nucleoli are frequently electron-dense and may exhibit irregular shapes. Typically, the chromatin is relegated to the peripheries. Infrequently, intranuclear inclusions may be observed. The inclusions comprise a spherical aggregation of electron-dense material near the nucleoli. Shapiro, a TEM scientist, examined the dimensions of nuclear pores [80]. The average was 100 nm, with no discernible variation in the level of distinction. The variation in nuclear pore size among patients ranged from 97 to 108 nm, with an overall specific range of 80 to 140 nm. The weakly differentiated osteosarcoma cells have a scarcity of organelles, whereas the highly differentiated osteosarcoma reveals dilated rough endoplasmic reticulum with extensive, intact, and repeatedly anastomosing lakes. Moderate electron-dense homogeneous material is present in the dilated cisternae of the rough endoplasmic reticulum. Cells in a less differentiated state exhibit endoplasmic reticulum characterized by thin lamellae arranged in parallel or circular formations. Neither mitochondria nor the Golgi apparatus is noticeable. Intracellular filaments, approximately 7 nm in diameter, are observed in malignant cells and may occasionally condense into parallel structures. Glycogen and lipid inclusions are hardly observed. Glycogen is often distributed broadly throughout the cytoplasm rather than concentrated in specific areas. This final trait may help differentiate osteosarcoma cells from Ewing sarcoma cells, as filaments are localized to specific cytoplasmic regions in

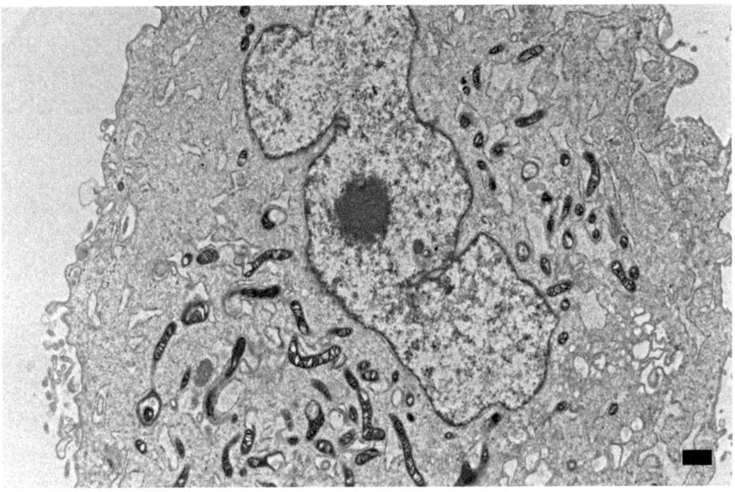

Figure 1.
Depicts an osteosarcoma cell exhibiting a degree of differentiation, characterized by dilated rough endoplasmic reticulum, a prominent nucleus, and an abundance of mitochondria, indicating matrix densification. Bar: 500 nm.

osteosarcoma cells. Typically, intercellular junctions of the zonula adherens (intermediate junction, also known as a belt desmosome) type are observed in poorly differentiated or early-stage osteosarcoma cells. Osteoid is located within the extracellular matrix. The osteoid is generally in a woven configuration, while occasional clusters of parallel fibers may also be observed. Cross-banded collagen is present [1, 3, 22, 35, 78–81]. This collagen exhibits a periodicity of 57–62 nm, with fiber diameters ranging from 30 to 90 nm. Giant cells may be observed in specific locations. These cells resemble uninuclear osteosarcoma cells. The cytoplasm has dilated rough endoplasmic reticulum, dispersed mitochondria, and flattened rough endoplasmic reticulum. This characteristic contrasts markedly with that of osteoclasts, which possess many mitochondria. The small-cell variant of osteosarcoma exhibits an immunohistochemical profile characterized by positivity for vimentin and S100. This reactivity is also negative for keratin, EMA, factor VIII-related antigen, desmin, synaptophysin, LeuM1, and CD45/leukocyte common antigen, which poses significant challenges, primarily due to the combination of the blue round form and size. The tiny cell variant is highly relevant to the differential diagnosis of small round blue cell tumors and must be considered. The challenge arises because the small-cell variety may contain CD99-positive cells in the cytoplasmic membrane [82]. CD99 is a transmembrane glycoprotein encoded by the MIC2 gene. CD99 is regulated by the osteoblast-specific transcription factor Cbfa1 (RUNX2) in osteoblasts. CD99 has been implicated in pathological situations, particularly in Ewing sarcoma cells, where it facilitates cell–cell adhesion and apoptotic signaling. Elevated CD99 expression is observable in lymphoblastic lymphoma/leukemia, synovial sarcoma, mesenchymal chondrosarcoma, and rhabdomyosarcoma. Consequently, dependence on CD99, despite suitable light morphology, presents a drawback. FLI-1 is implicated in cellular proliferation, cancer, and embryonic angiogenesis. FLI-1 is regarded as a specific and sensitive biomarker for Ewing sarcoma; however, it is available at only a limited number of immunohistochemistry facilities. FLI-1 has been shown to identify 90% of Ewing sarcoma/PNET cases with the t(11;22)(q24;q12) translocation, which results in the EWS–FLI1 fusion [83]. Ewing sarcoma/PNET and mesenchymal chondrosarcoma typically exhibit robust CD99 immunoreactivity. However, without osteoid, distinguishing small-cell osteosarcoma from Ewing sarcoma/PNET can be challenging, especially when few samples are obtained by fine-needle aspiration. Conversely, TEM or ultrastructural analysis of small-cell osteosarcoma may be pivotal. This situation arises when we prefer not to depend solely on FLI-1 immunohistochemistry or when this immunohistochemical marker is unavailable in our laboratory [8, 84, 85]. These cells exhibit a high nucleus-to-cytoplasm ratio, weakly differentiated cytoplasm, abundant free ribosomes and mitochondria, and tiny junctions.

The past 30 years have witnessed a disheartening stalemate in the treatment of osteosarcoma. The insulin-like growth factor (IGF) enhances bone production by modulating the proliferation, differentiation, and death of osteoblasts through its interaction with the IGF receptor type I. The IGFBPs inhibit IGFs by blocking receptor binding and regulating the circulating IGF concentration accessible to local tissues [86]. IGFBP-3 is synthesized in human osteoblasts. Overexpression of IGFBP-3 has been linked to bone mineral density (BMD). This phenomenon arises from reduced IGF-I activity and bone resorption, potentially resulting from IGF-I suppression due to excessive sequestration by excess IGFBP-3 [86]. The study by Ressler et al. [66] investigates the disparity in the geographical distribution of IGFBP-3 between normal bone osteocytes and malignant osteosarcoma cells. The study demonstrated that

IGFBP-3 is predominantly cytoplasmic in osteosarcoma cells, in contrast to its nuclear localization in healthy bone osteocytes [65, 87]. Micutkova et al. observed, through visual examination using both confocal and electron microscopy, the accumulation of IGFBP-3 vesicles in the cytoplasm, with a limited presence in the nucleus, while demonstrating successful delivery of vesicles into the nucleoplasm. They noted the protein's seamless translocation into the nucleus. There appears to be a fast deterioration within the nucleus, indicating ubiquitin/proteasome-mediated proteolysis [88]. Santer et al. [68] established that ubiquitin/proteasome-mediated proteolysis directly modulates nuclear IGFBP-3. They noted that IGFBP-3 degradation is contingent on the presence of an active ubiquitin E1 ligase. They asserted that a specific 26S proteasome inhibitor could effectively stabilize nuclear IGFBP-3 and that its metabolic half-life is significantly shorter than that of cytoplasmic IGFBP-3. They additionally observed that nuclear IGFBP-3 is preserved through the mutation of two COOH-terminal lysine residues. Consequently, they proposed that nuclear expression of IGFBP-3 would lead to apoptotic cell death [68]. This data may suggest a malfunction in one of the nuclear proteins associated with IGFBP-3 functions within the nucleus. An investigation into the heightened ubiquitin/proteasome-dependent proteolysis in osteosarcoma relative to normal osteocytes is essential to elucidate the fast degradation of IGFBP-3 within the nucleus.

5. Electron microscopy versus molecular diagnostics

In current practice, molecular diagnostic methods have largely replaced electron microscopy for routine infectious disease diagnosis due to higher sensitivity and specificity, but TEM maintains a crucial, albeit specialized, role in specific non-neoplastic and neoplastic diseases, particularly when an undirected "open view" or ultrastructural detail is needed. Both methods serve as complementary ancillary techniques in modern pathology [89]. As indicated above, electron microscopy uses an electron beam to produce high-resolution, high-magnification images of a specimen's surface or internal structure.

The following paragraphs present the advantages and disadvantages of TEM versus molecular pathology techniques.

5.1 Electron microscopy pros and cons

Currently, the advantages of TEM can be summarized as direct visualization, "open-view," identification of the ultrastructural detail, and elemental analysis. In practice, electron microscopy is the only method capable of directly visualizing small pathogens, such as viruses, without the use of specific probes. Electron microscopy can detect unexpected or novel agents, including potential bioterrorism agents (e.g., in a smallpox scenario), even if genetically modified, because it relies on morphology rather than specific sequences. Electron microscopy is essential for diagnosing diseases based on fine structural changes, such as in certain glomerulopathies (e.g., Alport's syndrome, thin membrane disease) and muscle disorders, and for distinguishing between certain tumor types. Finally, electron microscopy can be combined with energy-dispersive X-ray spectroscopy (EDX) to determine the elemental composition of materials like kidney stones or foreign bodies. On the contrary, electron microscopy has several disadvantages, including costs and complexity, reduced sensitivity at lower loads, the inability to observe living samples, and the difficulty of distinguishing viable from non-viable organisms. In detail, the high initial cost and the requirement for highly trained personnel and sophisticated equipment are critical. Sample preparation is often time-consuming and labor-intensive (e.g., requires ultrathin sectioning for TEM and drying/coating for SEM), which can damage living samples. Moreover, it requires a high concentration of particles (e.g., 10^6–10^8 virus particles/mL) for detection in direct clinical specimens without concentration, and electron microscopy requires a vacuum environment.

Substantially, molecular diagnostics is overwhelmingly used in laboratories. It entails a battery of techniques (e.g., PCR, next-generation sequencing) used to identify genetic markers in a genome or proteome, providing insights into disease mechanisms and pathogen identification. Still, molecular diagnostics has advantages and disadvantages that need to be weighed when compared with electron microscopy. Advantages include high sensitivity and specificity, rapid and high-throughput capabilities, detailed typing and drug-resistance data, and a wide range of applications. In fact, molecular diagnostic platforms can detect minimal amounts of DNA or RNA with high accuracy, even from non-culturable organisms. They contain several molecular assays, which provide quick results (hours to days) and can be automated to process numerous samples. Molecular diagnostics can identify specific strains/genotypes and determine antibiotic resistance profiles, which are crucial for treatment decisions. Molecular diagnostics is used extensively in oncology (tumor profiling), infectious diseases, genetics, and personalized medicine. Disadvantages include the need to know the targets, the potential for false positives/contamination, the inability to distinguish viable from non-viable organisms, and, of course, the cost and the need for laboratory accreditation for molecular diagnostics. In fact, assays are specific to known gene sequences or protein markers; mutations in the target region may lead to false-negative results. High sensitivity requires strict quality control to avoid contamination issues. Most DNA-based PCR tests detect nucleic acids from both living and dead pathogens. Initial setup can be expensive, and highly specialized bioinformatics analysis may be required for complex methods such as sequencing.

Thus, the two methods (electron microscopy and molecular diagnostics) are generally complementary rather than in direct competition. Electron microscopy excels in morphological "discovery" applications where the pathogen or condition is unknown or where ultrastructural detail is critical for definitive diagnosis (e.g., certain renal or muscle diseases). Molecular methods are the front line for routine, rapid, sensitive, and specific detection of known targets and for providing detailed genetic information to guide therapy and monitor disease progression.

6. An overview of the treatment strategies for SRBCTs, including osteosarcoma

Standard treatment algorithms for major small round blue cell tumors (SRBCTs) involve a multimodal approach combining surgery, multi agent chemotherapy, and radiation therapy, with specific protocols varying by the tumor type, stage, location, and the patient's risk factors [34, 74, 90]. The treatment strategies are presented schematically and sequentially.

6.1 Ewing sarcoma

- **Approach:** Multimodal therapy is the standard for localized and metastatic disease. Patients should be treated at specialized centers by multidisciplinary teams.

- **Chemotherapy:** The preferred regimen in North America is vincristine, doxorubicin, and cyclophosphamide, alternating with ifosfamide and etoposide (VAC/IE) for several cycles before and after local control.

- **Local control:** It is critical that surgery be carried out to achieve broad, clear margins without significant morbidity. Radiation therapy is an alternative if surgery is not possible or as an adjuvant if margins are positive or the response to chemotherapy is poor.

- **Metastasis:** Treatment is administered with curative intent, often involving the same chemotherapy regimens as localized disease, potentially with the addition of whole-lung irradiation for pulmonary metastases [91–93].

6.2 Neuroblastoma

- **Approach:** Treatment is stratified by risk group (low, intermediate, high), determined by patient age, stage, and molecular markers (e.g., *MYCN* amplification).

- **Low-risk:** It may involve observation, surgery, or minimal chemotherapy.

- **Intermediate-risk** It often includes chemotherapy and surgery, with radiation therapy for tumors that progress or cannot be resected.

- **High-risk:** It entails an intensive three-phase approach:

  o **Induction:** Combination of chemotherapy and surgery.

  o **Consolidation:** High-dose chemotherapy with stem cell rescue and radiation therapy.

  o **Maintenance:** Immunotherapy (e.g., dinutuximab) and retinoid treatment (e.g., isotretinoin) [54, 94–96].

6.3 Rhabdomyosarcoma

- **Approach:** All patients receive multi-agent chemotherapy due to the high likelihood of micrometastasis, combined with surgery and/or radiation therapy.

- **Chemotherapy:** Standard frontline regimens include vincristine, actinomycin D, and cyclophosphamide (VAC) in the United States, or ifosfamide, vincristine, and actinomycin D (IVA) in Europe. Chemotherapy is given in cycles for 6 to 9 months for intermediate/high-risk disease and up to 24 months for low-risk disease.

- **Local control:** Surgery is used for diagnosis and complete removal, with a focus on preserving function, especially in sensitive areas like the head and neck. Radiation therapy is typically used for intermediate- and high-risk patients, often after several cycles of chemotherapy [97–101].

6.4 Wilms tumor (nephroblastoma)

- **Approach:** Two main international protocols exist, with similar outcomes but different initial strategies:

    - **Children's Oncology Group (North America):** Primary surgical removal of the kidney tumor first to determine the exact stage and histology, followed by risk-adapted adjuvant chemotherapy and, potentially, radiation therapy.

    - **International Society of Pediatric Oncology (Europe):** Neoadjuvant chemotherapy is given first to shrink the tumor and reduce the risk of rupture, followed by surgery, and then risk-adapted post-operative therapy.

- **Treatment components:** It involves a combination of surgery (nephrectomy), chemotherapy (vincristine, dactinomycin, doxorubicin, cyclophosphamide, etoposide, depending on risk), and radiation therapy [102–106].

6.5 Desmoplastic small round cell tumor

- **Approach:** This is a rare, aggressive tumor, and while there is no single standard protocol, treatment generally involves a combination of intensive multi-agent chemotherapy, aggressive cytoreductive surgery, and radiation therapy.

- **Chemotherapy:** Regimens often use agents similar to Ewing sarcoma protocols, such as the P6 regimen (high-dose cyclophosphamide, doxorubicin, and vincristine, alternating with ifosfamide and etoposide).

- **Local control** A complete cytoreductive surgery is a critical part of treatment and is associated with improved survival. Radiation to the abdominopelvic area is also a key component [107–110].

Current osteosarcoma therapies combine neoadjuvant chemotherapy with surgical resection, often using a combination of doxorubicin, cisplatin, and methotrexate. Emerging therapies include immunotherapies such as immune checkpoint inhibitors (ICIs) and CAR-T cell therapy, targeted therapies such as tyrosine kinase inhibitors, and innovative approaches such as gene therapy and ferroptosis induction [66, 73, 74]. The focus is on improving outcomes by enhancing cancer cell killing, reducing side effects, and overcoming treatment resistance [34, 73, 74, 111–114].

Current standard therapies [115–118]

- **Chemotherapy:** The standard approach is to use neoadjuvant chemotherapy to shrink the tumor before surgery. A typical regimen is the "MAP" combination of methotrexate, doxorubicin, and cisplatin, which provides a multi-faceted attack on cancer cells.

- **Surgery:** Surgical resection is crucial for removing the tumor, with limb-salvage surgery being the goal whenever possible.

- **Radiation therapy:** While osteosarcoma is relatively radioresistant, modern approaches like stereotactic radiotherapy, proton radiotherapy, and radiosensitizers are being explored to improve its use in specific cases [115–118].

6.6 Emerging and experimental therapies:

- **Immunotherapy** [34, 119–132]:

  - **Immune checkpoint blockade:** It targets proteins like PD-1/PD–L1 and CTLA-4 to prevent the immune system from being suppressed by cancer cells.

  - **Cellular therapy:**

    - **CAR-T cell therapy:** Modifying a patient's T-cells to target and kill cancer cells.

    - **CAR-NK cells:** A similar approach, but using natural killer (NK) cells.

  - **Dendritic cell vaccines:** Vaccines that train the immune system to recognize and attack cancer cells.

- **Targeted therapies:**

  - **Tyrosine kinase inhibitors (TKIs):** Drugs that block specific pathways essential for cancer growth, such as AXL inhibitors, which have shown promise in preclinical and early clinical studies.

  - **Other targeted agents:** Research is exploring other targets, including those that can be targeted with novel drug delivery systems to improve efficacy and reduce toxicity.

- **Gene therapy:** Aims to correct or target specific genetic mutations driving cancer growth.

- **Ferroptosis induction:** Inducing a form of programmed cell death called ferroptosis, which can be a new therapeutic strategy, sometimes used in combination with existing chemotherapy agents.

- **Autophagy inhibitors:** Compounds that inhibit the process of autophagy, which can help cancer cells survive chemotherapy. Combining these inhibitors with chemotherapy can enhance cell death and improve treatment effectiveness.

- **Radiosensitizers:** Drugs that make tumor cells more sensitive to radiation, allowing for more effective treatment with less damage to normal tissue [133–139].

Recent molecular, genomic, and single-cell sequencing findings in osteosarcoma emphasize its genomic complexity, driven by structural variations (especially *TP53* and *RB1* alterations), significant intratumoral heterogeneity, and a highly dynamic immunosuppressive tumor microenvironment (TME).

6.7 Molecular and genomic findings

- **Genomic instability and chromothripsis**: Whole-genome sequencing (WGS) has confirmed that osteosarcoma is characterized by complex chromosomal rearrangements (chromoanagenesis, including chromothripsis and breakage-fusion-bridge cycles) rather than simple point mutations. These catastrophic events are primary oncogenic drivers and often lead to high rates of whole-genome doubling and copy number variations (CNVs) [140].

- **Key driver genes**: The *TP53* and *RB1* tumor suppressor genes are almost universally affected (biallelic inactivation) in OS, playing pivotal roles in tumor development.

    - *TP53* alterations can occur through deletions, point mutations, or unique rearrangements in intron 1, which appear specific to OS and are an early event in the disease's genesis.

    - Amplifications or gains in oncogenes, such as *MDM2* and *CDK4* are also frequently observed.

- **Non-coding RNAs**: Research highlights the role of dysregulated micro-RNAs (miRNAs) and long noncoding RNAs (lncRNAs) in OS progression. For example, the lncRNA *LOC285194* acts as a tumor suppressor and is a *p53* target, while its downregulation promotes cell proliferation.

6.8 Single-cell sequencing findings

- **Intratumoral heterogeneity**: Single-cell RNA sequencing (scRNA-seq) has provided an unprecedented look at the diverse cell populations within individual tumors (intratumoral heterogeneity), which contribute to poor prognosis and therapy resistance [106, 125, 141, 142].

- **TME insights**: The scRNA-seq studies have identified numerous cell types within the TME, including osteoblastic cells, chondroblastic cells, immune cells (T cells, macrophages, myeloid-derived suppressor cells), endothelial cells, and mesenchymal stem cells [65, 71–74].

    - **Immunosuppression**: The TME is notably immunosuppressive. Cell–cell communication analyses have identified interactions (e.g., involving myeloid-derived suppressor cells) that upregulate pathways such as NF-κB, thereby promoting immune evasion and tumor progression.

- o **Cell communication networks**: Significant cellular communication networks involving pathways such as SPP1, FGF, and NOTCH are crucial in TME regulation.

- o **Subtype differences**: The chondroblastic osteosarcoma subtype is usually associated with a poorer prognosis, exhibits higher levels of hypoxia markers, and reduced immune infiltration compared to other osteosarcoma subtypes [34, 74, 113].

- **Biomarkers and potential targets**: Analysis has revealed specific "hub genes" (e.g., *Skp2*, *TK1*, *KIF20A*, *JUN*) associated with metastasis and prognosis. These findings help in developing novel classification models for patient stratification and potential new therapeutic targets, such as inhibitors for MDM2 or HIF1A, which are currently being explored in clinical trials [143–145].

Recent clinical trials for osteosarcoma immunotherapy focus on combinations of ICIs, such as nivolumab and ipilimumab, and on exploring CAR-T cell therapy targeting HER2. While single-agent ICI therapy shows low efficacy, combination trials have demonstrated improved response rates, although it is still considered an "immune cold" tumor. Other approaches include developing dendritic cell (DC) vaccines and exploring new targets and treatment strategies.

7. Current clinical trial focus areas

- **Immune checkpoint inhibitors:**

  - o **Combination therapy:** Recent research is testing combinations of ICIs, such as nivolumab and ipilimumab, in trials for metastatic sarcoma. An Alliance trial reported a 16% response rate in the combination group compared with 5% in the nivolumab-only group, according to this article on aacrjournals.org.

  - o **Limited efficacy as monotherapy:** Trials with single agents like pembrolizumab and nivolumab have shown limited success, with low response rates (around 5%) in osteosarcoma patients, according to this article from the National Institutes of Health (NIH) [146].

- **CAR-T cell therapy:**

  - o **HER2-targeted CAR-T:** Trials are investigating the use of CAR-T cells engineered to target the HER2 protein, which is present in some osteosarcoma cases.

  - o **Safety and efficacy:** Early studies are evaluating both the persistence of the CAR-T cells and the potential for severe side effects, such as pulmonary toxicity, which may be caused by the T-cells attacking HER2 in normal lung tissue.

- **DC vaccines:**
    - o **Mechanism:** These vaccines are designed to train the patient's immune system to recognize and fight osteosarcoma cells by exposing it to tumor-associated antigens.
    - o **Combination with other therapies:** Researchers are exploring combining DC vaccines with other immunotherapy agents, such as checkpoint inhibitors and oncolytic viruses, to improve efficacy.
    - o **Safety:** DC-based vaccines have generally shown a good safety profile, though their clinical effectiveness remains limited.

Other immunotherapy approaches:

- Trials are also exploring the use of genetically modified bacteria, such as an investigational agent called OST31-164, for maintenance therapy.
- Researchers are looking into new targets and strategies, as osteosarcoma is often considered "immune cold" due to low immune cell infiltration in tumors.

7.1 Limitations and challenges

- **Low tumor mutational burden:** Osteosarcoma has a low tumor mutational burden, which means fewer neoantigens are available for the immune system to recognize, limiting the effectiveness of current immunotherapies like ICIs.
- **TME:** The TME in osteosarcoma can suppress immune responses, further hindering the effectiveness of immunotherapies.
- **Need for biomarkers:** A lack of predictive biomarkers makes it challenging to identify which patients are most likely to benefit from immunotherapy [34, 74].

8. Conclusion

In conclusion, we assert that TEM remains a reliable and valid technique in pathology. TEM serves as a supplementary tool for examining tiny, round, blue cell cancers, providing definitive evidence to support the immunohistochemical findings. When implemented in a contemporary facility, it can yield substantial interindividual agreement, elevated validity, and effective dependability. It may be essential for comprehending certain contemporary single-cell studies. Emerging medicines for osteosarcoma show great promise, thanks to ongoing advances in medical science. One of the most cutting-edge new approaches to cancer treatment is gene therapy, which aims to stop the disease in its tracks by destroying cancer cells at their molecular and genetic bases. Some common targets include genes that reduce tumor growth, pathways that make drugs more effective, and gene-editing tools such as CRISPR/Cas9 that help repair damaged DNA. To restore normal cell cycle regulation and physiological apoptosis, gene therapy can target tumor suppressor genes. This allows for the introduction of functional gene copies into the host genome. The G1 cell cycle checkpoint is disrupted by mutations in the tumor suppressor gene *TP53*, which is frequently mutated in osteosarcoma. In addition to encouraging tumor growth, this makes the tumor more dependent on the G2 checkpoint, which is responsible for preserving DNA integrity. Many osteosarcoma cells acquire mutations or express proteins that make them more resistant to drugs; therefore, gene therapies that aim to modulate drug-sensitization pathways are also showing some promise. The exosome, a tiny vesicle outside cells that often regulates the environment and communicates between cells, is a key player in this resistance. To aid in the propagation of resistance, exosomes in cancer cells can release doxorubicin and other chemotherapeutic drugs, transport or upregulate drug efflux pumps such as P-glycoprotein (P–gp), and transport multidrug-resistant mRNA from resistant to sensitive cells. What makes exosomes so intriguing as potential gene therapy targets is the same factor that renders them effective resistance vectors. Miniaturization, excellent solubility, low toxicity, and a long half-life are among the advantageous properties of exosomes. Studies have shown that programmed exosomes are often more selective and less toxic than current miRNA-delivery methods, possibly because of interactions between exosome membrane proteins and tumor cell membranes. In 2022, researchers found that miR-665-loaded exosomes inhibited osteosarcoma development *in vivo* and *in vitro*, with acceptable safety and efficacy profiles [23, 65, 147]. Although exosomes have many benefits, they also have drawbacks, including limited understanding of which exosomes are most effective against different types of cancer and the difficulty of isolating them in adequate numbers and with sufficient purity. Also, whether hypercell-permeable micelles or any other nanoparticle delivery strategy ultimately works better is still up in the air. The selectivity of lab-engineered nanoparticles is lacking in exosomes, despite their many advantageous features and numerous on-going projects not limited to a specific type of pathology [148–152]. Through gene therapy, scientists can also use CRISPR/Cas9 technology to precisely modify genomes and identify genes that cause drug resistance. As a result, therapeutic outcomes can be improved by targeting genes that drive osteosarcoma and drug resistance. Definitely, osteosarcoma therapy will be reshaped in this decade, and the advent of quantum computing will add value to the computation and interpretation of the single-cell transcriptomic data we are accumulating.

Acknowledgments

The author has obtained research funding from the Canadian Women and Children's Health Research Institute (WCHRI), the Canadian Foundation for Women's Health (CFWH), the Austrian Tyrolean Cancer Research Institute, the Austrian Research Fund (Fonds zur Förderung der wissenschaftlichen Forschung, FWF), and the Saudi Cultural Bureau of Saudi Arabia.

Conflict of Interest

The authors declare no conflict of interest. He receives royalties from several publishers. All royalties are donated to family and children's charities.

DOI: http://dx.doi.org/10.5772/intechopen.1014243

Author details

Consolato M. Sergi

1 Anatomic Pathology Division; Pediatric Pathologist, Children's Hospital of Eastern Ontario (CHEO), Ottawa, ON, Canada

2 Department of Pathology & Pediatrics, University of Alberta & University of Ottawa, Ottawa, ON, Canada

*Address all correspondence to: csergi@cheo.on.ca

References

[1] Kim NR, Ha SY, Cho HY. Utility of transmission electron microscopy in small round cell tumors. Journal of Pathology and Translational Medicine. 2015;**49**(2):93–101. DOI: 10.4132/jptm.2015.01.30

[2] Llombart-Bosch A, Contesso G, Peydro-Olaya A.Histology, immunohistochemistry, and electron microscopy of small round cell tumors of bone. Seminars in Diagnostic Pathology. 1996;**13**(3):153–170

[3] Peydro-Olaya A, Llombart-Bosch A, Carda-Batalla C, Lopez-Guerrero JA. Electron microscopy and other ancillary techniques in the diagnosis of small round cell tumors. Seminars in Diagnostic Pathology. 2003;**20**(1):25–45

[4] Abd El-Aziz YM, Sobh MS, Saad HM, Morsy MHE, El-Haroun E, Abass KS, Abdul Kari Z, Mathew RT, Eissa MEH, Eissa EH. Mastering the art of sectioning: A comprehensive guide to slide-microtome technology and histological applications. Frontiers in Veterinary Science. 2025;**12**:1635706. DOI: 10.3389/fvets.2025.1635706

[5] Ayadi L, Khabir A. Pediatric angiosarcoma of soft tissue: A rare clinicopathologic entity. Archives of Pathology & Laboratory Medicine. 2010;**134**(3):481–485. DOI: 10.5858/134.3.481

[6] Caruso R, Caruso V, Rigoli L. Eosinophil ETosis and Cancer: Ultrastructural Evidence and Oncological Implications. Cancers (Basel). 2025;**17**(19):3250. DOI: 10.3390/cancers17193250

[7] Dehner LP. Primitive Neuroectodermal Tumor and Ewing's Sarcoma. The American Journal of Surgical Pathology. 1993;**17**(1):1–13. DOI: 10.1097/00000478-199301000-00001

[8] Dickersin GR, Rosenberg AE.The ultrastructure of small-cell osteosarcoma, with a review of the light microscopy and differential diagnosis. Human Pathology. 1991;**22**(3):267–275

[9] Erlandson RA, Woodruff JM.Role of electron microscopy in the evaluation of soft tissue neoplasms, with emphasis on spindle cell and pleomorphic tumors. Human Pathology. 1998;**29**(12):1372–1381

[10] Fishbein GA, Bois MC, d'Amati G, Glass C, Masuelli L, Rodriguez ER, Seidman MA. Ultrastructural cardiac pathology: The wide (yet so very small) world of cardiac electron microscopy. Cardiovascular Pathology. 2024;**73**:107670. DOI: 10.1016/j.carpath.2024.107670

[11] Fletcher JA.Laboratory investigation, genetics, and experimental models in sarcomas. Current Opinion in Oncology. 1991;**3**(4):665–670

[12] Hadfield MG, Quezado MM, Williams RL, Luo VY. Ewing's Family of Tumors Involving Structures Related to the Central Nervous System: A Review. Pediatric and Developmental Pathology. 2000;**3**(3):203–210. DOI: 10.1007/s100249910026

[13] Hicks J, Mierau GW. The spectrum of pediatric tumors in infancy, childhood, and adolescence: A comprehensive review with emphasis on special techniques in diagnosis.

Ultrastructural Pathology. 2005;**29**(3-4):175–202. DOI: 10.1080/01913120590951185

[14] Holscher DL, Bulow RD, Strauch M, Boor P. Advances in computational nephropathology. Kidney International. 2025;**108**(6):1031–1044. DOI: 10.1016/j.kint.2025.06.029

[15] Hornick JL, Fletcher CDM. Soft tissue perineurioma: Clinicopathologic analysis of 81 cases including those with atypical histologic features. American Journal of Surgical Pathology. 2005;**29**(7):845–858. DOI: 10.1097/01.pas.0000155166.86409.d2

[16] Llombart-Bosch A, Lacombe MJ, Contesso G, Peydro-Olaya A.Small round blue cell sarcoma of bone mimicking atypical Ewing's sarcoma with neuroectodermal features. An analysis of five cases with immunohistochemical and electron microscopic support. Cancer. 1987;**60**(7):1570–1582

[17] Llombart-Bosch A, Pellin A, Carda C, Noguera R, Navarro S, Peydro-Olaya A.Soft tissue Ewing sarcoma–peripheral primitive neuroectodermal tumor with atypical clear cell pattern shows a new type of EWS-FEV fusion transcript. Diagnostic Molecular Pathology. 2000;**9**(3):137–144

[18] Madero M, Parameswaran S. Chronic kidney disease of unknown origin, a tubulointerstitial disease. Advances in Kidney Disease and Health. 2025;**32**(4):350–356. DOI: 10.1053/j.akdh.2025.06.004

[19] Mori D, Kagaku A, Wang KY, Tokunaga T, Kida Y, Shimozono Y, Nishiyama H, Kizaki K, Funakoshi N, Yamashita F, Kobayashi M. Histologic and ultrastructural degeneration of rotator cuff tendons in elderly patients with glenohumeral arthritis and cuff tear arthropathy. BMC Surgery. 2025;**25**(1):281. DOI: 10.1186/s12893-025-03002-8

[20] Price D, Cramer J, Rogers CB, Prajapati P, Shakhashiro Y, Nelson PT, Wang W-X. Immunoelectron microscopy and biochemical studies using three anti-tau antibodies in human brains: Associations between pTau and ribosomes. Acta Neuropathologica Communications. 2025;**13**(1):150. DOI: 10.1186/s40478-025-02072-2

[21] Sulman M, Aboubechara JP, Abu-Asab MS, Aboud O. Understanding glioma pathogenesis through ultrastructural analysis. Ultrastructural Pathology. 2025;**49**(6):528–536. DOI: 10.1080/01913123.2025.2558625

[22] Williams AH, Schwinn CP, Parker JW.The ultrastructure of osteosarcoma. A review of twenty cases. Cancer. 1976;**37**(3):1293–1301

[23] Wu J, Su B, Gu L, Zhang J, Shi Q, Hu D. Immunoelectron microscopy: A comprehensive guide from sample preparation to high-resolution imaging. Discover Nano. 2025;**20**(1):154. DOI: 10.1186/s11671-025-04346-z

[24] Gordon RE. Electron microscopy: A brief history and review of current clinical application. Methods in Molecular Biology. 2014;**1180**:119–135. DOI: 10.1007/978-1-4939-1050-2_7

[25] Moser TH, Mehta H, Park C, Kelly RT, Shokuhfar T, Evans JE. The role of electron irradiation history in liquid cell transmission electron microscopy. Science Advances. 2018;**4**(4):eaaq1202. DOI: 10.1126/sciadv.aaq1202

[26] Bahitham W, Liao X, Peng F, Bamforth F, Chan A, Mason A, Stone B, Stothard P, Sergi C. Mitochondriome and cholangiocellular carcinoma. PLoS One. 2014;**9**(8):e104694. DOI: 10.1371/journal.pone.0104694

[27] Chan BYH, Roczkowsky A, Cho WJ, Poirier M, Sergi C, Keschrumrus V, Churko JM, Granzier H, Schulz R. MMP inhibitors attenuate doxorubicin cardiotoxicity by preventing intracellular and extracellular matrix remodelling. Cardiovascular Research. 2021;**117**(1):188–200. DOI: 10.1093/cvr/cvaa017

[28] Garcia E, Ladak Z, Landry T, Wollin M, Persad ARL, Sergi CM, Huynh HQ, Persad R, Persad S. Epithelial-mesenchymal transition, regulated by β-catenin and Twist, leads to esophageal wall remodeling in pediatric eosinophilic esophagitis. PLoS One. 2022;**17**(3):e0264622. DOI: 10.1371/journal.pone.0264622

[29] Glueckert R, Rask-Andersen H, Sergi C, Schmutzhard J, Mueller B, Beckmann F, Rittinger O, Hoefsloot LH, Schrott-Fischer A, Janecke AR. Histology and synchrotron radiation-based microtomography of the inner ear in a molecularly confirmed case of CHARGE syndrome. American Journal of Medical Genetics Part A. 2010;**152A**(3):665–673. DOI: 10.1002/ajmg.a.33321

[30] Hall AR, Le H, Arnold C, Brunton J, Bertolo R, Miller GG, Zello GA, Sergi C. Aluminum exposure from parenteral nutrition: early bile canaliculus changes of the hepatocyte. Nutrients. 2018;**10**(6):723. DOI: 10.3390/nu10060723

[31] Johnson Chacko L, Sergi C, Eberharter T, Dudas J, Rask-Andersen H, Hoermann R, Fritsch H, Fischer N, Glueckert R, Schrott-Fischer A. Early appearance of key transcription factors influence the spatiotemporal development of the human inner ear. Cell and Tissue Research. 2020;**379**(3):459–471. DOI: 10.1007/s00441-019-03115-6

[32] Kehar M, Klaassen RJ, Sergi CM. Heterozygous missense mutation of the fibrinogen gene associated with cryptogenic liver disease in a 15-months-old Canadian caucasian child. Ultrastructural Pathology. 2025;**49**(2):235–242. DOI: 10.1080/01913123.2024.2447853

[33] McKillop SJ, Belletrutti MJ, Lee BE, Yap JY, Noga ML, Desai SJ, Sergi C. Adenovirus necrotizing hepatitis complicating atypical teratoid rhabdoid tumor. Pediatrics International. 2015;**57**(5):974–977. DOI: 10.1111/ped.12674

[34] Sergi CM, Burnett M, Jantuan E, Hakoum M, Beug ST, Leng R, Shen F. Digging through the complexities of immunological approaches in emerging osteosarcoma therapeutics: A comprehensive narrative review with updated clinical trials. Biomedicines. 2025;**13**(3):664. DOI: 10.3390/biomedicines13030664

[35] Sergi CM, Patry J, Coenraad H, McClintock J, Nicholls R, Steiner HJ, Mikuz G. Transmission Electron Microscopy: A Surgical Pathology Tool for Neuroblastoma. Journal of Visualized Experiments. 2022;**185**. DOI: 10.3791/63994

[36] Yogasundaram H, Paterson ID, Graham M, Sergi C, Oudit GY.Glycogen storage disease because of a PRKAG2 mutation causing severe biventricular hypertrophy and high-grade atrio-ventricular block. Circulation:

Heart Failure. 2016;**9**(8). DOI: 10.1161/CIRCHEARTFAILURE.116.003367

[37] Alfaro-Cervello C, Soriano-Navarro M, Cebrian-Silla A, Forteza-Vila J. Annulate Lamellae in a Desmoplastic Small Round Cell Tumor. International Journal of Surgical Pathology. 2016;**24**(7):623–624. DOI: 10.1177/1066896916644324

[38] Chen Q, Gu Y, Liu B. Clinicopathological characteristics of kidney mucinous tubular and spindle cell carcinoma. International Journal of Clinical and Experimental Pathology. 2015;**8**(1):1007–1012

[39] Das DK.Fine-needle aspiration (FNA) cytology diagnosis of small round cell tumors: Value and limitations. Indian Journal of Pathology and Microbiology. 2004;**47**(3):309–318

[40] Hes O, de Souza TG, Pivovarcikova K, Grossmann P, Martinek P, Kuroda N, Kacerovska D, Svajdler M, Straka L, Petersson F, Hora M, Michal M. Distinctive renal cell tumor simulating atrophic kidney with 2 types of microcalcifications. Report of 3 cases. Annals of Diagnostic Pathology. 2014;**18**(2):82–88. DOI: 10.1016/j.anndiagpath.2013.12.003

[41] Kakkar S, Gupta D, Kaur G, Rana V. Primary primitive neuroectodermal tumor of kidney: a rare case report with diagnostic challenge. Indian J Pathol Microbiol. 2014;**57**(2):298–300. DOI: 10.4103/0377-4929.134723

[42] Kano T, Sasaki A, Tomizawa S, Shibasaki T, Tamura M, Ohye C. Primary Ewing's sarcoma of the orbit: Case report. Brain Tumor Pathology. 2009;**26**(2):95–100. DOI: 10.1007/s10014-009-0256-x

[43] Maly B, Maly A, Reinhartz T, Sherman Y. Primitive neuroectodermal tumor of the kidney. Report of a case initially diagnosed by fine needle aspiration cytology. Acta Cytologica. 2004;**48**(2):264–268. DOI: 10.1159/000326329

[44] Shenjere P, Eyden B, Banerjee SS, Chakrabarty B, Shanks JH, Sikand KA, Menasce LP. Ultrastructurally confirmed myofibrosarcoma: A series of 10 new cases, with a discussion on diagnostic criteria. International Journal of Surgical Pathology. 2013;**21**(1):29–36. DOI: 10.1177/1066896912454568

[45] Tamada H, Kobayashi M, Sano K, Uehara T, Matsumoto Y, Tateishi A, Ohya M, Kito M, Aoki K, Kanno H. Ultrastructure of CIC-DUX4 sarcoma: The first pathological report. Ultrastructural Pathology. 2020;**44**(2):237–244. DOI: 10.1080/01913123.2020.1737610

[46] Trautmann M, Hartmann W. Molecular approaches to diagnosis in Ewing sarcoma: Fluorescence in situ hybridization (FISH). Methods in Molecular Biology. 2021;**2226**:65–83. DOI: 10.1007/978-1-0716-1020-6_6

[47] Veeramachaneni R, Herrera GA, Turbat-Herrera EA.Hepatoblastoma in a 15-month-old male: Cytomorphology, electron microscopy, and differential diagnosis. Ultrastructural Pathology. 2003;**27**(5):369–373

[48] Zhang H-Y, Yang G-H, Chen H-J, Wei B, Ke Q, Guo H, Ye L, Bu H, Yang K, Zhang Y-H.Clinicopathological, immunohistochemical, and ultrastructural study of 13 cases of melanotic schwannoma. Chinese Medical Journal. 2005;**118**(17):1451–1461

[49] Zhang W, Yu W, Wang Q, Jiang Y, Li Y. The clinicopathological, ultrastructural, genetic features and diagnosis of small cell variant renal oncocytoma. Acta Histochemica. 2015;**117**(6):505–511. DOI: 10.1016/j.acthis.2014.11.013

[50] Duan J, Guan X, Xue J, Wang J, Wang Z, Chen X, Jiang W, Sui W, Song Y, Li T, Rao D, Wu X, Lu M. RAB37 suppresses the EMT, migration and invasion of gastric cancer cells by mediating autophagic degradation of β-catenin. Cellular Oncology. 2024;**47**(6):2407–2421. DOI: 10.1007/s13402-024-01028-3

[51] Gong X, Qiu T, Zhou J, Yang K, Xiang S, Zhang Z, Lan Y, Zhang X, Zhou Z, Yang C, Zhang Y, Chen S, Ji Y. TGF-β1 promotes angiogenesis via endothelial-to-mesenchymal transition in infantile hemangioma. Arteriosclerosis, Thrombosis, and Vascular Biology. 2025;**45**(10):1912–1927. DOI: 10.1161/ATVBAHA.125.322793

[52] Pang Y, Guo T, Zhou Y, Jiang S, Li Y, Ni J, Chu X, Chu L, Chen F, Yang X, Zhu Z. Radiation-induced extracellular vesicles from cancer-associated fibroblasts drive oesophageal squamous cell carcinoma metastasis via the miR-193a-3p/PTEN/Akt pathway. Clinical and Translational Medicine. 2025;**15**(10):e70483. DOI: 10.1002/ctm2.70483

[53] Zhao N, Powell RT, Yuan X, Bae G, Roarty KP, Stossi F, Strempfl M, Toneff MJ, Johnson HL, Mani SA, Jones P, Stephan CC, Rosen JM. Morphological screening of mesenchymal mammary tumor organoids to identify drugs that reverse epithelial-mesenchymal transition. Nature Communications. 2021;**12**(1):4262. DOI: 10.1038/s41467-021-24545-3

[54] Geiger K, Hagenbuchner J, Rupp M, Fiegl H, Sergi C, Meister B, Kiechl-Kohlendorfer U, Muller T, Ausserlechner MJ, Obexer P. FOXO3/FKHRL1 is activated by 5-aza-2-deoxycytidine and induces silenced caspase-8 in neuroblastoma. Molecular Biology of the Cell. 2012;**23**(11):2226–2234. DOI: 10.1091/mbc.E11-06-0535

[55] Hagenbuchner J, Rupp M, Salvador C, Meister B, Kiechl-Kohlendorfer U, Muller T, Geiger K, Sergi C, Obexer P, Ausserlechner MJ. Nuclear FOXO3 predicts adverse clinical outcome and promotes tumor angiogenesis in neuroblastoma. Oncotarget. 2016a;**7**(47):77591–77606. DOI: 10.18632/oncotarget.12728

[56] Schultz TD, Sergi C, Grundy P, Metcalfe PD. Papillary renal cell carcinoma: Report of a rare entity in childhood with review of the clinical management. Journal of Pediatric Surgery. 2011;**46**(6):e31–34. DOI: 10.1016/j.jpedsurg.2011.03.080

[57] Brisigotti M, Cozzutto C, Fabbretti G, Sergi C, Callea F. Metanephric adenoma. Histology and Histopathology. 1992;7(4):689–692

[58] Osasan S, Zhang M, Shen F, Paul PJ, Persad S, Sergi C. Osteogenic Sarcoma: A 21st Century Review. Anticancer Research. 2016;**36**(9):4391–4398. DOI: 10.21873/anticanres.10982

[59] Méndez-Vilas A. Microscopy and Imaging Science: Practical Approaches to Applied Research and Education. Méndez-Vilas A, Ed. Spain: Formatex Research Center; 2017

[60] Johnson E, Kaufmann R. Correlative in-resin super-resolution fluorescence and electron microscopy of cultured cells. Methods in Molecular Biology. 2017;**1663**:163–177. DOI: 10.1007/978-1-4939-7265-4_14

[61] Kim JY, Lee H, Park T, Park J, Kim M-H, Cho H, Youn W, Kang SM, Choi IS. Artificial Spores: Cytocompatible Coating of Living Cells with Plant-Derived Pyrogallol. Chemistry – An Asian Journal. 2016;**11**(22):3183–3187. DOI: 10.1002/asia.201601237

[62] Takigawa T, Endo Y.Effects of glutaraldehyde exposure on human health. Journal of Occupational Health. 2006;**48**(2):75–87

[63] Weakley BS.How dangerous is sodium cacodylate? Journal of Microscopy. 1977;**109**(2):249–251

[64] Ali N, Venkateswaran G, Garcia E, Landry T, McColl H, Sergi C, Persad A, Abuetabh Y, Eisenstat DD, Persad S. Osteosarcoma progression is associated with increased nuclear levels and transcriptional activity of activated β-Catenin. Genes & Cancer. 2019;**10**(3-4):63–79. DOI: 10.18632/genesandcancer.191

[65] Burnett M, Abuetabh Y, Wronski A, Shen F, Persad S, Leng R, Eisenstat D, Sergi C. Graphene oxide nanoparticles induce apoptosis in wild-type and CRISPR/Cas9-IGF/IGFBP3 knocked-out Osteosarcoma Cells. Journal of Cancer. 2020;**11**(17):5007–5023. DOI: 10.7150/jca.46464

[66] Mojiri A, Stoletov K, Carrillo MA, Willetts L, Jain S, Godbout R, Jurasz P, Sergi CM, Eisenstat DD, Lewis JD, Jahroudi N. Functional assessment of von Willebrand factor expression by cancer cells of non-endothelial origin. Oncotarget. 2017;**8**(8):13015–13029. DOI: 10.18632/oncotarget.14273

[67] Ressler S, Radhi J, Aigner T, Loo C, Zwerschke W, Sergi C.Insulin-like growth factor-binding protein-3 in osteosarcomas and normal bone tissues. Anticancer Research. 2009;**29**(7):2579–2587

[68] Santer FR, Bacher N, Moser B, Morandell D, Ressler S, Firth SM, Spoden GA, Sergi C, Baxter RC, Jansen-dürr P, Zwerschke W. Nuclear insulin-like growth factor binding protein-3 induces apoptosis and is targeted to ubiquitin/proteasome–dependent proteolysis. Cancer Research. 2006;**66**(6):3024–3033. DOI: 10.1158/0008-5472.CAN-05-2013

[69] Sergi C, Shen F, Liu S-M. Insulin/IGF-1R, SIRT1, and FOXOs pathways—an intriguing interaction platform for bone and osteosarcoma. Frontiers in Endocrinology. 2019;**10**:93. DOI: 10.3389/fendo.2019.00093

[70] Sergi C, Zwerschke W. Osteogenic sarcoma (osteosarcoma) in the elderly: Tumor delineation and predisposing conditions. Experimental Gerontology. 2008;**43**(12):1039–1043. DOI: 10.1016/j.exger.2008.09.009

[71] Sergi CM.Targeting the 'garbage-bin' to fight cancer: HDAC6 inhibitor WT161 has an anti-tumor effect on osteosarcoma and synergistically interacts with 5-FU. Bioscience Reports. 2021;**41**(8). DOI: 10.1042/BSR20210952

[72] Sergi CM.Commentary on: SMARCB1 as a novel diagnostic and prognostic biomarker for osteosarcoma. Bioscience Reports. 2022;**42**(6). DOI: 10.1042/BSR20220040

[73] Sergi CM. The role of SPARC/ON in human osteosarcoma. Advances in Protein Chemistry and Structural Biology. 2023b;**133**:181–192. DOI: 10.1016/bs.apcsb.2022.10.007

[74] Sergi CM. Pediatric cancer—pathology and microenvironment influence: A perspective into osteosarcoma and non-osteogenic mesenchymal malignant neoplasms. Discover Oncology. 2024;**15**(1):358. DOI: 10.1007/s12672-024-01240-5

[75] Strasser BJ. Sickle Cell Anemia, a Molecular Disease. Science. 1999;**286**(5444):1488–1490. DOI: 10.1126/science.286.5444.1488

[76] Fujinuma A.Ultrastructural study of osteosarcoma. Nihon Seikeigeka Gakkai Zasshi. 1987;**61**(6):667–679

[77] Gupta P, Siraj F, Shankar KB, Rawat M, Mankotia DS, Yadav V, Dagar A. Clinical and histopathological spectrum of cranial small round cell tumors: An experience from a tertiary care center. Journal of Cancer Research and Therapeutics. 2024;**20**(1):238–242. DOI: 10.4103/jcrt.jcrt_383_22

[78] Komiya S.Electron microscopy of bone tumors--osteosarcoma, chondrosarcoma, giant cell tumor of bone. Nihon Seikeigeka Gakkai Zasshi. 1982;**56**(7):635–657

[79] Rajwanshi A, Srinivas R, Upasana G. Malignant small round cell tumors. Journal of Cytology. 2009;**26**(1):1–10. DOI: 10.4103/0970-9371.54861

[80] Shapiro F.Ultrastructural observations on osteosarcoma tissue: A study of 10 cases. Ultrastructural Pathology. 1983;**4**(2-3):151–161

[81] Park SH, Kim I. Small cell osteogenic sarcoma of the ribs: Cytological, immunohistochemical, and ultrastructural study with literature review. Ultrastructural Pathology. 1999;**23**(2):133–140. DOI: 10.1080/019131299281770

[82] Manara MC, Bernard G, Lollini P-L, Nanni P, Zuntini M, Landuzzi L, Benini S, Lattanzi G, Sciandra M, Serra M, Colombo MP, Bernard A, Picci P, Scotlandi K. CD99 acts as an oncosuppressor in osteosarcoma. Molecular Biology of the Cell. 2006;**17**(4):1910–1921. DOI: 10.1091/mbc.e05-10-0971

[83] Cho U, Cha HJ, Kim HJ, Min SK, Kim HK, Jung HR, Park G, Kim JE. FLI-1 is expressed in a wide variety of hematolymphoid neoplasms: A special concern in the differential diagnosis. Clinical and Experimental Medicine. 2024;**24**(1):18. DOI: 10.1007/s10238-023-01284-x

[84] Bishop JA, Shum CH, Sheth S, Wakely Jr PE, Ali SZ. Small cell osteosarcoma: Cytopathologic characteristics and differential diagnosis. American Journal of Clinical Pathology. 2010;**133**(5):756–761. DOI: 10.1309/AJCPO07VGDZCBRJF

[85] Mills SE, Fechner RE."Undifferentiated" neoplasms of the sinonasal region: Differential diagnosis based on clinical, light microscopic, immunohistochemical, and ultrastructural features. Seminars in Diagnostic Pathology. 1989;**6**(4):316–328

[86] Silha JV, Mishra S, Rosen CJ, Beamer WG, Turner RT, Powell DR, Murphy LJ. Perturbations in bone formation and resorption in insulin-like growth factor binding protein-3

transgenic mice. Journal of Bone and Mineral Research. 2003;**18** (10):1834–1841. DOI: 10.1359/jbmr.2003.18.10.1834

[87] Jin L, Shen F, Weinfeld M, Sergi C. Insulin growth factor binding protein 7 (IGFBP7)-related cancer and IGFBP3 and IGFBP7 crosstalk. Frontiers in Oncology. 2020;**10**:727. DOI: 10.3389/fonc.2020.00727

[88] Micutkova L, Hermann M, Offterdinger M, Hess MW, Matscheski A, Pircher H, Muck C, Ebner H-L, Laich A, Ferrando-May E, Zwerschke W, Huber LA, Jansen-Dürr P. Analysis of the cellular uptake and nuclear delivery of insulin-like growth factor binding protein-3 in human osteosarcoma cells. International Journal of Cancer. 2012;**130**(7):1544–1557. DOI: 10.1002/ijc.26149

[89] Erlandson RA. Role of electron microscopy in modern diagnostic surgical pathology. Modern Surgical Pathology. 2009;71–84. DOI: 10.1016/b978-1-4160-3966-2.00005-9

[90] Sergi CM. Pathology of Childhood and Adolescence. Springer; 2020

[91] Bruce A, Anchondo G, Carter R, Guerrero Pacheco S, Kambala HS, Cortez E, Parker K, Su L. Targeting RNA polymerase I in ewing sarcoma treatment. Cancer Science. 2025;**116** (8):2317–2319. DOI: 10.1111/cas.70047

[92] Molina ER, Chim LK, Barrios S, Ludwig JA, Mikos AG. Modeling the tumor microenvironment and pathogenic signaling in bone sarcoma. Tissue Engineering Part B: Reviews. 2020;**26**(3):249–271. DOI: 10.1089/ten.teb.2019.0302

[93] Zetouni NC, Sergi CM. Features of Metastatic Ewing Sarcoma. In Sergi CM, editor. Metastasis. Exon; 2022. DOI: 10.36255/exon-publications.metastasis.metastatic-ewing-sarcoma

[94] Donato I, Velpula KK, Tsung AJ, Tuszynski JA, Sergi CM. Demystifying neuroblastoma malignancy through fractal dimension, entropy, and lacunarity. Tumori Journal. 2023;**109** (4):370–378. DOI: 10.1177/03008916221146208

[95] Hagenbuchner J, Rupp M, Salvador C, Meister B, Kiechl-Kohlendorfer U, Muller T, Geiger K, Sergi C, Obexer P, Ausserlechner MJ. Nuclear FOXO3 predicts adverse clinical outcome and promotes tumor angiogenesis in neuroblastoma. Oncotarget. 2016b;7:77591–77606. DOI: 10.18632/oncotarget.12728

[96] Sergi CM. In situ neuroblastoma: the intriguing "Tumor" of neuroectodermal origin and the putative cancer stem cells. In Sergi CM, editor. Advancements in Cancer Research. 2023a. p. 10.36255/neuroblastoma–in–situ

[97] Corradini N, Andre N, Orbach D. Maintenance therapy for pediatric sarcoma: Full throttle ahead? Current Opinion in Oncology. 2025;**37**(4):347–357. DOI: 10.1097/CCO.0000000000001148

[98] Hassan C-H, Kerimian M, Even C, Moya-Plana A, Verillaud B, Malard O, Michel J, Favier V, Mortuaire G, Moriniere S, Baujat B, Rumeau C, Vergez S, Righini C, Patron V, Dupin C, Loffler A, Benard A, Digue L, Thariat J. Survival rates and prognostic factors of 118 sinonasal sarcomas among adolescents and adults: A national database REFCOR study. European

Journal of Surgical Oncology. 2025;**51**(9):110247. DOI: 10.1016/j.ejso.2025.110247

[99] McCarville MB, Wu S, Li Y, Kaste SC, Bishop M, Doubrovin M, Pappo AS, Krasin M, Hillenbrand CM. Comparing Whole-Body Diffusion-weighted MRI to Conventional Imaging: Staging Pediatric Bone and Soft-Tissue Sarcomas. Radiology: Imaging Cancer. 2025;**7**(5):e240475. DOI: 10.1148/rycan.240475

[100] Metts J, Ginn K, He Z, Keesari R, Cook JC, Senn S, Schink M, Sansil S, Yin H, Cash T. A phase i trial of nab-paclitaxel in combination with gemcitabine for relapsed/refractory pediatric solid tumors. Pediatric Blood & Cancer. 2025;e32102. DOI: 10.1002/pbc.32102

[101] Mohas A, Horvath K, Jakab Z, Csoka M. Multi-targeted kinase inhibitor therapy in pediatric bone and soft tissue sarcoma patients—a single centre experience. Cancer Medicine. 2025;**14**(9):e70951. DOI: 10.1002/cam4.70951

[102] Botta L, Didone F, Lopez-Cortes A, Nieto AC, Desandes E, Hjalgrim LL, Jakab Z, Stiller CA, Zeller B, Gatta G, Pritchard-Jones K, Group BPW. International benchmarking of stage at diagnosis for six childhood solid tumours (the BENCHISTA project): A population-based, retrospective cohort study. The Lancet Child & Adolescent Health. 2025;**9**(2):89–99. DOI: 10.1016/S2352-4642(24)00302-X

[103] Epperly R, Gottschalk S, DeRenzo C. CAR T cells redirected to B7-H3 for pediatric solid tumors: Current status and future perspectives. EJC Paediatric Oncology. 2024;**3**. DOI: 10.1016/j.ejcped.2024.100160

[104] Li T, Zhou J, Wu H, Gao X, Shen Q, Cheng R, Zhang M. Single-cell transcriptomes of kidneys in a 6-month-old boy with Denys-Drash syndrome reveal stromal cell heterogeneity in the tumor microenvironment. Clinical Kidney Journal. 2024;**17**(1):sfad277. DOI: 10.1093/ckj/sfad277

[105] Wens F, Zonca F, van Tinteren H, Timmermann B, Laprie A, Boterberg T, Gaze M, Lim P, Jazmati D, Dieckmann K, Vennarini S, Melchior P, Weber B, Albiac MR, Szulc A, Grigorenko V, Magelssen H, van Beek K, Graf N, Papadakis V. Late toxicity after upper abdominal radiotherapy in pediatric Wilms tumor and neuroblastoma survivors. A systematic review on behalf of SIOPEN and SIOP-RTSG. Radiotherapy and Oncology. 2025;**209**:110961. DOI: 10.1016/j.radonc.2025.110961

[106] Zhang R, Zhou X, Shen C. Inflammation-driven prognostic model and immune landscape profiling in osteosarcoma. Discover Oncology. 2025;**16**(1):2061. DOI: 10.1007/s12672-025-03691-w

[107] Bodea J, Caldwell KJ, Federico SM. Bevacizumab, with sorafenib and cyclophosphamide provides clinical benefit for recurrent or refractory osseous sarcomas in Children and Young Adults. Frontiers in Oncology. 2022;**12**:864790. DOI: 10.3389/fonc.2022.864790

[108] Davis JL, Cheesman E. Emerging round cell sarcomas in children. Virchows Archiv. 2025;**486**(1):117–126. DOI: 10.1007/s00428-024-03979-2

[109] Thway K, Fisher C. A practical approach to small round cell tumors involving the gastrointestinal tract and abdomen. Surgical Pathology Clinics. 2023;**16**(4):765–778. DOI: 10.1016/j.path.2023.05.012

[110] Underdown MJ, Kappa S, Metts J, Cash T. Ewing sarcoma, desmoplastic small round cell Tumor, and other round cell sarcomas. Hematology/Oncology Clinics of North America. 2025;**39**(4):709–726. DOI: 10.1016/j.hoc.2025.04.003

[111] Mitxelena-Iribarren O, Lizarbe-Sancha S, Campisi J, Arana S, Mujika M. Different microfluidic environments for in vitro testing of lipid nanoparticles against osteosarcoma. Bioengineering (Basel, Switzerland). 2021;**8**(6). DOI: 10.3390/bioengineering8060077

[112] Orel VE, Diedkov AG, Ostafiichuk VV, Lyalkin SA, Tkachenko IO, Kolesnyk DL, Orel VB, Dasyukevich OY, Rykhalskyi OY, Movchan OV, Galkin AY, Prosvietova AB. Combination treatment with free doxorubicin and inductive moderate hyperthermia for sarcoma saos-2 cells. Pharmaceuticals (Basel). 2025;**18**(6):852. DOI: 10.3390/ph18060852

[113] Taylor AM, Sheng J, Ng PKS, Harder JM, Kumar P, Ahn JY, Cao Y, Dzis AM, Jillette NL, Goodspeed A, Bodlak A, Wu Q, Isakoff MS, George J, Grassmann JDS, Luo D, Flynn WF, Courtois ET, Robson P, Lau CC. Immunosuppressive tumor microenvironment of osteosarcoma. Cancers (Basel). 2025;**17**(13). DOI: 10.3390/cancers17132117

[114] Trujillo-Paolillo A, Tesser-Gamba F, Seixas Alves MT, Filho RJG, Oliveira R, Petrilli AS, Toledo SRC. Pharmacogenetics of the primary and metastatic osteosarcoma: gene expression profile associated with outcome. International Journal of Molecular Sciences. 2023;**24**(6):5607. DOI: 10.3390/ijms24065607

[115] Cillo AR, Mukherjee E, Bailey NG, Onkar S, Daley J, Salgado C, Li X, Liu D, Ranganathan S, Burgess M, Sembrat J, Weiss K, Watters R, Bruno TC, Vignali DAA, Bailey KM. Ewing sarcoma and osteosarcoma have distinct immune signatures and intercellular communication networks. Clinical Cancer Research. 2022;**28**(22):4968–4982. DOI: 10.1158/1078-0432.CCR-22-1471

[116] Evdokimova V, Gassmann H, Radvanyi L, Burdach SEG.Current state of immunotherapy and mechanisms of immune evasion in ewing sarcoma and osteosarcoma. Cancers (Basel). 2022;**15**(1). DOI: 10.3390/cancers15010272

[117] Hussein MO, Abdulhameed AS. Design of bionanomaterial of chitosan carbohydrate polymer composited with broccoli extract and zinc oxide nanoparticles: Anticancer activity in human osteosarcoma. Applied Biochemistry and Biotechnology. 2025;**197**(2):1073–1089. DOI: 10.1007/s12010-024-05066-3

[118] van Ewijk R, Cleirec M, Herold N, le Deley M-C, van Eijkelenburg N, Boudou-Rouquette P, Risbourg S, Strauss SJ, Palmerini E, Boye K, Kager L, Hecker-Nolting S, Marchais A, Gaspar N. A systematic review of recent phase-II trials in refractory or recurrent osteosarcoma: Can we inform future trial design? Cancer Treatment Reviews. 2023;**120**:102625. DOI: 10.1016/j.ctrv.2023.102625

[119] Chen Y, Cheng X, Zhu C, Chen M, Wang Y, Liu C, Sun J, Shen H, Niu J,

Yang H, Liu X, Cui W, Shi Q. A microsphere-vesicle hybrid system for tumor treatment through enhancement of innate and adaptive immune responses. Biomaterials. 2026;**325**:123587. DOI: 10.1016/j.biomaterials.2025.123587

[120] Cui Y, Wu Y, Jiang D, Ding T. Single-cell and spatial transcriptomics reveal post-translational modifications in osteosarcoma progression and tumor microenvironment. PLoS One. 2025;**20**(10):e0333809. DOI: 10.1371/journal.pone.0333809

[121] Dong Y, Wang L, Zhang H, Li M, Luo Z, Hu Y, Cai C. Engineering Osteoimmune Responses with Functionalized Orthopedic Implants for Post-Operative Osteosarcoma Treatment. Advanced Science. 2025; e12363. DOI: 10.1002/advs.202512363

[122] Gu Z, Zhang S, Hu X, Xu N, Wang Y, Ruan J, Ma W, Chen H. Deciphering the Role of KIF18A in Osteosarcoma Progression: An Integrative Analysis and Experimental Validation. Frontiers in Bioscience-Landmark. 2025;**30**(10):44663. DOI: 10.31083/FBL44663

[123] Jiang G, Zhang F, Wu Z, Zhang X, Xu J, Peng Z, Li G, Zhu G, Wang X, Xie W. Targeting Mitochondrial Oxidative Stress by Calcium/Copper/Elesclomol Tri-Overloaded Nanocages for Osteosarcoma Immunotherapy via Immunogenic Cell Death. ACS Nano. 2025;**19**(43):37600–37616. DOI: 10.1021/acsnano.5c08243

[124] Lei P, Li L. Neurotrophic factors as double-edged swords in osteosarcoma: Drivers of tumour growth and immune remodelling. Frontiers in Immunology. 2025;**16**:1666343. DOI: 10.3389/fimmu.2025.1666343

[125] Li J, Chang C, Ma Y, Zhuang B, Ma Q, Wang Y, Ji Y. Identification and validation of stemness-related gene signatures to predict prognosis and immune infiltration in osteosarcoma reveals a critical role for S100A13. BMC Cancer. 2025;**25**(1):1734. DOI: 10.1186/s12885-025-14939-7

[126] Liu X, Xu J, Zhu J, Wang Z, Fang H, Guo W, Cao L, Cheng YY, Song K. Multimodal therapy process engineering mediated by 3D-printed scaffolds for enhanced postoperative osteosarcoma regeneration. Tissue and Cell. 2026;**98**:103212. DOI: 10.1016/j.tice.2025.103212

[127] Luker ME, York D, Al-Nadaf S, Johnson EG, Withers SS, Cruz SM, Lejeune A, Skorupski KA, Young J, Cohen-Davidyan T, Sparger EE, Culp WT, Murphy WJ, Kent MS, Canter RJ, Rebhun RB. Evaluating the impact of doxorubicin preconditioning on the efficacy of inhaled recombinant human IL-15 immunotherapy in dogs with pulmonary metastasis. Veterinary Oncology. 2025;**2**(1):23. DOI: 10.1186/s44356-025-00040-5

[128] Madsen PJ, Schlitter AM, Flemmig C, Dickson C, Harvey K, Wilson C, Beaubien E, Patterson L, Stern A, Griffin C, Joshi N, Hajeebu S, Martinez D, Storm PB, Resnick AC, Hillemanns P, Stanulla M, Faber J, Wingerter A, Gaida MM. Claudin 6 is a suitable target for CAR T-cell therapy in atypical teratoid/rhabdoid brain tumors and other pediatric solid tumors. Journal for ImmunoTherapy of Cancer. 2025;**13**(10):e011709. DOI: 10.1136/jitc-2025-011709

[129] Nirala BK, Yustein JT. The Role of MYC in Tumor Immune Microenvironment Regulation: Insights and Future Directions. Frontiers in Bioscience-Landmark. 2025;**30**(9):37304. DOI: 10.31083/FBL37304

[130] Schmidt AA, Prasad A, Huisman AR, Wakefield MR, Fang Y. Exploring the Tumor Microenvironment in Osteosarcoma: Driver of Resistance and Progression. Cancers (Basel). 2025;**17**(19). DOI: 10.3390/cancers17193106

[131] Su W, Li Y, Yang G, Zhao Y, Zhou X, Liu G, Huang X, Sohail MF, Hussain I, Liu Q, Chen F. Nanotechnology-Driven Strategies in Osteosarcoma Advances in Treatment: Immunotherapy and Drug Delivery. International Journal of Nanomedicine. 2025;**20**:12913–12937. DOI: 10.2147/IJN.S549587

[132] Yan S, Zhu X, Xiao Y. CD70-targeted CAR-T/NK therapy: Rationale, advances, and future directions. Translational Oncology. 2025;**62**:102555. DOI: 10.1016/j.tranon.2025.102555

[133] Che W, Luo X, Xu X, Qi J. A prognostic model of platinum resistance in osteosarcoma: Key roles of BNIP3, MYC, and ACTA2. Computers in Biology and Medicine. 2025;**197**(Pt A):111001. DOI: 10.1016/j.compbiomed.2025.111001

[134] Chen X, Li M, Hu Z, Sun D, Xu Y, Dong W, Zhu T, Zhang W, Liu S. Thiazolidinones as Potential PGK1 Inhibitors for Treatment of Osteosarcoma Growth and Metastasis. Journal of Medicinal Chemistry. 2025;**68**:22216–22245. DOI: 10.1021/acs.jmedchem.5c00738

[135] Deng Z, Zhang Q, Zhu J, Li J, Zhang M, Yuan J, Wu Z, Zhang Q, Liu R, Ma B. Novel cyclometalated iridium(III) complexes with a π-expansive benzothiophene ligand for enhanced photodynamic therapy against human osteosarcoma by disrupting Iron homeostasis. Bioorganic Chemistry. 2025;**166**:109121. DOI: 10.1016/j.bioorg.2025.109121

[136] Gyau BB, Wang J, Wu W, Scull B, Major AM, Jin W, Cates JMM, Hicks J, Man T-K.Multiplex Imaging Mass Cytometry Reveals Prognostic Immunosuppressive Subpopulations and Macrophage-Driven Metastasis in Osteosarcoma. Cancers (Basel). 2025;**17**(17). DOI: 10.3390/cancers17172780

[137] He X, Cao W, Wang J, and Zhong H. Emerging research themes in drug resistance in osteosarcoma: A 25-year bibliometric and visualized analysis. Naunyn-Schmiedeberg's Archives of Pharmacology. 2025:41055716. DOI: 10.1007/s00210-025-04683-x

[138] Liu G, Tang R, Wang C, Yu D, Wang Z, Yang H, Wei J, Zhu S, Gao F, Yuan F, Pan B. Bimetallic nanoconjugate hijack Fe-S clusters to drive a closed-loop cuproptosis-ferroptosis strategy for osteosarcoma inhibition. Journal of Colloid and Interface Science. 2026;**703**(Pt 1):139052. DOI: 10.1016/j.jcis.2025.139052

[139] Savadkouhi Ghoudjanaki M, Bahadorani F, Hosseini M, Panta R, Karimi B. Metal-Based Categorization of Recent Metal Organic Frameworks with Application in Bone Disease Treatment. ACS Biomaterials Science & Engineering. 2025;**11**:6895–6929. DOI: 10.1021/acsbiomaterials.5c00830

[140] Reimann E, Koks S, Ho XD, Maasalu K, Martson A. Whole exome sequencing of a single osteosarcoma case--integrative analysis with whole transcriptome RNA-seq data. . Human Genomics. 2014;**8**:20. DOI: 10.1186/s40 246-014-0020-0

[141] Ramesh S, Qin Q, Li Z, Cherief M, Zhong L, Archer M, Xing X, Thottappillil N, Balaji D, Bae S, Gomez-Salazar M, Xu M, Zhu M, Uniyal A, Chang L, Mazhar K, Mittal M, Birbrair A, McCarthy EF, Morris CD. Single-cell sequencing uncovers sensory neuron–mediated CGRP signaling as a driver of sarcoma progression. Proceedings of the National Academy of Sciences of the United States of America. 2025;**122**(43):e2500161122. DOI: 10.1073/pnas.2500161122

[142] Zhou L, Tang Y, Chen C, Jiang J. Paraptosis landscape reveals distinct prognoses and immune microenvironments in osteosarcoma: Experimental validation of key regulator TNK2. European Journal of Pharmacology. 2025;**1007**:178304. DOI: 10.1016/j.ejphar.2025.178304

[143] El Motassime A, Vitiello R, Comodo RM, Capece G, Bocchino G, Bocchi MB, Maccauro G, Meschini C. Osteosarcoma: A Comprehensive Morphological and Molecular Review with Prognostic Implications. Biology (Basel). 2025;**14**(10). DOI: 10.3390/biology14101407

[144] Reale ML, Chiari R, Tiseo M, Vitiello F, Barbieri F, Cortinovis D, Ceresoli GL, Finocchiaro G, Romano GD, Piovano PL, Del Conte A, Borra G, Verderame F, Scotti V, Nonnis D, Galetta D, Sergi C, Migliorino MR, Tonini G, Cecere F. Be-TeaM: An Italian real-world observational study on second-line therapy for EGFR-mutated NSCLC patients. Lung Cancer. 2020;**140**:71–79. DOI: 10.1016/j.lungcan.2019.12.006

[145] Shen F, Zailaie SA, Chiu B, Magliocco A, Sergi CM. Liquid biopsy – A narrative review with an update on current US governmental clinical trials targeting immunotherapy. Future Science OA. 2025;**11**(1):2527598. DOI: 10.1080/20565623.2025.2527598

[146] Clemente O, Ottaiano A, Di Lorenzo G, Bracigliano A, Lamia S, Cannella L, Pizzolorusso A, Di Marzo M, Santorsola M, De Chiara A, Fazioli F, Tafuto S. Is immunotherapy in the future of therapeutic management of sarcomas? Journal of Translational Medicine. 2021;**19**(1):173. DOI: 10.1186/s12967-021-02829-y

[147] Fu H, Wu Y, Chen J, Hu X, Wang X, Xu G. Exosomes and osteosarcoma drug resistance. Frontiers in Oncology. 2023;**13**:1133726. DOI: 10.3389/fonc.2023.1133726

[148] Rana V, Gupta D, Kaur G, Rana V. Primary primitive neuroectodermal tumor of kidney: A rare case report with diagnostic challenge. Indian Journal of Pathology and Microbiology. 2014;**57**(2):298–300. DOI: 10.4103/0377-4929.134723

[149] Zhang SD, He LJ, Chen L. [Interpretation of the soft tissue specific tumors in the 5th WHO classification of pediatric tumors]. Zhonghua Bing Li Xue Za Zhi = Chinese Journal of Pathology. 2025;**54**(6):568–574. DOI: 10.3760/cma.j.cn112151-20240930-00650

[150] Sergi C, Patry J, Kehar M. Collagenous gastritis, hyperplastic polyp, and intraepithelial duodenal lymphocytosis in a 15-year-old child: An

iconographic case report. Medicine (Baltimore). 2025;**104**(46):e45993. DOI: 10.1097/MD.0000000000045993

[151] Wu X, Deng W, Zhao Q, Xiong J. Single-cell analysis links DCUN1D5 to immune remodeling and cisplatin resistance in recurrent osteosarcoma. Communications Biology. 2025;**8** (1):1019. DOI: 10.1038/s42003-025-08 409-w

[152] Su Z, Fang X, Duan H. The paradoxical role of stem cells in osteosarcoma: From pathogenesis to therapeutic breakthroughs. Frontiers in Oncology. 2025;**15**:1643491. DOI: 10.33 89/fonc.2025.1643491

Section 2

Bone Tumors: Management

Chapter 6

Decoding Bone Cancer Pain: Pathological Mechanisms and Targeted Interventions

Mingzhu Zhai, Yanni Luo and Wuping Sun

Abstract

Bone cancer pain (BCP) is one of the most prominent and disabling symptoms in patients with primary bone malignancies (e.g. osteosarcoma, Ewing's sarcoma) and metastatic bone tumors (e.g. multiple myeloma), severely impacting quality of life and treatment efficacy. Conventional analgesic approaches are often limited in effectiveness or associated with significant side effects. This chapter will delve into the complex pathological mechanisms underlying the development and persistence of BCP. It will focus on elucidating the intricate interactions within the tumor micro-environment involving cancer cells, immune cells (e.g. macrophages, T cells), osteoclasts, osteoblasts, and sensory neurons. Key mechanisms include sensitization of nociceptors by allogeneic mediators (protons, nerve growth factor, cytokines, chemokines) released from tumor and stromal cells; activation of nerve terminals by factors (e.g. ATP, acid) released during bone matrix destruction; tumor and immune cell infiltration of nerves; and peripheral and central nervous system sensitization and remodeling. Building upon this mechanistic understanding, the chapter will systematically review current and emerging targeted therapeutic strategies. These include monoclonal antibodies, small molecule inhibitors, gene therapies, and neuromodulation techniques targeting key pain-signaling pathways (e.g. NGF/TrkA, GDNF, CXCL12/CXCR4, RANK/RANKL). The aim is to provide the theoretical foundation and translational insights necessary for developing more effective and better-tolerated precision treatments for BCP.

Keywords: bone cancer pain, pathological mechanisms, tumor-neural crosstalk, tumor microenvironment, targeted therapy

1. Introduction

Cancer pain is a type of refractory chronic pain, characterized by severe symptoms that persist throughout the lifetime of cancer patients, and has long been one of the serious disorders endangering human health. Among the various types of cancer pain, bone cancer pain (BCP) is the most common and presents the most severe pain symptoms after onset [1]. BCP is a chronic condition caused by bone metastasis in common cancers such as lung and breast cancer. Its pathogenesis is highly complex and variable, evolving with disease progression [2]. Statistics show that 75.7% of cancer patients experience bone metastasis-related pain, with approximately 40% of early-to-mid-stage cases and 90% of advanced-stage patients suffering moderate to severe pain, significantly impacting their quality of life [3, 4]. Characterized by persistent, sudden-onset spontaneous pain accompanied by hyperalgesia, this complex condition typically results from bone metastases or primary bone tumors. It causes severe discomfort, substantially reduces patients' quality of life, and diminishes confidence in overcoming the disease [5, 6].

The pathogenesis of bone metastasis-induced pain is complex, involving intricate interactions between tumor cells, osteoblasts, osteoclasts, immune cells, and sensory neurons [7]. BCP, caused by primary bone tumors or secondary bone metastases from other tumors, is the most common type of cancer pain in clinical practice. Among affected patients, those with primary bone tumors and approximately one-third of those with bone metastases experience bone pain of varying degrees, and this pain – along with associated conditions such as hypercalcemia, pathological fractures, and increased susceptibility to infections – severely impairs patients' quality of life. This chapter will explore the multifaceted pathological mechanisms underlying BCP development, with particular focus on the dynamic interplay among tumor microenvironment components: sensitization of nociceptors by tumor and stromal-derived mediators (protons, nerve growth factors (NGFs), cytokines, chemokines); activation of nerve endings through bone matrix degradation products (e.g. ATP, acidic substances); neural infiltration by tumor and immune cells; and peripheral/central nervous system sensitization and remodeling. Building on these mechanisms, this chapter systematically reviews current and emerging targeted therapies, including monoclonal antibodies, small molecule inhibitors, gene therapies, and neuromodulatory techniques targeting critical pain pathways (e.g. NGF/TrkA, GDNF, CXCL12/CXCR4, RANK/RANKL). These insights aim to establish theoretical foundations and translational strategies for developing more effective, less-irritating precision treatment regimens for BCP.

2. Clinical features

The clinical manifestations of BCP are relatively complex, including two forms: persistent mild-to-severe pain (also referred to as background pain) and intermittent moderate-to-severe spontaneous pain or movement-induced pain (also known as breakthrough pain). In the early stage of cancer pain, it mainly presents as background pain, characterized by persistent dull pain. As the disease progresses, transient yet intense breakthrough pain emerges on the basis of stable background pain. Breakthrough pain is often characterized by acute onset, severe intensity, and unpredictability; it can occur spontaneously or be induced by mechanical stimuli such as movement or bone weight-bearing. Approximately 75% of BCP patients experience breakthrough pain, which significantly impacts their quality of life: it severely disrupts normal sleep, restricts physical activity, reduces mobility and work capacity, and exacerbates emotional distress, making it the most challenging issue in the management of cancer pain.

3. Pathogenesis of BCP

Osteolysis caused by tumor invasion and stimulation of nociceptors at nerve endings by various cellular factors leads to peripheral nerve sensitization (see **Figure 1**). Peripheral injury signals via the dorsal root ganglion (DRG) are transmitted to the dorsal horn of the spinal cord, where primary processing and integration of information activate relevant brain regions, leading to the development of BCP.

3.1 Sensitization of nociceptors by tumor and stromal cells releasing pain mediators

Neurotrophic factors are a group of molecules, including NGF, brain-derived neurotrophic factor (BDNF), and neurotrophin-3 (NT-3) [8]. Tumor-associated stroma, inflammation, and tumor cells release NGF. NGF binds to TrkA on

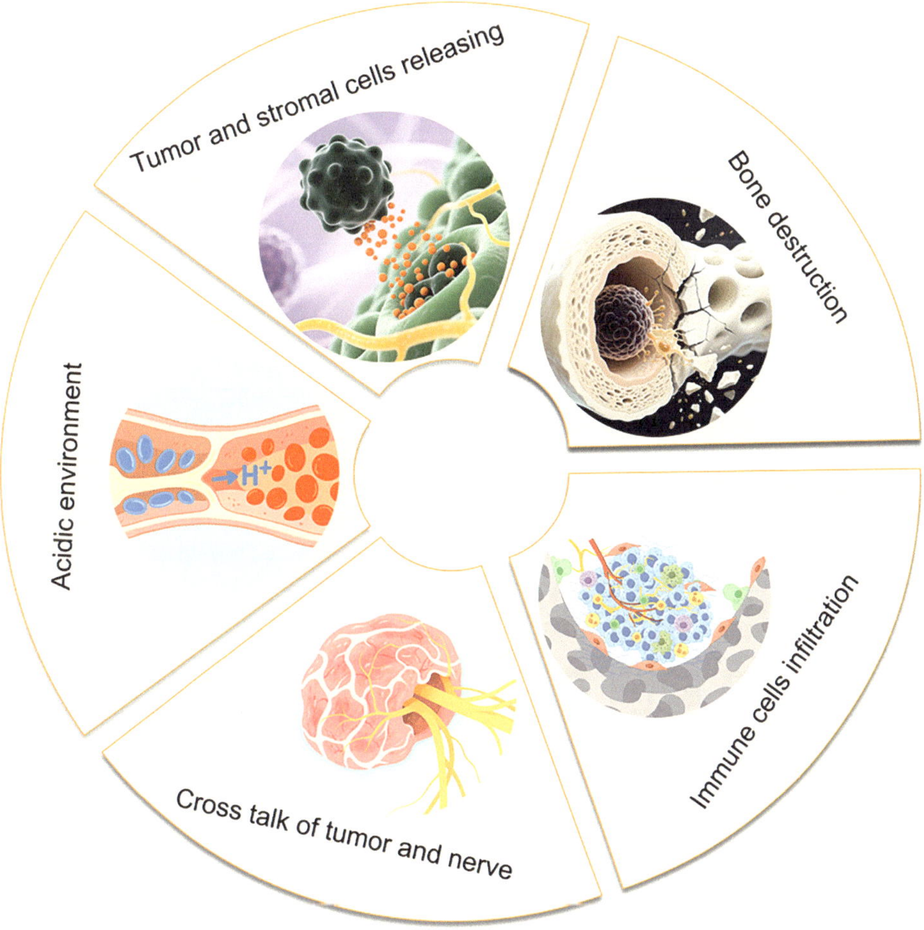

Figure 1.
The pathological mechanism of the generation and development of bone cancer pain.

nociceptors, activating the NGF/TrkA signaling pathway in peripheral nociceptor terminals and dorsal root ganglia (DRGs). This enhances the activity of nociceptive channels, receptors, and peptide-like substances, leading to peripheral sensitization of primary nociceptors and central sensitization of dorsal horn neurons in the spinal cord. Concurrently, NGF may increase the local density of nociceptors at bone metastases through TrkA-mediated neuroblasting, ultimately strengthening pain signal transmission from the dorsal horn to higher brain structures [9]. A novel immunoreactive prostate cancer bone metastasis model was established, revealing reduced mechanical claw withdrawal thresholds, abnormal motor-related emotional responses, and osteolytic and osteoblastic changes. The study further confirmed that NGF and p75 neurotrophic factor receptor (p75NTR) play roles in chronic pain following bone metastasis [10].

BDNF, a member of the neurotrophic family, is a key molecule in pathological pain states observed in various pain models [11]. It also plays a crucial role in pain regulation. When MRMT-1 breast cancer cells were implanted into rat tibias, BDNF expression was significantly upregulated in DRG neurons, particularly in smaller neurons. Notably, NGF-TrkA signaling may contribute to the elevated BDNF levels observed in chronic inflammatory pain syndrome [12].

Previous studies have demonstrated that the chemokine CXCL12 and its receptor CXCR4 are crucial for pain sensitization. The CXCL12/CXCR4 signaling pathway promotes BCP by sensitizing neurons and activating astrocytes and microglia [13]. Research indicates that the spinal RhoA/ROCK2 pathway may serve as a key downstream target in CXCR4-mediated BCP, particularly in neuronal sensitization and hyperalgesia, potentially representing a promising therapeutic target for pain management [14].

3.2 Factors released by bone destruction activate nerve endings

Bone undergoes continuous reorganization and remodeling through the coordinated action of osteoclasts (bone-absorbing cells) and osteoblasts (bone-forming cells). Under normal conditions, these two cell types maintain a balanced interaction to preserve stable bone density [15]. However, tumor invasion or bone metastasis disrupts the bone metabolic balance, accelerating bone resorption and acidification of the bone marrow cavity microenvironment, which is one of the important causes of BCP (see **Figure 2**).

3.2.1 Osteoclasts

Bone marrow-derived cancer cells (e.g. breast cancer) migrate to the bone marrow and begin secreting factors that promote osteoclast formation, including epidermal growth factor (EGF), osteoclast-stimulating factor (OSF), tumor necrosis factors (TNFs), and activated insulin A. Simultaneously, these cancer cells secrete factors that promote osteoclast differentiation, such as nuclear factor κB receptor ligand (RANKL), macrophage colony-stimulating factor (M-CSF), and interleukins 1, 6, and 11. These factors facilitate the differentiation of pre-osteoclasts into osteoclasts [8]. Osteoclasts exhibit significant variability, originate from the monocyte lineage, and can regulate T-cell activation like other monocyte-lineage-derived immune cells such as monocytes, macrophages, and dendritic cells [16]. Studies have found that osteoclasts activate acid-sensitive receptors, including

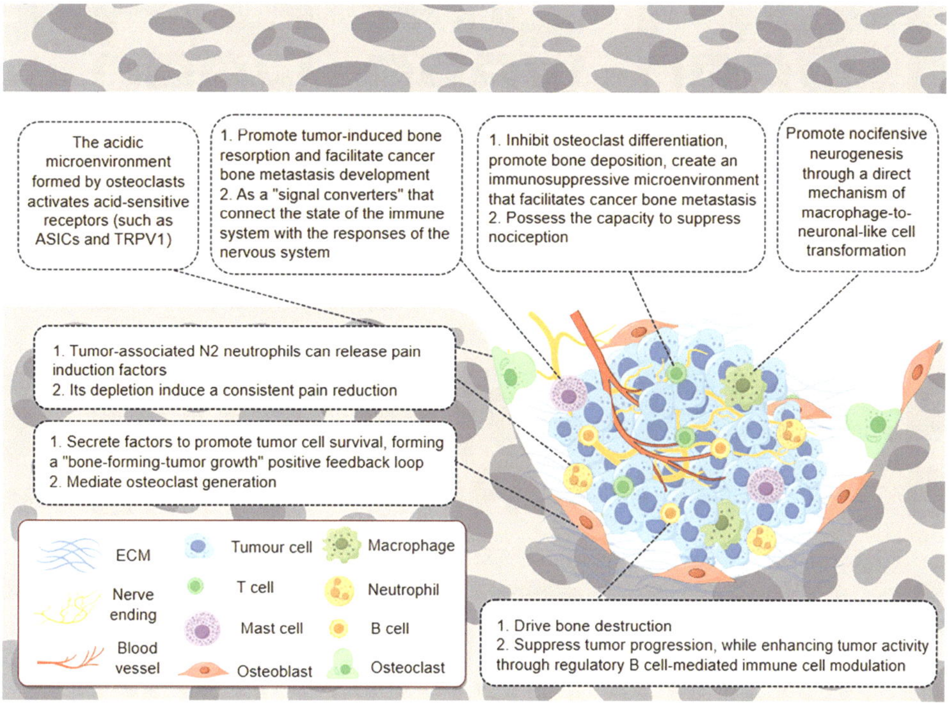

Figure 2.
The schematic diagram illustrating the roles of osteocytes and immune cells in the tumor microenvironment for the development of bone cancer pain.

acid-sensing intracellular receptors (ASICs) and transient receptor vanilloid 1 (TRPV1) [17]. In addition, rat model studies revealed that the acidic microenvironment generated by osteoclasts partially induces hyperalgesia through upregulation of acid-sensitive ion channels (ASIC1a and ASIC1b) in DRGs, suggesting that the acidic microenvironment formed by osteoclasts is associated with tumor implantation-related bone pain [18]. Osteoclasts and tumor cells generate acidic environments (H^+) and release ATP through mechanisms like the Warburg effect. Simultaneously, processes such as bone formation, bone resorption, and fractures activate nociceptive receptors within bones (e.g. primary afferent neurons expressing Trk receptors and prostaglandin receptors). These nociceptive signals are transmitted from the DRGs to the spinal cord, ultimately reaching the brain to produce pain sensations.

3.2.2 Osteoblasts

Osteoblasts, the key functional cells in bone formation, primarily differentiate from mesenchymal stem cells and are present in regions such as the periosteum and bone marrow [19]. Tumor cells secrete factors like BMP and WNT to directly activate osteoblasts, leading to abnormal bone formation. Conversely, factors secreted by osteoblasts, such as IGF-1 and ET-1, promote tumor cell survival, forming a “bone-forming-tumor growth” positive feedback loop [20]. RANKL, secreted by osteoblasts, is a critical factor in osteoclast differentiation, while OPG acts as a decoy receptor to inhibit RANKL activity. Studies have shown that RANKL also activates TNF receptor-related factor (TRAF)-6, which involves c-Src and subsequently mediates osteoclast generation through the phosphoinositide 3-kinase (PI3K)/Akt signaling pathway [21]. By upregulating RANKL in osteoblasts or modulating osteoprotegerin secretion, tumor cells promote excessive activation of osteoclasts, exacerbating bone destruction and pain [22].

3.3 Tumor-associated immune cell infiltration

As a vital central immune organ, BCP development is significantly influenced by immune cells and cytokines. Key players include macrophages, neutrophils, and T lymphocytes within tumor stromal cells, which secrete various cytokines such as prostaglandins, endothelin, interleukin-1 (IL-1), interleukin-6 (IL-6), EGF, and transforming growth factor.

3.3.1 Tumor-associated macrophages

Tumor-associated macrophages (TAMs) in the tumor microenvironment can promote nocifensive neurogenesis through a direct mechanism of macrophage-to-neuronal-like cell transformation (MNT) [23]. It has been reported that macrophage-specific Smad3 acts as a pivotal genomic regulator to promote macrophage-neuron crosstalk. Disrupting macrophage-specific Smad3 effectively blocked tumor innervation and cancer-induced nocifensive behaviors *in vivo* [23]. Macrophages within ganglia play a variety of roles in chronic pain. Ganglia-associated macrophages fall into two primary categories: infiltrated macrophages and tissue-resident macrophages. Resident ganglionic macrophages reside in peripheral ganglia rather than the central nervous system (CNS). After nerve injury, infiltrated macrophages migrate to damaged nerves and accumulate in the DRG to initiate and maintain neuropathic pain [24]. Sciatic nerve injury leads to an increase in resident CX3CR1+ macrophages in sensory ganglia, which are involved in the development of neuropathic pain [25]. Conversely, depleting infiltrated macrophages reduces the development of mechanical and thermal hypersensitivity caused by injury in mice and pain induced by knee osteoarthritis in rats [26]. As the predominant infiltrating immune cell type in tumors, TAMs are typically classified into two functionally contrasting subtypes: classically activated M1 macrophages and alternatively activated M2 macrophages [27]. M1 macrophages play a crucial role in tumor suppression by activating the immune system to produce a large number of pro-inflammatory cytokines (such as IL-1, IL-6, and IL-12), assisting in the maturation of T helper 1 (Th1) cells, and inducing the production of inducible nitric oxide synthase (iNOS) [28, 29]. Numerous studies have shown that in most solid malignant tumors, the significant infiltration of M2 macrophages, which are associated with immunosuppression, matrix degradation, and tumor angiogenesis and promote tumor growth and metastasis, is strongly correlated with poor prognosis [16]. DRG neurons recruit M2 macrophages and translocate mitochondria to neurons to alleviate chronic inflammatory pain [30]. However, M1 macrophages expressing Cx3cr1 can infiltrate the DRG and promote nociceptive neuron activation, resulting in rheumatoid arthritis-associated pain [31]. Microglia, a subset of macrophages, serve as primary immune effector cells in the CNS, exhibiting characteristic phagocytic functions and immunomodulatory roles. During BCP development, spinal microglia undergo enhanced M1 polarization and reduced M2 polarization, with concurrent detection of IL-1β suppression and upregulated IL-10 expression [32]. Neuronal complement mediates microglia activation via complement 3 receptor (C3R), thereby enhancing BCP [33]. The P2Y12R receptor in spinal microglia may activate both microglia and p38MAPK pathways to promote cancer-induced bone pain [34]. Studies reveal that in mouse models of malignant bone pain, microglia downregulate the CD47-SIRP-α signaling axis to regulate phagocytosis at dorsal horn inhibitory synapses, thereby modulating nociceptive behavior [35]. Research indicates that sustained activation of spinal astrocytes and their secreted interleukin-17A (IL-17A) promotes BCP progression in mice without gender bias [36]. Studies have shown that NFAT1-p38 signaling in microglia leads to BCP through IL-18-mediated central sensitization of spinal microglia [32].

3.3.2 T cells

Bone marrow, rich in blood vessels, serves as the primary component of the lymphocyte recirculation network, with billions of lymphocytes passing through it daily [37]. In CD4+ T cells, regulatory T cells (Tregs) are recognized as potent immune suppressors playing crucial roles in maintaining immune system homeostasis. Tregs promote tumor cell metastasis to bone via the CXCR4/CXCL12 signaling pathway or the RANK/RANKL axis [37]. Simultaneously, Tregs inhibit osteoclast differentiation and promote bone deposition, thereby creating an immunosuppressive microenvironment that facilitates cancer bone metastasis [38]. T cells have recently been recognized as key regulators in pain amplification processes [39]. Adoptive transfer of CD8+ T cells caused robust allodynia in females [40]. However, Treg cell ablation can trigger experimental autoimmune encephalomyelitis (EAE) and facial allodynia in immunized mice [41]. Treg cells suppress the development of neuropathic pain through the inhibition of the CD4 Th1 response and indirectly reduce neuronal damage and neuroinflammation in sensory ganglia [42]. Treg cells, in particular, possess the capacity to suppress nociception – and this inhibitory effect does not rely on their well-known functions in regulating immune activation or facilitating tissue repair. They inhibited nociception via producing the endogenous opioid enkephalin that acted on the delta opioid receptor expressed by MrgprD+ sensory neurons [43].

3.3.3 Neutrophils

Neutrophils are short-lived white blood cells containing neutrophilic granules in their cytoplasm, which are the first circulating inflammatory cells recruited to sites of injury. They originate from hematopoietic stem cells in the bone marrow, differentiate into neutrophil precursors through myeloid progenitor cells, and mature before entering the bloodstream. The CXCR4/SDF-1 axis regulates both the release of neutrophils from the bone marrow and their post-circulation chemotactic navigation [44]. Transforming growth factor β (TGFβ) plays a crucial role in determining neutrophil phenotypes, enabling the transition from tumor-suppressing (N1) to more tumor-promoting (N2) states [45]. Tumor-associated N2 neutrophils can release CXCR4, VEGF, and MMP9, thereby facilitating bone metastasis in tumors [37, 46]. Although these cytokines have been reported to play an important role in pain induction [47–49], the pooled meta-analysis of animal studies showed that neutrophil depletion induced a consistent pain reduction. Inflammatory, neuropathic, and visceral pain showed significant pain alleviation by neutrophil depletion. In addition, neutrophils had a larger impact on mechanical allodynia, followed by nociceptive behaviors and mechanical allodynia, with a smaller effect on thermal hyperalgesia [50].

3.3.4 Mast cells

Mast cells, a unique granular white blood cell in the immune system, play crucial roles in allergic reactions, inflammatory regulation, and tissue repair. Mast cells express Fcε RI and Fcγ R and sense a broad diversity of antigens through IgG and IgE, representing current immunity and memory of past B cell immune responses. They regulate various tumor biology events such as cell proliferation, survival, angiogenesis, invasiveness, and metastasis within the tumor microenvironment [51]. These highly adaptable cells coordinate inflammatory responses, induce ectodermal program expression, and reconstruct microenvironments resembling embryonic structures to promote cancer stem cell proliferation and invasion [52]. The tumor-induced growth factor β (Tyr-β) released by mast cells stimulates osteoclast activation through the RANKL pathway or directly induces osteoclast formation when M-CSF is present, thereby promoting tumor-induced bone resorption. This creates a "tumor growth–bone destruction" vicious cycle that ultimately facilitates gastric cancer bone metastasis development [53]. Recent studies have shown that mast cells are "signal converters" that connect the state of the immune system with the responses of the nervous system [54]. Mast cells express receptors to detect signals released during tissue insult or stress – such as infection, inflammation, or injury – including neuropeptides, peptide toxins, defensins, ATP, IL-33, and endothelin-1. They can convert these inputs into neurotransmitter-like output signals, which are easily sensed by sensory neurons. Key mediators derived from mast cells, including serotonin, histamine, cytokines, leukotrienes, and proteases, further induce action potentials in sensory neurons and reduce their activation threshold [54].

3.3.5 B cells

B cells exhibit dual roles in immune responses: they suppress tumor progression by secreting immunoglobulins, stimulating T-cell activation, and directly killing cancer cells, while enhancing tumor activity through regulatory B cell-mediated immune cell modulation [55]. Their development depends on the production and regulation of factors such as RANKL, osteoprotegerin (OPG), interleukin-7 (IL-7), and CXCL12, which are generated by bone marrow stromal cells and osteoblasts [56]. Studies using mouse models and patient-derived xenograft experiments have demonstrated that B-cell acute lymphoblastic leukemia (B-ALL) cells overexpress RANKL, driving bone destruction via the RANK-RANKL axis [57].

3.4 Crosstalk between tumor and nerve

Pathological fractures and peripheral injury signals generated by cell factors stimulating nerve fibers in the tumor microenvironment are transmitted to the spinal cord via the DRG. DRG neurons are the main entities responsible for the primary conduction of pain signals. DRG neurons are pseudounipolar neurons, whose peripheral axon terminals are distributed in different peripheral tissues innervated by them, and various ion channels and receptors are present on the nerve endings of their peripheral segments. The central axon terminals of DRG neurons form synapses with the dendritic terminals of spinal dorsal horn (SDH) neurons, thereby transmitting pain signals to the spinal cord center. After primary processing and integration, these signals activate relevant brain regions, thereby contributing to the development of BCP [58]. Under the influence of tumor cells, factors such as NGF, an "acidic environment", and "inflammatory mediators" trigger "nerve sprouting", leading to sensitization of peripheral nociceptive pathways [55]. Research has revealed that the core mechanism of BCP-induced peripheral sensitization involves Wnt5a/Ryk signaling mediated through the TRPV1 pathway via JNK, which sensitizes peripheral nociceptors [59]. Tumor-associated stromal cells release factors that sensitize and activate bone nociceptors, damage sensory nerve fibers, and release growth factors that promote ectopic nerve sprouting and neurofibroma formation – all contributing to both peripheral and central sensitization [60]. Abnormal signals generated by peripheral sensitization are transmitted through the DRG to the spinal cord, then further relayed to the brain, triggering central sensitization within the spinal cord and brain. This amplifies pain perception, collectively forming the pathophysiological basis of BCP [20].

The impact of denervation is known to reduce cancer growth. Recently, the investigation of nerve-cancer crosstalk has greatly advanced due to a few landmark discoveries. Particularly, exosome-induced neural reprogramming by tumors has shown that cancer-derived extracellular vesicles (EVs) play a role in cancer-related axonogenesis, which solidified the effect of reciprocal neural crosstalk [61]. In addition, cancer cells can induce increased nerve density and initiate adrenergic neurogenesis [59]. In bone cancer microenvironments, Netrin-1 can promote axonal growth of nociceptive neurons by activating deleted in colorectal cancer (DCC) signaling, thereby participating in the onset and progression of BCP [62]. During interactions between tumor cells (e.g. fibrosarcoma cells) and nociceptive neurons, fibrosarcoma cells exhibit high expression of autotaxin (ATX), which catalyzes the synthesis of lysophosphatidic acid (LPA). LPA not only promotes tumor proliferation but also activates LPA receptors (LPAR) on DRG nociceptive neurons and satellite cells, transforming them into pain signal molecules [63]. Recent research has demonstrated that neural transfer of mitochondria enhances cancer cell metabolic plasticity, stem cell characteristics, and resistance to metastatic stress, ultimately facilitating cancer metastasis[64]. BCP leads to mitochondrial ultrastructural damage, decreased ATP levels, and reduced mitochondrial membrane potential (MMP) in the spinal cord [65]. In addition, the interaction between melanoma cells and nociceptor neurons can drive enhanced neurite growth, which in turn increases the response to harmful ligands and the release of neuropeptides in neurons. It is worth noting that reducing the release of CGRP from tumor-innervating nociceptors could be a strategy to improve anti-tumor immunity – this is achieved by eliminating the immunomodulatory effect of CGRP on cytotoxic CD8+ T cells [66].

3.5 Acidic environment

The acidification of the tumor microenvironment in the bone marrow cavity is an important feature of cancerous lesions in bones. Under physiological conditions, osteoclasts release calcium ions and phosphate into the blood through bone resorption, a process that dissolves the mineralized portion of the bone matrix and increases the acidity within the bone marrow cavity [67]. Under normal physiological conditions of bone resorption, the pH value in the bone marrow remains stable due to the relatively small number of osteoclasts involved in bone remodeling; however, in cases of cancer invasion, cancer stimulates the proliferation of osteoclasts, and the acidity in the bone marrow cavity increases with the rise in the absolute number of osteoclasts. On the contrary, the bone marrow is also in a hypoxic environment (5% pO_2). Tumor cells promote the acidification of the microenvironment through the Warburg effect, stimulating cancer cells to shift toward glycolytic metabolism, thereby generating lactic acid and protons. Therefore, both osteoclast proliferation and glycolysis induced by cancer cells contribute to the acidity of the bone marrow [59]. Acid-sensing ion channel 3 (ASIC3) and TRPV1 are the main participants in acid-sensing within the bone marrow cavity during the occurrence and development of BCP [68]. ASIC3 is typically activated by a weakly acidic environment with a pH range of 6.7–7.3, indicating mild extracellular acidification in the bone marrow cavity. Experimental models of BCP revealed significantly upregulated mRNA and protein expression of acid-sensing ion channel 3 (ASIC3) on the ipsilateral DRGs, which correlates positively with pain-sensitizing behavior. ASIC3 may contribute to the occurrence and maintenance of cancer-related bone pain through increased expression in both small-diameter and large-diameter neurons [68]. Studies have demonstrated that the activation of ASIC3 is sufficient to induce nociceptive behaviors in various pain models [69]. Inhibiting ASIC3 can alleviate BCP caused by multiple myeloma [70, 71]. When the pH value is less than 6, indicating severe extracellular acidification of bone marrow cells, TRPV1 is activated and becomes sensitive to other irritants (such as capsaicin, heat, and some inflammatory mediators) [59]. Blocking TRPV1 with its antagonists can effectively alleviate BCP [72]. In addition, extracellular acidification caused by osteoclasts is another driving force of BCP. In particular, inhibiting vacuolar proton pumps (V-ATPase) through proton pump inhibitors (PPIs) can significantly reduce BCP in breast cancer and multiple myeloma [73]. Therefore, molecules with bone-protective effects can inhibit BCP by blocking the activation and proliferation of osteoclasts or promoting the apoptosis of osteoclasts.

4. Targeted therapy and strategy

Based on the peripheral mechanisms underlying BCP, drugs targeting specific receptors have demonstrated effective analgesic effects (see **Table 1**) [74]. Current treatment options for BCP include external beam radiation therapy, opioid analgesics (such as sufentanil citrate), nonsteroidal anti-inflammatory drugs (NSAIDs, including diclofenac diethylamine emulgel, ibuprofen, and parecoxib sodium), and bisphosphonates, such as alendronate sodium, zoledronic acid, and ibandronate sodium. However, opioid use carries multiple potential side effects. Recent studies indicate that transient receptor potential (TRP) channels may play a regulatory role in bone remodeling and participate in preclinical models of BCP, offering innovative analgesic strategies to overcome opioids' long-term adverse effects [75]. Bisphosphonates and denosumab, potent anti-bone-resorption agents, significantly reduce the risks of bone-related events associated with poor quality of life, bone pain, functional impairment, and decreased survival rates. While

Class	Target	Mechanism	Drug	Indications	Reference
Monoclonal antibodies	NGF/TrkA	Nerve growth factor (NGF) binds to TrkA on nociceptors, activating the NGF/TrkA signaling pathway. This enhances the activity of nociceptive channels, receptors, and peptide-like substances, leading to peripheral and central sensitization. The drug blocks the binding of NGF to TrkA, thereby inhibiting pain signal transmission.	Tanezumab	Bone metastasis-related cancer pain, osteoarthritis pain, and chronic low back pain.	[9, 77]
	GDNF	Inflammatory factors released by tumor and immune cells induce the expression of glial cell-derived neurotrophic factor (GDNF). GDNF activates non-peptidergic neurons, enhancing their sensitivity to mechanical stimuli. It also activates the ERK-Runx1 signaling cascade in dorsal root ganglion (DRG) neurons, increasing P2X3R gene transcription and neuronal excitability.	No specific marketed drug (under research).	Bone cancer pain	[78, 79]
	CXCL12/ CXCR4	The CXCL12/CXCR4 signaling pathway mediates neuronal sensitization and glial activation, regulates the spinal JNK-c-Jun pathway and the ALK5/Smad3 signaling pathway, and participates in central sensitization and cancer pain hypersensitivity.	mAb15G5	Metastatic osteosarcoma inhibits tumor cell chemotaxis and reduces bone resorption.	[80, 81]
	RANK/ RANKL	Receptor activator of nuclear factor-κB Ligand (RANKL) binds to RANK to promote osteoclast differentiation and activation, exacerbating bone destruction and pain. The drug specifically binds to RANKL, inhibiting osteoclast activation and reducing bone resorption.	Denosumab	Osteolytic bone metastases, chronic inflammatory bone diseases, and bone cancer pain.	[82, 83]
	MrgC	BAM8-22 activates spinal MrgC receptors, modulates mitochondrial unfolded protein response (UPRmt) activity, improves mitochondrial function, and alleviates bone cancer pain.	No specific marketed drug (under research).	Bone cancer pain	[84]
	DYRK1A	Haemine can inhibit the expression of Dual-Specificity Tyrosine Phosphorylation-Regulated Kinase 1A (DYRK1A) in the dorsal horn of the spinal cord, regulate the NF-κB pathway, and reduce bone cancer pain in a dose-dependent manner.	No specific marketed drug is currently under research.	Bone cancer pain	[85]

Class	Target	Mechanism	Drug	Indications	Reference
Small molecule inhibitors	PPARα/ CXCR2	Anwulignan exerts anti-tumor and analgesic effects by upregulating the expression of Peroxisome Proliferator-Activated Receptor α (PPARα) and inhibiting the activation of C–X–C chemokine receptor 2 (CXCR2).	Anwulignan	Bone cancer pain	[68, 86]
	RANKL/ RANK/OPG, PAR2/TRPV1	Quercetin regulates the RANKL/RANK/OPG signaling pathway to inhibit osteoclast activation and modulates the protease-activated receptor 2 (PAR2)/Transient Receptor Potential Vanilloid 1 (TRPV1) signaling pathway to suppress peripheral and central sensitization, thereby reducing bone destruction.	Quercetin	Bone cancer pain	[83, 87]
	Akt	GSK690693 inhibits Akt protein phosphorylation, reduces the expression of with-no-lysine kinase 1 (WNK1) in spinal cord tissues, blocks pain signal transmission, and improves pain threshold.	GSK690693	Bone cancer pain	[87]
	TNF-α/NF-κB/uPA/ PAR2	Pomelo extract (containing naringenin) inhibits the tumor necrosis factor-α (TNF-α)-mediated NF-κB/urokinase plasminogen activator (uPA)/PAR2 pathway, alleviating pain sensitization and bone damage.	Pomelo extract (Naringenin)	Bone cancer pain	[88]
	PI3K/Akt	LY294002 selectively inhibits the phosphoinositide 3-kinase (PI3K)/ Akt signaling pathway, restores mitochondrial function, inhibits spinal inflammation, and relieves bone cancer pain.	LY294002	Bone cancer pain	[89]

Class	Target	Mechanism	Drug	Indications	Reference
Gene therapy	PDGF	A herpes simplex virus vector carrying platelet-derived growth factor (PDGF) siRNA is used to reduce the levels of phosphorylated PDGFR α/β (pPDGFRα/β) in the dorsal horn of the spinal cord, inhibit the AKT-ERK signaling pathway, alleviate astrocyte hypertrophy, and decrease the expression of Substance P (SP) and calcitonin gene-related peptide (CGRP).	PDGF siRNA (viral vector-mediated)	Bone cancer pain	[90]
	STING	Stimulator of interferon genes (STING) agonists induce the production of type I interferon, which directly suppresses nociceptor excitability and osteoclast formation, enhances T-cell-mediated anti-tumor immunity, inhibits cancer pain in the short term, and reduces bone destruction and tumor burden in the long term.	STING agonists (under research)	Bone cancer pain	[91]
	GPR37	Activation of G protein-coupled receptor 37 (GPR37) promotes macrophages to release Interleukin-10 (IL-10) through NPD1 or ARU targeting, inhibits osteoclast formation, reduces the action potential frequency and spontaneous excitatory postsynaptic currents (sEPSCs) in DRGs and the spinal dorsal horn (SDH), and suppresses neuronal hyperexcitability.	No specific gene-drug (under research).	Bone cancer pain	[91]
Neuroregulation technology	TRP channels	Transient receptor potential (TRP) channels are involved in bone remodeling and BCP regulation; their inhibitors can modulate channel activity, relieve pain, and mitigate the long-term side effects of opioids.	N.A.	Bone cancer pain	[75]
	Ferroptosis-related pathways	Inhibiting ferroptosis-like cell death in spinal interneurons alleviates hyperalgesia and spontaneous pain associated with bone cancer.	N.A.	Bone cancer pain	[92]

Table 1.
Potential drug targets and mechanisms for the treatment of bone cancer pain.

long-term use in advanced malignancies generally demonstrates good tolerability, some severe side effects require regular monitoring and are partially preventable [76].

4.1 Monoclonal antibodies targeting key pain pathways

4.1.1 NGF/TrkA

NGF primarily originates from cancerous tissues, tumor cells, and related inflammatory (immune) cells, including macrophages, T lymphocytes, mast cells, and endothelial cells. It exhibits high affinity for its primary molecular target, TrkA, which is highly expressed in the nerve fibers of bones [19]. Studies have shown that elevated NGF levels correlate with enhanced mDOR expression through TrkA signaling. The activation of mDOR produces analgesic effects, which depend on upregulating the NGF/TrkA pathway by increasing mDOR levels under BCP conditions in mice [77]. Tanezumab, a monoclonal antibody against NGF, improves pain and function in chronic pain conditions such as osteoarthritis and chronic low back pain. Tanezumab 20 mg demonstrated short-term analgesic efficacy in patients with bone metastasis-related cancer pain [9].

4.1.2 GDNF

Studies using male Sprague-Dawley rats have demonstrated that tumor cells and immune cells in cancer microenvironments release inflammatory factors such as IL-1 and TNF-α, which induce increased expression of glial cell-derived neurotrophic factor (GDNF) family ligands (GFLs), including GDNF. This activates non-peptidergic neurons. Notably, GDNF enhances sensitivity to mechanical stimuli, such as tumor-induced bone compression, through sensitized non-peptidergic neurons expressing TRPV1 (a type of mechanoreceptor), ultimately leading to persistent bone pain. These findings suggest that GDNF may serve as a therapeutic target for BCP management [78]. Another study revealed that intrathecal administration of GDNF activates the ERK-Runx1 signaling cascade in rat DRG neurons, increasing P2X3R gene transcription and neuronal excitability, thereby inducing pain hypersensitivity in normal rats. Conversely, inhibiting ERK signaling or knocking down RunX1 can block these effects of GDNF while alleviating BCP-related symptoms [79].

4.1.3 CXCL12/CXCR4

The CXCL12/CXCR4 signaling pathway in the spinal cord plays a pivotal role in the development of BCP by mediating neuronal sensitization and glial activation [12]. CXCL12/CXCR4 serves as a potent molecular signal source during CIBP, with the spinal JNK-c-Jun pathway acting as a downstream target for CXCL12/CXCR4-mediated central sensitization and cancer pain hypersensitivity [93]. Studies have demonstrated that transactivation of the CXCR4-mediated ALK5/Smad3 signaling pathway significantly reduces pain-related behaviors in CIBP rat models when this pathway is blocked, suggesting that the CXCR4/ALK5/Smad3 signaling pathway may be an important therapeutic target [80]. Research has shown that the CXCR4 antibody mAb15G5 can markedly suppress lung micro-metastases by blocking

CXCR4/CXCL12 chemotaxis, while mildly inhibiting primary tumor growth and reducing bone resorption without affecting lung metastases. This indicates that the antibody could serve as a complementary agent to current (new) adjuvant chemotherapy for tumor cell chemotaxis inhibition in metastatic osteosarcoma treatment [81].

4.1.4 RANK/RANKL

Research indicates that RANKL is the most accurate biomarker [94]. Studies demonstrate that inhibiting the RANK/RANKL/OPG system and osteoclast activity not only improves bone resorption but also prevents tumor bone metastasis [82]. Given the multi-regulatory functions of the RANKL-RANK pathway, the monoclonal antibody denosumab, which targets this pathway, has been widely used in treating chronic inflammatory bone diseases and osteolytic bone metastases. In addition, preclinical data confirm denosumab's potential application value in broader cancer treatment fields [83]. Bisphosphonates inhibit osteoclast function by inducing osteoclast apoptosis, while denosumab is a monoclonal antibody that specifically targets receptor activator of NF-κB ligand (RANKL). It can inhibit osteoclast activation, thereby reducing bone resorption, and clinical studies have confirmed its effectiveness in the treatment of BCP.

4.1.5 New targets

Recent studies using BCP mouse models and cellular experiments have revealed that BAM8-22 activates spinal MrgC receptors, modulates mitochondrial unfolded protein response (UPRmt) activity, and improves mitochondrial function to alleviate BCP, providing a novel therapeutic target [84]. Nicotinamide riboside (NR) enhances UPRmt to restore mitochondrial function, reduces BCP-induced hypersensitivity, and activates transcription factor 5 (Atf5), indicating UPRmt as a potential clinical pain management target [65]. Research demonstrated that hemin exhibits analgesic effects in rats with BCP, significantly reducing fluorescence-labeled malignant atypical discrete breast cancer 106 cell line (LUC-MADB106)-induced BCP through dose-dependent mechanisms. This mechanism may involve inhibition of DYRK1A expression in the dorsal horn of the spinal cord and activation of NF-κB pathways, providing a foundation for BCP drug development [85].

4.2 Small molecule inhibitors

Research has identified Anwulignan as a potential anti-tumor and analgesic agent that exerts its effects by upregulating PPARα expression to inhibit CXCR2 activation, making it applicable for treating BCP [68]. Quercetin can suppress osteoclast activation and reduce bone destruction in BCP models by modulating the RANKL/RANK/OPG signaling pathway and inflammatory responses [83]. It also inhibits peripheral sensitization and central sensitization in BCP through regulation of the PAR2/TRPV1 signaling pathway. Studies have shown that administering GSK690693 – a novel Akt inhibitor – can alleviate pain by blocking pain signal transmission and improving pain workability (PWMT) when no Akt-mediated intermediate signals are present [87]. Notably, GSK690693 inhibits Akt protein phosphorylation, leading to a significant reduction in the expression of with-no-leucine kinase 1 (WNK1) in spinal cord tissues. In addition, pomelo extract has been found to mitigate pain sensitization and bone damage in bone cancer mice by inhibiting the TNF-α-mediated NF-κB/uPA/PAR2 pathway [88]. Intrathecal injection of LY294002, a selective inhibitor of PI3K/Akt signaling, can alleviate BCP by restoring mitochondrial function and inhibiting spinal inflammation [89].

4.3 Gene therapy and neuroregulation technologies

Inhibiting bone tissue sensory nerve activity may provide new therapeutic directions for cancer progression, metastasis, and pain caused by bone metastases [94]. A study developed a herpes simplex virus vector carrying PDGF small interfering RNA (siRNA) and administered it intrathecally to rats with BCP. The results showed that the vector could reduce SDH pPDGFRα/β levels, inhibit the AKT-ERK signaling pathway, alleviate astrocyte hypertrophy, and decrease neurochemical substances SP and CGRP expression. These effects reversed both thermal hyperalgesia and mechanical hyperalgesia, offering novel strategies for BCP management [90]. Researchers identified and proposed the STING mechanism: STING agonists induce robust production of type I interferon, which directly suppresses nociceptor excitability and osteoclast formation while enhancing T-cell-mediated anti-tumor immunity. They hypothesized that STING agonists could acutely inhibit cancer pain through direct action, while long-term relief of BCP might come from inhibiting osteoclast-mediated bone destruction and reducing local tumor burden [91]. Activation of GPR37 promotes macrophage-mediated release of IL-10 via NPD1 or ARU targeting and recruiting β-arrestin2, thereby suppressing cancer-induced osteoclast formation. Moreover, it reduces action potential frequency and sEPSCs in DRG and SDH, effectively inhibiting neuronal hyperexcitability through dual peripheral and neuronal mechanisms, thus alleviating BCP [86]. In addition, some studies have found that pharmacological inhibition of ferroptosis-like cells in spinal cord interneurons can relieve BCP in mice [92].

5. Conclusion

BCP, a chronic pain caused by bone metastases or primary bone tumors, has a complex pathogenesis involving dynamic interactions between tumor cells, osteoclasts, osteoblasts, immune cells (such as macrophages and T cells), and sensory neurons in the tumor microenvironment. Specifically, it includes the sensitization of nociceptors by mediators (such as NGF and CXCL12) released by tumor and stromal cells, the activation of nerve endings by bone matrix degradation products (such as ATP and acidic substances), the inflammatory response caused by immune cell infiltration into nerves, and peripheral and central sensitization induced by signaling pathways like Wnt5a/Ryk between tumors and nerves. Based on these mechanisms, current targeted therapeutic strategies include monoclonal antibodies (such as Tanezumab targeting NGF/TrkA and denosumab targeting RANK/RANKL), small molecule inhibitors (such as Anwulignan and quercetin), gene therapies (such as PDGF siRNA), and interventions on emerging targets (such as UPRmt and BAM8-22/MrgC receptors). Although these strategies show potential in relieving pain and reducing bone destruction, they still face challenges such as the need for multi-target synergistic intervention due to the complex pathological mechanism, the need to optimize long-term safety, and the impact of individual differences on treatment response. In the future, further exploration of multi-pathway regulation, development of drugs with dual effects, and promotion of personalized medicine are required to improve treatment efficacy.

Acknowledgments

This work was supported by the Shenzhen Science and Technology Program (JCYJ20240813152049062) and the National Natural Science Foundation of China (82401438).

Conflict of interest

The authors declare no conflicts of interest.

Author details

Mingzhu Zhai[1]*, Yanni Luo[1,2] and Wuping Sun[2]*

1 Center for Medical Experiments (CME), Shenzhen Guangming District People's Hospital, Shenzhen, China

2 Department of Clinical Laboratory Medicine, Fifth Affiliated Hospital of Southern Medical University, Guangzhou, China

*Address all correspondence to: mingzhu.zhai@foxmail.com, wuping.sun@foxmail.com

References

[1] Goblirsch MJ, Zwolak PP, Clohisy DR.Biology of bone cancer pain. Clinical cancer research :an official journal of the American Association for Cancer Research. 2006;**12**(20 Pt 2):6231s–5s

[2] Huifen Y, Tang L, Anjiale YM, Ling Q, Guifang Z. Research advances in the pathogenesis of bone cancer pain. Journal of Jilin University - Medicine Edition. 2018;**39**(5):385–388

[3] Sulistio M, Ling N, Finkelstein T, Tee HJ, Gorelik A, Kissane D, et al. The Edmonton Classification System for Cancer Pain in Patients with Bone Metastasis: A descriptive cohort study. Support Care Cancer Off J Multinatl Assoc Support Care Cancer 2023;**31**:305

[4] Paley CA, Johnson MI, Tashani OA, Bagnall AM. Acupuncture for cancer pain in adults. Cochrane Database Syst Rev. 2015;**2015**(10):CD007753

[5] Yang L, Liu B, Zheng S, Xu L, Yao M. Understanding the initiation, delivery and processing of bone cancer pain from the peripheral to the central nervous system. Neuropharmacology. 2023;**237**:109641

[6] Tahara RK, Brewer TM, Theriault RL, Ueno NT. Bone metastasis of breast cancer. Advances in Experimental Medicine and Biology. 2019;**1152**:105–129

[7] Takei D, Tagami K. Management of cancer pain due to bone metastasis. Journal of Bone and Mineral Metabolism. 2023;**41**(3):327–336

[8] Aielli F, Ponzetti M, Rucci N.Bone metastasis pain, from the bench to the bedside. International Journal of Molecular Sciences. 2019;**20**(2):280

[9] Fallon M, Sopata M, Dragon E, Brown MT, Viktrup L, West CR, et al. A randomized placebo-controlled trial of the anti-nerve growth factor antibody tanezumab in subjects with cancer pain due to bone metastasis. The Oncologist 2023;**28**:e1268–78

[10] Liu Z, Murphy SF, Huang J, Zhao L, Hall CC, Schaeffer AJ, et al. A novel immunocompetent model of metastatic prostate cancer-induced bone pain. The Prostate 2020;**80**:782–794

[11] Tomotsuka N, Kaku R, Obata N, Matsuoka Y, Kanzaki H, Taniguchi A, et al. Up-regulation of brain-derived neurotrophic factor in the dorsal root ganglion of the rat bone cancer pain model. Journal of Pain Research. 2014;**7**:415–423

[12] Shen W, Hu XM, Liu YN, Han Y, Chen LP, Wang CC, et al. CXCL12 in astrocytes contributes to bone cancer pain through CXCR4-mediated neuronal sensitization and glial activation in rat spinal cord. Journal of Neuroinflammation. 2014;**11**:75

[13] Xu H, Peng C, Chen XT, Yao YY, Chen LP, Yin Q, et al. Chemokine receptor CXCR4 activates the RhoA/ROCK2 pathway in spinal neurons that induces bone cancer pain. Molecular Pain. 2020;**16**:1744806920919568

[14] Zajączkowska R, Kocot-Kępska M, Leppert W, Wordliczek J.Bone pain in cancer patients: Mechanisms and current treatment. International Journal of Molecular Sciences. 2019;**20**(23):6047

[15] Zhang W, Wang M, Ji C, Liu X, Gu B, Dong T. Macrophage polarization in

the tumor microenvironment: Emerging roles and therapeutic potentials. Biomed Pharmacother Biomedecine Pharmacother. 2024;**177**:116930

[16] Sergi CM, Burnett M, Jantuan E, Hakoum M, Beug ST, Leng R, et al. Digging through the complexities of immunological approaches in emerging osteosarcoma therapeutics: A comprehensive narrative review with updated clinical trials. Biomedicines 2025;**13**:664

[17] Nagae M, Hiraga T, Wakabayashi H, Wang L, Iwata K, Yoneda T. Osteoclasts play a part in pain due to the inflammation adjacent to bone. Bone. 2006;**39**(5):1107–1115

[18] Khasabova IA, Khasabov SG, Johns M, Juliette J, Zheng A, Morgan H, et al. Exosome-associated lysophosphatidic acid signaling contributes to cancer pain. Pain 2023;**164**:2684–2695

[19] Tanaka Y, Nakayamada S, Okada Y. Osteoblasts and osteoclasts in bone remodeling and inflammation. Current Drug Target -Inflammation & Allergy. 2005;**4**(3):325–328

[20] Saad F, Lipton A. SRC kinase inhibition: Targeting bone metastases and tumor growth in prostate and breast cancer. Cancer Treatment Reviews. 2010;**36**(2):177–184

[21] Wong BR, Besser D, Kim N, Arron JR, Vologodskaia M, Hanafusa H, et al. TRANCE, a TNF family member, activates Akt/PKB through a signaling complex involving TRAF6 and c-Src. Molecular Cell 1999;**4**:1041–1049

[22] Zhou D, Yang D. [miRNAIs Involved in the Pathogenesis of Multiple Diseases by Targeting Osteoprotegerin]. Journal Of Sichuan University (Medical Sciences). 2024;**55**(3):777–782

[23] Tang PCT, Chung JYF, Liao J, Chan MKK, Chan ASW, Cheng G, et al. Single-cell RNA sequencing uncovers a neuron-like macrophage subset associated with cancer pain. Science Advances. 2022;**8**(40):eabn5535

[24] Yu X, Liu H, Hamel KA, Morvan MG, Yu S, Leff J, et al. Dorsal root ganglion macrophages contribute to both the initiation and persistence of neuropathic pain. Nature Communications 2020;**11**:264

[25] Guimarães RM, Aníbal-Silva CE, Davoli-Ferreira M, Gomes FIF, Mendes A, Cavallini MCM, et al. Neuron-associated macrophage proliferation in the sensory ganglia is associated with peripheral nerve injury-induced neuropathic pain involving CX3CR1 signaling. eLife. 2023;**12**:e78515

[26] Raoof R, Martin Gil C, Lafeber FPJG, de Visser H, Prado J, Versteeg S, et al. Dorsal root ganglia macrophages maintain osteoarthritis pain. The Journal Of Neuroscience Officially in journal of the Society for Neuroscience. 2021;**41**:8249–8261

[27] Tu H, Chu H, Guan S, Hao F, Xu N, Zhao Z, et al. The role of the M1/M2 microglia in the process from cancer pain to morphine tolerance. Tissue and Cell. 2021;**68**:101438

[28] Mirabello L, Zhu B, Koster R, Karlins E, Dean M, Yeager M, et al. Frequency of pathogenic germline variants in cancer-susceptibility genes in patients with osteosarcoma. JAMA Oncology 2020;**6**:724–734

[29] Sergi C, Shen F, Liu SM. Insulin/IGF-1R, SIRT1, and FOXOs pathways—

an intriguing interaction platform for bone and osteosarcoma. Frontiers in Endocrinology. 2019;**10**:93

[30] van der Vlist M, Raoof R, Hldm W, Prado J, Versteeg S, Martin Gil C, et al. Macrophages transfer mitochondria to sensory neurons to resolve inflammatory pain. Neuron 2022;**110**:613–626.e9

[31] Oggero S, Cecconello C, Silva R, Zeboudj L, Sideris-Lampretsas G, Perretti M, et al. Dorsal root ganglia CX3CR1 expressing monocytes/macrophages contribute to arthritis pain. Brain, Behavior, and Immunity. 2022;**106**:289–306

[32] Chen X, Zeng Y, Wang Z, Zhu J, Liu F, Zhu M, et al. NFAT1 signaling contributes to bone cancer pain by regulating IL-18 expression in spinal microglia. CNS Neuroscience & Therapeutics. 2025;**31**:e70222

[33] Huang X, Li J, Xie J, Li Y, Gao Y, Li X, et al. Neuronal complement cascade drives bone cancer pain via C3R mediated microglial activation. Brain Research. 2018;**1698**:81–88

[34] Liu M, Yao M, Wang H, Xu L, Zheng Y, Huang B, et al $P2Y_{12}$ receptor-mediated activation of spinal microglia and p38MAPK pathway contribute to cancer-induced bone pain. Journal of Pain Research. 2017;**10**:417–426

[35] Zhang Z, Mao Y, Huang S, Xu R, Huang Y, Li S, et al. Microglia promote inhibitory synapse phagocytosis in the spinal cord dorsal horn and modulate pain-like behaviors in a murine cancer-induced bone pain model. Anesthesia & Analgesia. 2024;**139**:411–419

[36] Liu H, Lv X, Zhao X, Yi L, Lv N, Xu W, et al. Spinal astrocyte-derived interleukin-17A promotes pain hypersensitivity in bone cancer mice. Acta Pharmaceutica Sinica B 2024;**14**:5249–5266

[37] Xiang L, Gilkes DM.The contribution of the immune system in bone metastasis pathogenesis. International Journal of Molecular Sciences. 2019;**20**(4):999

[38] Zhao E, Wang L, Dai J, Kryczek I, Wei S, Vatan L, et al. Regulatory T cells in the bone marrow microenvironment in patients with prostate cancer. Oncoimmunology. 2012;**1**:152–161

[39] Ino Y, Maruyama M, Shimizu M, Morita R, Sakamoto A, Suzuki H, et al. TSLP in DRG neurons causes the development of neuropathic pain through T cells. Journal of Neuroinflammation. 2023;**20**:200

[40] Fan CY, McAllister BB, Stokes-Heck S, Harding EK, Pereira de Vasconcelos A, Mah LK, et al. Divergent sex-specific pannexin-1 mechanisms in microglia and T cells underlie neuropathic pain. Neuron. 2025;**113**:896–911.e9

[41] Duffy SS, Keating BA, Perera CJ, Lees JG, Tonkin RS, Makker PGS, et al. Regulatory T Cells and Their Derived Cytokine, Interleukin-35, Reduce Pain in Experimental Autoimmune Encephalomyelitis. The Journal Of Neuroscience Officially Society For Neuroscience. 2019;**39**:2326–2346

[42] Davoli-Ferreira M, de Lima KA, Fonseca MM, Guimarães RM, Gomes FI, Cavallini MC, et al. Regulatory T cells counteract neuropathic pain through inhibition of the Th1 response at the site

of peripheral nerve injury. Pain. 2020;**161**:1730–1743

[43] Midavaine É, Moraes BC, Benitez J, Rodriguez SR, Braz JM, Kochhar NP, et al. Meningeal regulatory T cells inhibit nociception in female mice. Science. 2025;**388**:96–104

[44] Suratt BT, Petty JM, Young SK, Malcolm KC, Lieber JG, Nick JA, et al. Role of the CXCR4/SDF-1 chemokine axis in circulating neutrophil homeostasis. Blood. 2004;**104**:565–571

[45] Shaul ME, Levy L, Sun J, Mishalian I, Singhal S, Kapoor V, et al. Tumor-associated neutrophils display a distinct N1 profile following TGFβ modulation: A transcriptomics analysis of pro- vs. antitumor TANs. Oncoimmunology. 2016;**5**(11):e1232221

[46] Schernberg A, Blanchard P, Chargari C, Deutsch E. Neutrophils, a candidate biomarker and target for radiation therapy?. Acta Oncologica. 2017;**56**(11):1522–1530

[47] VEGF-A/VEGFR-1 signalling and chemotherapy-induced neuropathic pain: Therapeutic potential of a novel anti-VEGFR-1 monoclonal antibody – PubMed [Internet]. Available from: https://pubmed.ncbi.nlm.nih.gov/34649573/ [Accessed: 2025-August-23]

[48] Khabbazi S, Hassanshahi M, Hassanshahi A, Peymanfar Y, Su YW, Xian CJ. Opioids and matrix metalloproteinases: The influence of morphine on MMP-9 production and cancer progression. Naunyn-Schmiedeberg's Archives of Pharmacology. 2019;**392**(2):123–133

[49] Deng X, Ma P, Wu M, Liao H, Song XJ. Role of matrix metalloproteinases in myelin abnormalities and mechanical allodynia in rodents with diabetic neuropathy. Aging and Disease. 2021;**12**(7):1808–1820

[50] Huerta MÁ, Molina-Álvarez M, García MM, Tejada MA, Goicoechea C, Ghasemlou N, et al. The role of neutrophils in pain: Systematic review and meta-analysis of animal studies. Pain. 2025;**166**:1230–1249

[51] Aponte-López A, Muñoz-Cruz S. Mast cells in the tumor microenvironment. Advances in Experimental Medicine and Biology. 2020;**1273**:159–173

[52] Aller MA, Arias A, Arias JI, Arias J. Carcinogenesis: The cancer cell-mast cell connection. Inflammation Research is the official journal of the European Histamine Research Society. 2019;**68**(2):103–116

[53] Leporini C, Ammendola M, Marech I, Sammarco G, Sacco R, Gadaleta CD, et al. Targeting mast cells in gastric cancer with special reference to bone metastases. World Journal of Gastroenterology. 2015;**21**:10493–10501

[54] Plum T, Feyerabend TB, Rodewald HR. Beyond classical immunity: Mast cells as signal converters between tissues and neurons. Immunity. 2024;**57**(12):2723–2736

[55] Tokunaga R, Naseem M, Lo JH, Battaglin F, Soni S, Puccini A, et al. B cell and B cell-related pathways for novel cancer treatments. Cancer Treatment Reviews. 2019;**73**:10–19

[56] Nagasawa T.Microenvironmental niches in the bone marrow required for B-cell development. Nature Reviews. Immunology. 2006;**6**(2):107–116

[57] Rajakumar SA, Papp E, Lee KK, Grandal I, Merico D, Liu CC, et al. B cell

acute lymphoblastic leukemia cells mediate RANK-RANKL-dependent bone destruction. Science Translational Medicine. 2020;**12**(561):eaba5942

[58] Wang X, Li L, Wang Y. Mechanisms of cancer-induced bone pain. Journal of Pain Research. 2025;**18**:315–326

[59] Zhai M, Peng B, Zhu H, Xiao J, Xu L, Song XJ. Wnt5a/Ryk signaling contributes to bone cancer pain by sensitizing the peripheral nociceptors through JNK-mediated TRPV1 pathway in rats. Pain. 2025;**166**(3):680–692

[60] Mantyh PW.Bone cancer pain: From mechanism to therapy. Current Opinion in Supportive & Palliative Care. 2014;**8**(2):83–90

[61] Amit M, Takahashi H, Dragomir MP, Lindemann A, Gleber-Netto FO, Pickering CR, et al. Loss of p53 drives neuron reprogramming in head and neck cancer. Nature. 2020;**578**:449–454

[62] Gong Z, Zhang Y, Wang W, Li X, Wang K, You X, et al. Netrin-1 role in nociceptive neuron sprouting through activation of DCC signaling in a rat model of bone cancer pain. Journal of Integrative Neuroscience 2024;**23**:47

[63] Xiaotao H, Yanyan W, Yunqing L, Yulin D.Research status of the occurrence and development of bone cancer pain. Journal Neuroanatomy. 2015;**31**(3):374–378

[64] Hoover G, Gilbert S, Curley O, Obellianne C, Lin MT, Hixson W, et al. Nerve-to-cancer transfer of mitochondria during cancer metastasis. Nature. 2025;**644**:252–262

[65] Li D, Xie M, Zeng H, Yu J, Xu R, Wang Z, et al. UPRmt alleviates bone cancer pain through the restoration of mitochondrial function. Experimental Cell Research. 2025;**448**(2):114568

[66] Balood M, Ahmadi M, Eichwald T, Ahmadi A, Majdoubi A, Roversi K, et al. Nociceptor neurons affect cancer immunosurveillance. Nature. 2022;**611**:405–412

[67] Teti A, Zallone A.Do osteocytes contribute to bone mineral homeostasis? Osteocytic osteolysis revisited. Bone. 2009;**44**(1):11–16

[68] Qiu F, Wei X, Zhang S, Yuan W, Mi W. Increased expression of acid-sensing ion channel 3 within dorsal root ganglia in a rat model of bone cancer pain. Neuroreport. 2014;**25**(12):887–893

[69] Deval E, Gasull X, Noël J, Salinas M, Baron A, Diochot S, et al. Acid-sensing ion channels (ASICs): Pharmacology and implication in pain. Pharmacology & Therapeutics. 2010;**128**:549–558

[70] Carattino MD, Montalbetti N. Acid-sensing ion channels in sensory signaling. American Journal of Physiology-Renal Physiology. 2020;**318** (3):F531–43

[71] Hiasa M, Okui T, Allette YM, Ripsch MS, Sun-Wada GH, Wakabayashi H, et al. Bone pain induced by multiple myeloma is reduced by targeting V-ATPase and ASIC3. Cancer Research. 2017;**77**: 1283–1295

[72] Niiyama Y, Kawamata T, Yamamoto J, Furuse S, Namiki A. SB366791, a TRPV1 antagonist, potentiates analgesic effects of systemic morphine in a murine model of bone cancer pain. British Journal of Anaesthesia. 2009;**102**(2):251–258

[73] Di Pompo G, Lemma S, Canti L, Rucci N, Ponzetti M, Errani C, et al. Intratumoral acidosis fosters cancer-induced bone pain through the activation of the mesenchymal tumor-associated stroma in bone metastasis from breast carcinoma. Oncotarget. 2017;**8**:54478–54496

[74] Yang Y, Yang W, Zhang R, Wang Y.Peripheral mechanism of cancer-induced bone pain. Neuroscience Bulletin. 2024;**40**(6):815–830

[75] Coluzzi F, Scerpa MS, Alessandri E, Romualdi P, Rocco M.Role of TRP channels in cancer-induced bone pain. International Journal of Molecular Sciences. 2025;**26**(3):1229

[76] Ventura C, Núñez SV, Gonçalves A, Abreu C, Costa L. Bone health in metastatic cancer. Seminars in Oncology Nursing. 2022;**38**(2):151278

[77] Kan BF, Liu XY, Han MM, Yang CW, Zhu X, Jin Y, et al. Nerve growth factor/tyrosine kinase A receptor pathway enhances analgesia in an experimental mouse model of bone cancer pain by increasing membrane levels of δ-opioid receptors. Anesthesiology. 2024;**140**:765–785

[78] Nencini S, Ringuet M, Kim DH, Greenhill C, Ivanusic JJ. GDNF, neurturin, and artemin activate and sensitize bone afferent neurons and contribute to inflammatory bone pain. The Journal Of Neuroscience Official Journal of the Society For Neuroscience. 2018;**38**(21):4899–4911

[79] Yuan ZL, Liu XD, Zhang ZX, Li S, Tian Y, Xi K, et al. Activation of GDNF-ERK-Runx1 signaling contributes to P2X3R gene transcription and bone cancer pain. iScience. 2022;**25**(9):104936

[80] Peng C, Chen XT, Xu H, Chen LP, Shen W. Role of the CXCR4/ALK5/Smad3 signaling pathway in cancer-induced bone pain. Journal of Pain Research. 2020;**13**:2567–2576

[81] Brennecke P, Arlt MJE, Campanile C, Husmann K, Gvozdenovic A, Apuzzo T, et al. CXCR4 antibody treatment suppresses metastatic spread to the lung of intratibial human osteosarcoma xenografts in mice. Clinical & Experimental Metastasis. 2014;**31**:339–349

[82] Zhang Y, Liang J, Liu P, Wang Q, Liu L, Zhao H. The RANK/RANKL/OPG system and tumor bone metastasis: Potential mechanisms and therapeutic strategies. Frontiers in Endocrinology. 2022;**13**:1063815

[83] Sobacchi C, Menale C, Villa A. The RANKL-RANK axis: a bone to thymus round trip. Frontiers in Immunology. 2019;**10**:629

[84] BAM8-22 targets spinal MrgC receptors to modulate UPRmt activity in the mechanism of bone cancer pain - PubMed [Internet]. Available from: https://pubmed.ncbi.nlm.nih.gov/40230701/ [Accessed: 2025-August-4]

[85] Zhang S, Zheng S, Jin J, Li Y, Chen L, Lin J, et al. Harmine-mediated reduction of bone cancer pain in rats correlates with suppressed DYRK1A/NF-κB signaling axis. Journal of Integrative Neuroscience. 2025;**24**(6):38100

[86] Wang Y, Liu Q, Jiang Y, Mao L, Zoubaa M, Wang J, et al. Anwulignan alleviates bone cancer pain by modulating the PPARα/CXCR2 signaling pathway in the rat spinal cord. CNS Neuroscience and Therapeutics. 2025;**31**(3):e70302

[87] Li Z, Zhang J, Ren X, Liu Q, Yang X. The mechanism of quercetin in regulating osteoclast activation and the PAR2/TRPV1 signaling pathway in the treatment of bone cancer pain. International Journal of Clinical and Experimental Pathology. 2018;**11** (11):5149–5156

[88] Li Y, Zheng G, Tang Y, Chen Y, Yang M, Zheng Q, et al. Naringenin alleviates bone cancer pain via NF-κB/uPA/PAR2 pathway in mice. Journal of Orthopaedic Surgery Hong Kong. 2024;**32**(2):10225536241266671

[89] Zhao J, Yan Y, Zhen S, Yu L, Ding J, Tang Q, et al. LY294002 alleviates bone cancer pain by reducing mitochondrial dysfunction and the inflammatory response. International Journal of Molecular Medicine 2023;**51**:42

[90] Xu Y, Liu J, He M, Liu R, Belegu V, Dai P, et al. Mechanisms of PDGF siRNA-mediated inhibition of bone cancer pain in the spinal cord. Scientific Reports. 2016;**6**:27512

[91] Wang K, Zhang Y, Shu R, Yuan L, Tu H, Wang S, et al. GPR37 activation alleviates bone cancer pain via the inhibition of osteoclastogenesis and neuronal hyperexcitability. Advanced science Weinheim,Baden-Wurttemberg, Germany. 2025;**12**: e2417367

[92] Ding Z, Liang X, Wang J, Song Z, Guo Q, Schäfer MKE, et al. Inhibition of spinal ferroptosis-like cell death alleviates hyperalgesia and spontaneous pain in a mouse model of bone cancer pain. Redox Biology. 2023;**62**:102700

[93] Duan C, Zhu Y, Zhang Z, Wu T, Shen M, Xu J, et al. Esketamine inhibits the c-Jun N-terminal kinase pathway in the spinal dorsal horn to relieve bone cancer pain in rats. Molecular Pain. 2024;**20**:17448069241239231

[94] Ibrahim T, Ricci M, Scarpi E, Bongiovanni A, Ricci R, Riva N, et al. RANKL: A promising circulating marker for bone metastasis response. Oncology Letters. 2016;**12**:2970–2975

[95] Yoneda T, Hiasa M, Okui T, Hata K.Cancer-nerve interplay in cancer progression and cancer-induced bone pain. Journal of Bone and Mineral Metabolism. 2023;**41**(3):415–427

[96] Middlemiss T, Laird BJA, Fallon MT.Mechanisms of cancer-induced bone pain. Clinical Oncology. 2011;**23** (6):387–392

Chapter 7

Evolving Role of Radiotherapy in the Treatment of Bone Tumors

Shraddha Srivastava and Shally Batham

Abstract

Radiotherapy plays a pivotal role in the management of bone tumors, both primary and metastatic. While surgery remains the cornerstone for many primary bone malignancies, such as osteosarcoma and chondrosarcoma, radiotherapy is increasingly utilized in selected cases where surgical resection is not feasible or as an adjunct for local control. In particular, Ewing sarcoma is highly radiosensitive, and radiotherapy forms a key component of its multimodal treatment approach. For metastatic bone disease, radiotherapy is the primary modality for pain palliation, prevention of pathological fractures, and spinal cord compression management. Technological advances such as intensity-modulated radiotherapy (IMRT), stereotactic body radiotherapy (SBRT), and image-guided radiotherapy (IGRT) have enhanced treatment precision, minimizing toxicity to surrounding healthy tissues. Emerging evidence also supports the potential role of radiotherapy in modifying the tumor microenvironment and enhancing systemic immunotherapeutic effects. Overall, radiotherapy remains an indispensable tool in the multidisciplinary management of bone tumors, contributing to both symptom relief and disease control.

Keywords: bone tumors, intensity-modulated radiotherapy (IMRT), osteosarcoma, chondrosarcoma, metastasis

1. Introduction

Bone tumors embody a complex spectrum of lesions, either originating in the bone itself (primary tumors) or spreading to the bone from elsewhere in the body (secondary or metastatic tumors).

Primary bone tumors can indeed be broadly classified into benign and malignant categories, each with distinct characteristics, symptoms, and treatment outcomes. Benign tumors, like osteochondromas or giant cell tumors, often have a more favorable prognosis, whereas malignant tumors, such as osteosarcoma or Ewing sarcoma, require aggressive treatment due to their potential for metastasis and recurrence. The distinction between these two categories is crucial for determining the most effective treatment approach.

Osteosarcoma is the most frequent primary malignant bone tumor, typically occurring in adolescents and young adults during periods of rapid growth. It is distinguished by the production of immature bone or osteoid tissue by cancerous cells, most commonly found in the long bones of the extremities, such as the femur, tibia, and humerus [1].

Ewing sarcoma is marked by small, round, blue cells and often occurs in the pelvis, femur, humerus, ribs, and spine. It typically affects children and young adults. In contrast, chondrosarcoma, a cartilage-producing malignancy, more commonly affects adults, frequently arising in the pelvis, femur, and shoulder girdle [2].

2. Incidence and etiology

Primary bone cancers exhibit significant clinical diversity and can be curable with appropriate treatment. According to the National Comprehensive Cancer Network (NCCN), in adults, the most common types are chondrosarcoma (over 40%), osteosarcoma (around 25%), chordoma (10%), and Ewing sarcoma (8%), with other rare types including giant cell tumor and undifferentiated pleomorphic sarcoma. In contrast, children and adolescents are more likely to develop osteosarcoma and Ewing sarcoma, with chondrosarcoma and chordoma being less common in this age group.

3. Pathogenesis

The pathogenesis of most bone cancers remains unclear, but specific genetic alterations have been identified. Ewing sarcoma is associated with gene rearrangements between FET (EWSR1) and ETS (FLI1) family genes [3]. In osteosarcoma, germline mutations, such as those found in Li-Fraumeni syndrome (TP53 gene mutation) and retinoblastoma (RB1 gene mutation), increase the risk of developing this cancer [4]. Additionally, osteosarcoma is the most common radiation-induced bone sarcoma and has been linked to other genetic mutations and inherited syndromes.

The molecular mechanisms driving chondrosarcoma are not fully understood, but research suggests the involvement of various genes and pathways, including TP53, hedgehog signaling, insulin-like growth factor, cyclin-dependent kinase 4, hypoxia-inducible factor, matrix metalloproteinases, SRC, and AKT [5].

Environmental factors, such as ionizing radiation (therapeutic or accidental) and treatment with alkylating agents, contribute to the development of bone sarcomas, accounting for around 3% of cases [6].

4. Diagnosis

Diagnosing bone tumors typically involves a combination of imaging tests (X-rays, MRI, computed tomography [CT] scans), laboratory tests, and tissue biopsies to confirm the presence, type, and extent of the tumor. A biopsy is essential for a definitive diagnosis and determining the tumor's grade.

The most common symptoms of bone cancer are localized pain, tenderness, and limited range of motion in the affected area; hence, history and clinical examination become critical for bone cancer diagnosis.

X-rays can reveal characteristic findings, such as osteolytic, osteoblastic, or mixed changes; a "moth-eaten" appearance, indicating rapid bone destruction (common in Ewing sarcoma and telangiectatic osteosarcoma); a permeative appearance, suggesting tumor progression through bone (often seen in small cell tumors like Ewing sarcoma); "Onion skinning," where the tumor lifts partially formed periosteal bone (classically associated with Ewing sarcoma); "Codman triangle," where the periosteum is lifted and osteoid is deposited; and a "sunburst" appearance, characterized by vertical osteoid calcification due to significant periostitis [7].

MRI is the gold standard for evaluating local tumor extent, providing detailed images of the entire anatomical compartment, bone, and soft tissue. It is essential for biopsy planning, defining neurovascular structures, and assessing tumor response to chemotherapy, which is critical for limb salvage surgery. Advanced MRI techniques, such as dynamic MRI, can also help identify high-grade tumor areas [8].

Bone scans and CT of the chest are useful in evaluating metastasis.

PET scans are useful in detecting metastases and tumor recurrence in bone cancer, and PET-CT can help plan biopsies or evaluate lesions when MRI is not feasible. Its role in the initial workup is still being established [9].

Biopsies for bone tumors should be performed under the guidance of a specialist surgeon at a bone tumor unit to minimize errors and complications. A biopsy is crucial for determining the lesion's grade and diagnosis. Techniques include percutaneous, incisional, or excisional biopsy, with excisional biopsy typically reserved for lesions with low malignant potential or small, potentially malignant lesions that require wide local excision [10].

5. Staging

After completing diagnostic studies, oncologic staging is performed using the TNM system, as outlined by the American Joint Committee on Cancer (AJCC) [11], to conclude the pretreatment evaluation.

The stage of cancer directly impacts prognosis, which is crucial for discussing expected outcomes with patients and their families.

6. Management of Ewing sarcoma and osteosarcoma

6.1 Ewing sarcoma

Ewing sarcoma treatment involves a multimodal approach combining the following:

(1) Systemic chemotherapy: to downstage or reduce the size of the tumor and address potential spread.

(2) Local treatment: surgery to excise the tumor, radiotherapy (RT), or both.

(3) Adjuvant chemotherapy: to eliminate the remaining cancer burden.

This approach targets both the primary tumor and systemic disease.

6.1.1 Systemic therapy

The advent of systemic chemotherapy marked a significant turning point in the treatment of Ewing sarcoma, transforming a once-poor prognosis into a more hopeful outcome. Historically, the cure rate for Ewing sarcoma was dismal, with less than 10% of patients achieving long-term survival, even among those with localized disease [12].

In contrast, modern multiagent chemotherapy regimens have dramatically improved outcomes, with approximately 70% of patients presenting with localized disease achieving long-term event-free survival (EFS) [13]. However, the prognosis varies significantly depending on the extent of disease at diagnosis.

For patients with lung metastases, long-term EFS rates range from 30% to 50%, highlighting the challenges of treating disease that has spread beyond the primary site. Unfortunately, patients with metastases to distant bones or bone marrow face an even more daunting prognosis, with long-term EFS rates of less than 20% [14].

These statistics underscore the importance of early detection and aggressive treatment, as well as the need for continued research into more effective therapies for patients with advanced disease.

Current standard chemotherapy approaches for Ewing sarcoma involve:

For localized disease: A regimen that alternates between vincristine, doxorubicin, and cyclophosphamide (VAC) and ifosfamide and etoposide (I/E), known as the VAC-I/E regimen.

For metastatic disease: A regimen consisting of vincristine, doxorubicin, and cyclophosphamide (VAC).

These chemotherapy regimens are cornerstone treatments for Ewing sarcoma, tailored to the extent of the disease at diagnosis [15].

Recurrence of Ewing sarcoma after initial treatment is associated with a dismal prognosis, with fewer than 5% of patients surviving beyond two years. This highlights the urgent need for effective salvage therapies. Despite the challenges, several chemotherapy combinations have shown promise in treating relapsed Ewing sarcoma, including cyclophosphamide and topotecan, irinotecan and temozolomide, and gemcitabine and docetaxel [16, 17].

These regimens offer potential options for patients with recurrent disease, although ongoing research is crucial to improve outcomes for this high-risk population.

6.1.2 Radiotherapy

RT plays an essential role in the multidisciplinary management of Ewing sarcoma, as it is a highly radiosensitive tumor. It is used in the following settings:

(1) **Definitive treatment:**

When surgical resection is not feasible due to the tumor's location (e.g., spine, pelvis, or skull), RT combined with chemotherapy serves as the primary local control modality.

(2) **Adjuvant (post-operative) treatment:**

Adjuvant RT is given following surgery with positive or close margins, or incomplete resection, to reduce the risk of local recurrence by sterilizing microscopic residual disease.

(3) Pre-operative (neoadjuvant) RT:

It is occasionally used to shrink large, unresectable tumors to facilitate surgery.

(4) Palliative RT:

Palliative RT is given for symptom relief in metastatic or recurrent disease.

RT techniques in Ewing sarcoma

Ewing sarcoma can arise in various sites (pelvis, spine, extremity, chest wall, skull). Beam arrangement is tailored according to the site, target volume, and nearby critical organs. The following RT techniques can be used in the treatment of Ewing sarcoma.

6.1.2.1 Three-dimensional conformal RT

In the three-dimensional conformal RT (3D-CRT) technique, multiple photon beams are shaped using MLCs to conform around the 3D target volume. For pelvic or extremity tumors typically three to five coplanar beams (e.g., 0°, 120°, 240°) are used, avoiding entry through critical structures such as the bowel, bladder, and joints. In spinal and paraspinal tumors, posterior–oblique fields (e.g., 210° and 150°) are usually employed to spare the anterior abdominal viscera. In the case of chest wall lesions, anterior oblique beams are used to minimize lung dose. **Figure 1a** shows a case of Ewing sarcoma in the iliac bone in the right leg of a patient, displaying the PTV and different OARs. **Figure 1b** shows the same patient planned with the 3D-CRT technique. Three beams consisting of an anterior-posterior beam, a right posterior oblique beam, and a left anterior oblique beam at gantry angles of 0°, 220°, and 300° respectively have been used. A dose of 50.4 Gy in 28 fractions has been prescribed.

6.1.2.2 Intensity-Modulated RT

Intensity-modulated RT (IMRT) delivers variable beam intensities from multiple fixed angles, inverse-planned to optimize target coverage and organ sparing. IMRT helps in better sparing of organs at risk (OARs). Typically, five to nine beam angles spaced around the patient (e.g., 0°, 40°, 80°, 120°, 160°, 200°, 240°, 280°, 320°) are used to avoid entry through critical OARs (bowel, kidneys, heart), achieve uniform target dose distribution, and reduce hot/cold spots.

For example, in the case of Ewing sarcoma in the pelvic region, the beam is spread in an arc-like distribution posteriorly and laterally to minimize the anterior bowel dose. In spinal/paraspinal tumors, predominantly posterior and posterior–oblique beams are used, avoiding entry through the lungs or abdomen, while in the chest wall/scapular region, multiple anterior and oblique fields are employed to minimize contralateral lung dose. The IMRT technique provides better conformity and homogeneity, as well as improved sparing of OARs dose (e.g., bladder, bowel, rectum) compared to 3D-CRT.

Figure 2a, **Figure 2b** show axial and frontal sections of a patient with Ewing sarcoma in the right posterior thigh, with PTV and OARs contoured. **Figure 2c** shows the same patient planned with the IMRT technique using seven beams at different gantry angles. A dose of 66 Gy in 33 fractions was prescribed in three phases, wherein 50, 10, and 6 Gy were delivered in phase 1, phase 2, and phase 3, respectively.

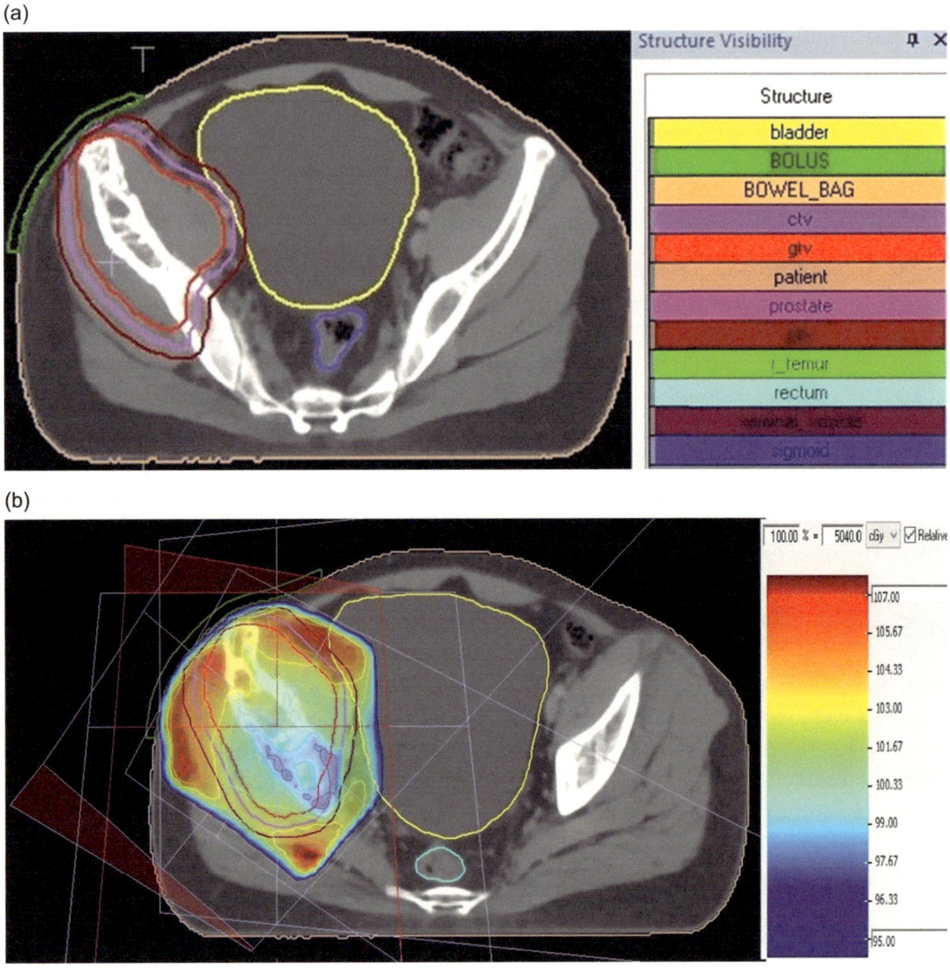

Figure 1.
(a) Axial section of a patient with Ewing sarcoma in the iliac bone in the right leg. (b) Patient with Ewing sarcoma planned using the 3D-CRT technique with three beams.

6.1.2.3 Volumetric modulated arc therapy (VMAT)

In volumetric modulated arc therapy (VMAT), beam intensity, gantry speed, and dose rate are modulated continuously as the gantry rotates around the patient (one or two arcs). Beam angles are delivered in an arced manner. In single-arc VMAT, the gantry rotates from 181° to 179° (clockwise or counterclockwise), while in dual-arc VMAT, two complementary arcs (e.g., 181° to 179° and back 179° to 181°) are used to enhance conformity and homogeneity. Partial arcs (e.g., 200° to 160°) can be used to spare critical organs anteriorly (e.g., bowel, lungs).

In pelvic or chest wall Ewing sarcoma, dual partial arcs sparing the anterior bowel or contralateral lung are used. In the case of head and neck or spinal Ewing tumor, partial arcs are placed posteriorly to reduce the dose to anterior OARs. VMAT is advantageous for shorter treatment time, high conformity, and achieving good homogeneity even in irregular shapes.

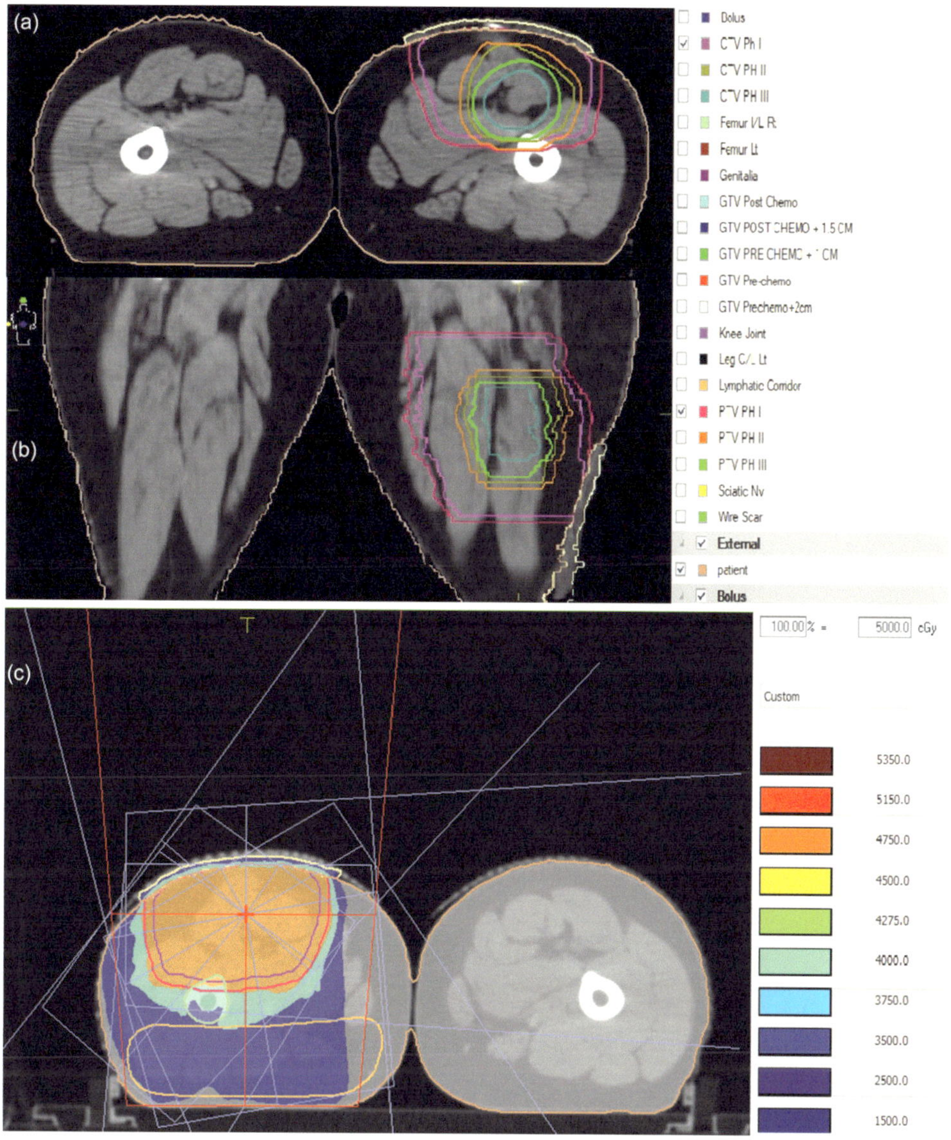

Figure 2.
(a) The axial and (b) frontal sections of a patient with Ewing sarcoma in the right posterior thigh. (c) An Ewing sarcoma patient planned with the IMRT technique using seven beams at different gantry angles.

Figure 3a shows an axial section of a patient with Ewing sarcoma of the left lung, with the PTV and OARs contoured. **Figure 3b** shows the same patient planned with the VMAT technique using three arcs of 230 degrees. A dose of 45 Gy in 25 fractions was prescribed to the PTV.

6.1.2.4 Image-guided RT

Image-guided RT (IGRT) technique involves the use of on-board imaging (kV X-rays, cone-beam CT [CBCT]) before each fraction to verify patient positioning

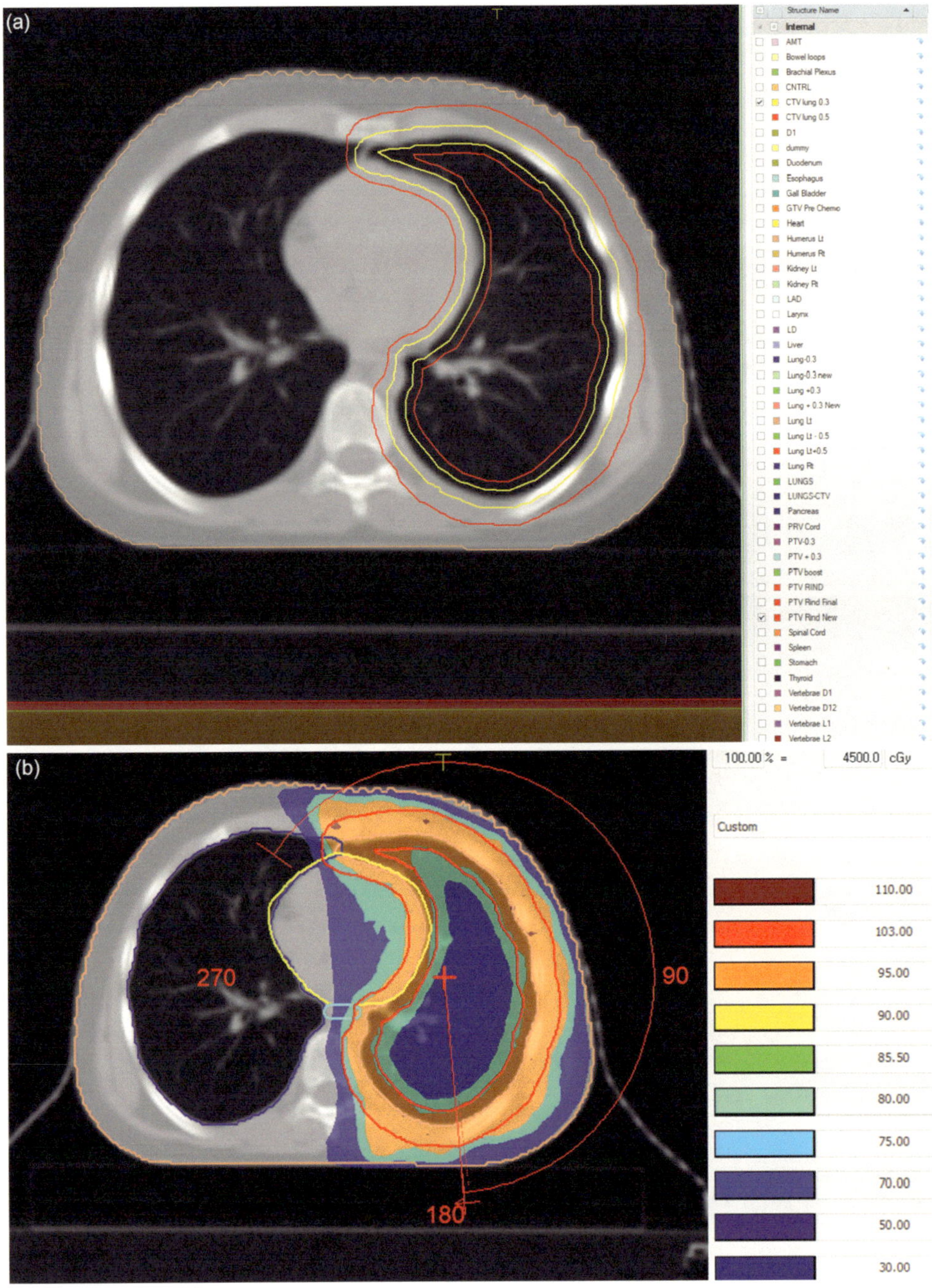

Figure 3.
(a) Axial section of a patient with Ewing sarcoma of the left lung, with the PTV and OARs contoured. (b) Patient with Ewing sarcoma of the left lung, planned with the VMAT technique using three arcs of 230 degrees.

and tumor localization. It improves precision through daily image verification and adaptive corrections for setup errors and tumor motion.

It is used for Ewing sarcoma for pelvic, paraspinal, and chest wall lesions where motion or setup variability can lead to geographic misses. In pelvic and sacral tumors, large daily setup variations due to bowel filling, bladder volume, and pelvic rotation can occur. Daily CBCT ensures consistent target localization and minimizes bowel dose.

In chest wall lesions, respiratory motion management (with 4D-CBCT or gating) prevents target motion blur. Real-time surface monitoring helps maintain a reproducible breath-hold or free-breathing setup.

6.2 Osteosarcoma

The management of osteosarcoma requires a comprehensive and multidisciplinary approach, integrating:

(1) Surgery: To remove the tumor and surrounding tissue.

(2) Chemotherapy: To control microscopic disease and reduce tumor size.

(3) Radiation therapy: In select cases, it is used to target tumors that cannot be fully resected or to alleviate symptoms.

The primary objectives are to eradicate the tumor, prevent disease spread, and preserve limb function and quality of life whenever feasible.

6.2.1 Systemic therapy

The prognosis for osteosarcoma has undergone a significant transformation. Historically, before the advent of systemic therapy, the cure rate for osteosarcoma was starkly low, with fewer than 20% of patients achieving long-term survival. This dismal outcome persisted even among patients who presented with localized disease without clinically detectable metastasis.

The introduction of multiagent chemotherapy marked a paradigm shift in osteosarcoma treatment, dramatically improving patient outcomes. The probability of cure has increased substantially, with approximately 60% to 70% of patients achieving long-term survival [18].

The standard first-line chemotherapy regimen for osteosarcoma typically consists of a combination of three key agents:

- Doxorubicin: A potent anthracycline chemotherapeutic agent.
- Cisplatin: A platinum-based agent that interferes with DNA replication.
- High-dose methotrexate: A folate antagonist that inhibits DNA synthesis.

This multiagent regimen, commonly referred to as the MAP regimen, is widely used as the initial chemotherapy approach for osteosarcoma, aiming to maximize treatment efficacy and improve patient outcomes [19].

6.2.2 Radiotherapy

RT has an important role to play in the treatment of osteosarcoma. It is delivered in situations like unresectable or inoperable tumors (e.g., spine, pelvis, skull base), positive or close surgical margins after resection, palliative treatment for pain, bleeding, or metastases, and local control when wide surgical margins cannot be achieved.

Historically, osteosarcoma has been considered radioresistant, but with modern high-precision techniques and dose escalation, RT can achieve meaningful tumor control while sparing adjacent normal tissues.

6.2.2.1 Conventional external beam RT

In conventional external beam RT (EBRT) technique, generally, two-dimensional planning and bony landmarks are used. Doses, usually around 60–70 Gy, are given depending on the tumor site. Limitations of conventional RT are that it provides poor conformity, delivers a high dose to normal tissues, and offers limited local control in radioresistant tumors like osteosarcoma.

6.2.2.2 3D conformal RT

3D-CRT technique is based on 3D CT simulation to create precise target volumes (GTV, CTV, PTV). Multileaf collimators (MLCs) shape the beam to conform to tumor geometry. Usually, three to five static beams are selected to minimize the dose to nearby organs (lungs, bowel, spinal cord, etc.). The advantage of 3D-CRT over conventional two-dimensional (2D) RT is improved conformity and better dose distribution around irregularly shaped bone tumors. However, 3D-CRT shows less conformality than IMRT or VMAT.

6.2.2.3 Intensity-modulated RT

IMRT is used to achieve conformal dose around complex tumor shapes while minimizing dose to OARs. Five to nine coplanar fields spaced around the patient are used. It is advantageous as it offers better dose conformity and homogeneity, allows dose escalation (≥70 Gy) to resistant bone lesions, and reduces exposure to surrounding soft tissues (muscle, skin, marrow). It is used in pelvic osteosarcoma, where it helps in minimizing bowel and bladder dose. In the case of spinal/paraspinal tumors, it helps in sparing the spinal cord and kidneys. For head and neck/skull base tumors, it helps in protecting the brainstem and optic nerves.

6.2.2.4 Volumetric modulated arc therapy

In VMAT, single or dual arcs (e.g., 181° → 179°) are used. Partial arcs are used to avoid critical structures. It offers faster treatment delivery compared to IMRT. Furthermore, good conformity and sparing of normal tissue can be achieved with VMAT. It is ideal for irregular targets (pelvic, scapular, or chest wall osteosarcomas).

6.2.3 Surgery in bone tumors

The surgical management of bone tumors involves a range of techniques aimed at removing the tumor while preserving limb function and achieving optimal oncologic and functional outcomes. Surgical approaches may include:

- Limb-salvage surgery: Removing the tumor along with a margin of healthy tissue to preserve the limb, often followed by reconstruction.

- Amputation: In cases where the tumor is extensive or limb preservation is not feasible.

Common surgical procedures for bone tumors include:

(1) Wide resection: Removing the tumor with a wide margin of surrounding healthy tissue, often used for aggressive or malignant tumors.

(2) Curettage: Scraping out the tumor tissue, typically used for benign tumors.

(3) Reconstruction: Using prosthetic devices or bone grafts to restore limb function and stability.

(4) Adjuvant techniques: Such as cryosurgery or local chemotherapy to destroy any residual tumor cells.

The choice of surgical approach is tailored to each patient based on factors such as tumor size and type (benign or malignant), location, and the patient's overall health status.

A multidisciplinary team collaborates to develop a personalized surgical plan, ensuring the most effective and suitable treatment strategy for each individual case [20].

The main objective of surgical management in bone sarcomas is to achieve complete tumor excision with negative margins (R0 resection).

Limb salvage surgery may not be suitable for all patients, and relative contraindications include major neurovascular involvement, very immature skeletal age, infection, limited reconstructive or soft tissue coverage options, biopsy-related contamination, inability to achieve acceptable margins, and pathologic fracture.

The most common reason for recommending amputation is significant neurological involvement by the tumor, which can compromise the effectiveness and safety of limb salvage procedures.

For patients with Ewing sarcoma, especially those with extremity lesions, surgical resection is often a key component of treatment. When surgical margins are negative, it may be possible to avoid adjuvant radiation therapy, thereby reducing the risk of long-term complications such as growth arrest and deformity, skin and soft tissue induration, lymphedema, arthrofibrosis, osteonecrosis, fracture, and secondary malignancy.

By achieving negative margins through surgery, patients may benefit from a more favorable risk–benefit profile, minimizing the potential side effects associated with radiation therapy.

7. Palliation

Palliative care for bone tumors prioritizes alleviating pain and enhancing quality of life rather than seeking a cure. Treatment strategies often involve:

(1) Radiation therapy: Utilizing external beam radiation or brachytherapy to target tumor sites and reduce pain.

(2) Radiopharmaceuticals: Systemic treatments that selectively target bone metastases to provide pain relief, for example, Samarium-153.

(3) Minimally invasive procedures: Techniques like cementoplasty to stabilize bones and prevent fractures.

(4) Ablative therapies: Methods such as microwave ablation or cryoablation are used to reduce tumor burden and alleviate pain.

A multidisciplinary palliative care team provides comprehensive support, addressing not only physical symptoms but also emotional, social, and psychological needs to improve the overall quality of life for patients with advanced disease [21].

Author details

Shraddha Srivastava* and Shally Batham
Department of Radiation Oncology, King George's Medical University, Lucknow, India

*Address all correspondence to: shraddha686@gmail.com

References

[1] Yoshikawa H, Nakase T, Myoui A, et al. Bone morphogenetic proteins in bone tumors. Journal of Orthopaedic Science. 2004;**9**:334–340

[2] Grünewald TGP, Cidre-Aranaz F, Surdez D, et al. Ewing sarcoma. Nature Reviews Disease Primers. 2018;**4**(5). DOI: 10.1038/s41572-018-0003-x

[3] Denny CT. Gene rearrangements in Ewing's sarcoma. Cancer Investigation. 1996;**14**:83–88

[4] Ottaviani G, Jaffe N. The etiology of osteosarcoma. Cancer Treatment and Research. 2009;**152**:15–32

[5] Bovée JV, Hogendoorn PC, Wunder JS, et al. Cartilage tumours and bone development: Molecular pathology and possible therapeutic targets. Nature Reviews Cancer 2010;**10**:481–488

[6] Kalra S, Grimer RJ, Spooner D, et al. Radiation-induced sarcomas of bone: Factors that affect outcome. The Journal of Bone and Joint Surgery. British Volume 2007;**89**:808–813

[7] Kundu ZS. Classification, imaging, biopsy and staging of osteosarcoma. Indian Journal of Orthopaedics. 2014;**48**(3):238–246. DOI: 10.4103/0019-5413.132491

[8] Gerrand C, Athanasou N, Brennan B, Grimer R, Judson I, Morland B, Peake D, Seddon B, Whelan J; British Sarcoma Group. UK guidelines for the management of bone sarcomas. Clinical Sarcoma Research. 2016;**6**:7. DOI: 10.1186/s13569-016-0047-1

[9] Ferguson JL, Turner SP. Bone cancer: Diagnosis and treatment principles. American Family Physician. 2018;**98**(4):205–213

[10] Mankin HJ, Mankin CJ, Simon MA. Members of the musculoskeletal tumor society. The hazards of the biopsy, revisited. The Journal of Bone & Joint Surgery. 1996;**78**:656–663

[11] Tanaka K, Ozaki T. New TNM classification (AJCC eighth edition) of bone and soft tissue sarcomas: JCOG bone and soft tissue tumor study group. Japanese Journal of Clinical Oncology. 2019;**49**(2):103–107. DOI: 10.1093/jjco/hyy157

[12] Nesbit M. Bone tumors in infants and children. Paediatrician. 1972;**1**:273–287

[13] Granowetter L, Womer R, Devidas M, et al. Dose-intensified compared with standard chemotherapy for nonmetastatic Ewing sarcoma family of tumors: A children's oncology group study. Journal of Clinical Oncology. 2009;**27**:2536–2541

[14] Grier HE, Krailo MD, Tarbell NJ, et al. Addition of ifosfamide and etoposide to standard chemotherapy for Ewing's sarcoma and primitive neuroectodermal tumor of bone. New England Journal of Medicine. 2003;**348**:694–701

[15] Kolb EA, Kushner BH, Gorlick R, Laverdiere C, Healey JH, LaQuaglia MP, et al. Long-term event-free survival after intensive chemotherapy for Ewing's family of tumors in children and young adults. Journal of Clinical Oncology. 2003;**21**:3423–3430

[16] Casey DA, Wexler LH, Merchant MS, et al. Irinotecan and temozolomide for Ewing sarcoma: The memorial sloan-kettering experience. Pediatric Blood & Cancer. 2009;**53**:1029–1034

[17] Hunold A, Weddeling N, Paulussen M, et al. Topotecan and cyclophosphamide in patients with refractory or relapsed Ewing tumors. Pediatric Blood & Cancer. 2006;**47**: 795–800

[18] Link MP, Goorin AM, Miser AW, et al. The effect of adjuvant chemotherapy on relapse-free survival in patients with osteosarcoma of the extremity. New England Journal of Medicine. 1986;**314**:1600–1606

[19] Strauss SJ, Frezza AM, Abecassis N, Bajpai J, Bauer S, Biagini R, Bielack S, Blay JY, Bolle S, Bonvalot S, et al. Bone sarcomas: ESMO-EURACAN-GENTURIS-ERN paedcan clinical practice guideline for diagnosis, treatment and follow-up. Annals of Oncology. 2021;**32**:1520–1536

[20] Bläsius F, Delbrück H, Hildebrand F, Hofmann UK. Surgical treatment of bone sarcoma. Cancers (Basel). 2022;**14**(11):2694. DOI: 10.3390/cancers14112694

[21] Gangi A, Tsoumakidou G, Buy X, Quoix E. Quality improvement guidelines for bone tumour management. CardioVascular and Interventional Radiology. 2010;**33**(4):706–713. DOI: 10.1007/s00270-009-9738-9

Chapter 8

Rotationplasty of the Knee

Lizz van der Heijden, Jonneke Kuperus and Michiel van de Sande

Abstract

Rotationplasty is a biological limb-salvage procedure originally developed for tuberculosis and congenital femoral deficiency and later adopted in orthopedic oncology for malignant bone tumors around the knee. The technique involves a 180° rotation of the distal limb and fusion to the proximal femur, allowing the ankle joint to function as a neo-knee and enabling use of a below-knee prosthesis with highly efficient gait mechanics. Compared with transfemoral amputation or endoprosthetic reconstruction, rotationplasty offers important advantages, including durability during growth, a low revision burden, excellent energy efficiency, and high long-term patient satisfaction. Primary oncologic indications include high-grade malignant tumors of the distal femur (Winkelmann type A1), proximal tibia (A2), and selected cases requiring total femur resection (B3). Non-oncologic indications include severe congenital femoral deficiency. Absolute contraindications are loss of tibial nerve function, irreparable vascular compromise, and severe ankle stiffness, while psychosocial intolerance and limited survival prognosis are considered relative contraindications. Optimal outcomes depend on multidisciplinary preparation, including psychosocial counseling, growth prediction, and early prosthetic planning. Surgical technique emphasizes meticulous neurovascular preservation or reconstruction, perpendicular osteotomies, and controlled rotation guided by preoperative alignment markings. Fixation is most commonly achieved using locking plates, with adapted reconstructive strategies for total femur cases. Postoperative management includes vascular monitoring, early mobilization, and structured rehabilitation. Long-term results demonstrate excellent functional outcomes, high levels of physical activity, and superior gait efficiency compared with transfemoral amputation. When carefully selected and precisely executed, rotationplasty remains a durable and effective reconstructive option that preserves function and quality of life in young patients undergoing limb-sparing tumor surgery.

Keywords: rotationplasty, pediatric limb-salvage surgery, bone sarcoma, growth (prediction), functional outcomes

1. Introduction: Background and rationale

Rotationplasty was first described by Borggreve (1927) for severe bone loss caused by tuberculosis and was later popularized by Van Nes (1950) for congenital femoral deficiency (CFD). The rotationplasty (Borggreve–Van Nes procedure) gained oncologic use in the 1980s for treating osteosarcoma and Ewing sarcoma. In orthopedic oncology, rotationplasty is a biological limb-salvage technique that enables durable reconstruction following the resection of malignant bone tumors around the knee. Rotationplasty is performed especially in pediatric patients with bone tumors but may also be preferred over megaprostheses in low- and middle-income countries due to cost and availability.

In rotationplasty surgery, the ankle is repurposed as a functional "knee" by rotating the distal limb 180° and fusing it to the proximal femur (**Figure 1**). The leg can be fitted with a below-knee-amputation-type prosthetic leg, where the ankle functions as the new "knee" and the foot functions as the tibia. In this manner, ankle plantar flexion acts as "knee" extension and ankle dorsiflexion as "knee" flexion. Advantages, compared with above-knee amputation or megaprostheses, include biological reconstruction, durability across growth, lower revision burden, efficient gait, and high long-term patient satisfaction when psychosocial preparation is adequate [1–4].

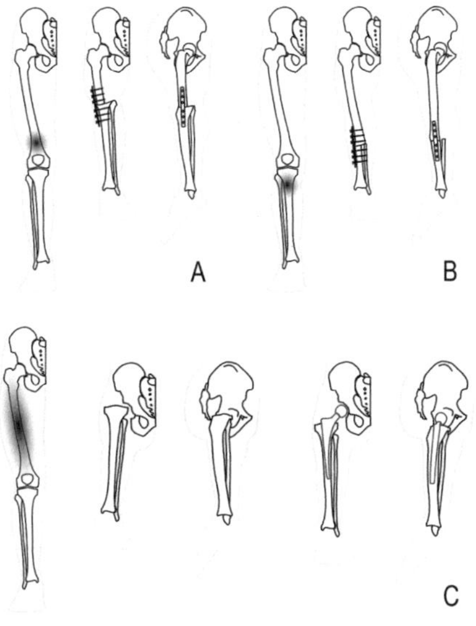

Figure 1.
Different types of rotationplasty about the knee. (a) Winkelmann type A1 for distal femur tumors. (b) Winkelmann type A2 for proximal tibia tumors. (c) Winkelmann type B3A/B for total femur resection, replacing the femoral head with the tibia in a very young patient or with a femoral prosthesis.

2. Indications and patient selection

2.1 Oncologic indications

The primary indications for rotationplasty of the knee are high-grade malignant tumors of the distal femur (Winkelmann Type A1) or proximal tibia (Winkelmann Type A2), and, less frequently, for total femoral resections (Winkelmann Type B3) [1].

Relative indications for rotationplasty are large tumor extensions outside and inside the knee joint, requiring extra-articular resection, or more than 40% of growth remaining in young children. Rotationplasty is also considered when expandable prostheses would carry an unacceptably high revision risk during growth, or when infection or a poor soft-tissue envelope precludes megaprosthetic reconstruction [4].

Unlike megaprosthetic reconstruction or amputation, rotationplasty offers the following:

- Durable, growth-adapted biomechanics without the revision burden of expandable prostheses.
- Efficient gait mechanics, as ankle plantarflexion substitutes for knee extension.
- Lower long-term complication rates, with fewer re-operations compared to prosthetic reconstructions.
- High patient satisfaction and psychosocial adaptation occur when adequate preoperative counseling is provided.

Modern series with over 30 years of follow-up demonstrate sustained functional capacity, confirming its role as a definitive solution in young, active patients [5].

2.2 Non-oncologic indications

Non-oncologic indications include CFD, especially severe proximal femoral focal deficiency (PFFD) [6], and, in selected cases, complex trauma or chronic osteoarticular infections resulting in severe lower limb bone loss [4]. Several variants of the rotationplasty techniques have been described for different types of PFFD by Paley but are not discussed in this chapter [6].

2.3 Contraindications

Absolute contraindications include irreparable vascular compromise (i.e., long-standing arterial occlusion or extensive deep venous thrombosis [DVT]), loss of tibial nerve function, or severely restricted ankle motion (**Table 1**). Tumor involvement of the artery and vein is not necessarily a contraindication for rotationplasty, as they can be resected and anastomosed proximally for Winkelmann A1 and, to a lesser extent, in Winkelmann A2 rotationplasty. Ankle function should minimally range from plantigrade to 90 degrees plantar flexion.

Absolute contraindications
• Irreparable vascular compromise (arterial occlusion, extensive venous thrombosis).
• Loss of tibial nerve function, precluding ankle motor control.
• Ankle stiffness or degenerative change preventing effective neo-knee function.
Relative contraindications
• Peroneal nerve function loss after resection.
• Severe psychosocial intolerance to cosmesis.
• Poor systemic health, precluding long rehabilitation.

Table 1.
Overview of absolute and relative contraindications for rotationplasty.

Relative contraindications include peroneal nerve function loss after resection, anticipated psychosocial distress, or very poor systemic therapy response and/or extensive pulmonary metastatic disease [4, 7, 8]. Peroneal nerve loss can sometimes be accepted in Winkelmann A2 rotationplasty, and to a lesser extent in Winkelmann A1 rotationplasty, if tibial nerve function, and thus the driving, extending motor unit of the ankle, remains intact. Rotationplasty is a life and limb-altering procedure with accompanying rehabilitation and acceptance, and poor survival prognosis can therefore be a relative contraindication.

3. Preparation

3.1 Multidisciplinary preparation

Optimal preparation includes preoperative counseling of patients and parents with illustrations, photos, and videos; psychosocial assessment; preoperative physiotherapy input; vascular imaging; and prosthetic planning. Preoperative peer support through meeting other patients and parents improves acceptance [1, 4].

3.2 Growth calculations and leg-length prediction

In children, predicting final leg length at the end of skeletal maturity is crucial (**Figure 2**). Anderson et al. (1963) quantified growth: ~70% of femoral growth arises from the distal femoral physis (~1.4 cm/year), and ~55% of tibial growth arises from the proximal physis (~1 cm/year) until skeletal maturity. Growth ceases by ~16 years in boys and ~14 years in girls. The multiplier method is also very frequently used to predict limb length discrepancies at the end of growth [9].

For example, a 10-year-old boy with osteosarcoma of the distal femur, losing the distal femoral physis after resection, will lose ~1.4 cm/year × 6 years = 8.4 cm. As the proximal tibia growth plates are also resected in most rotationplasty indications, an additional loss of 6 cm is expected. Surgical planning should, therefore, anticipate ~14.4 cm of overlength to achieve an equal knee joint line (of the affected rotationplasty leg and contralateral knee) and to equalize pelvic level at the end of growth [4, 10]. Relative distal tibia epiphysis overgrowth of about 2 cm compared to the contralateral side is to be expected after rotationplasty. Preoperative templating should aim to align contralateral trochanter–patella and trochanter–heel distances.

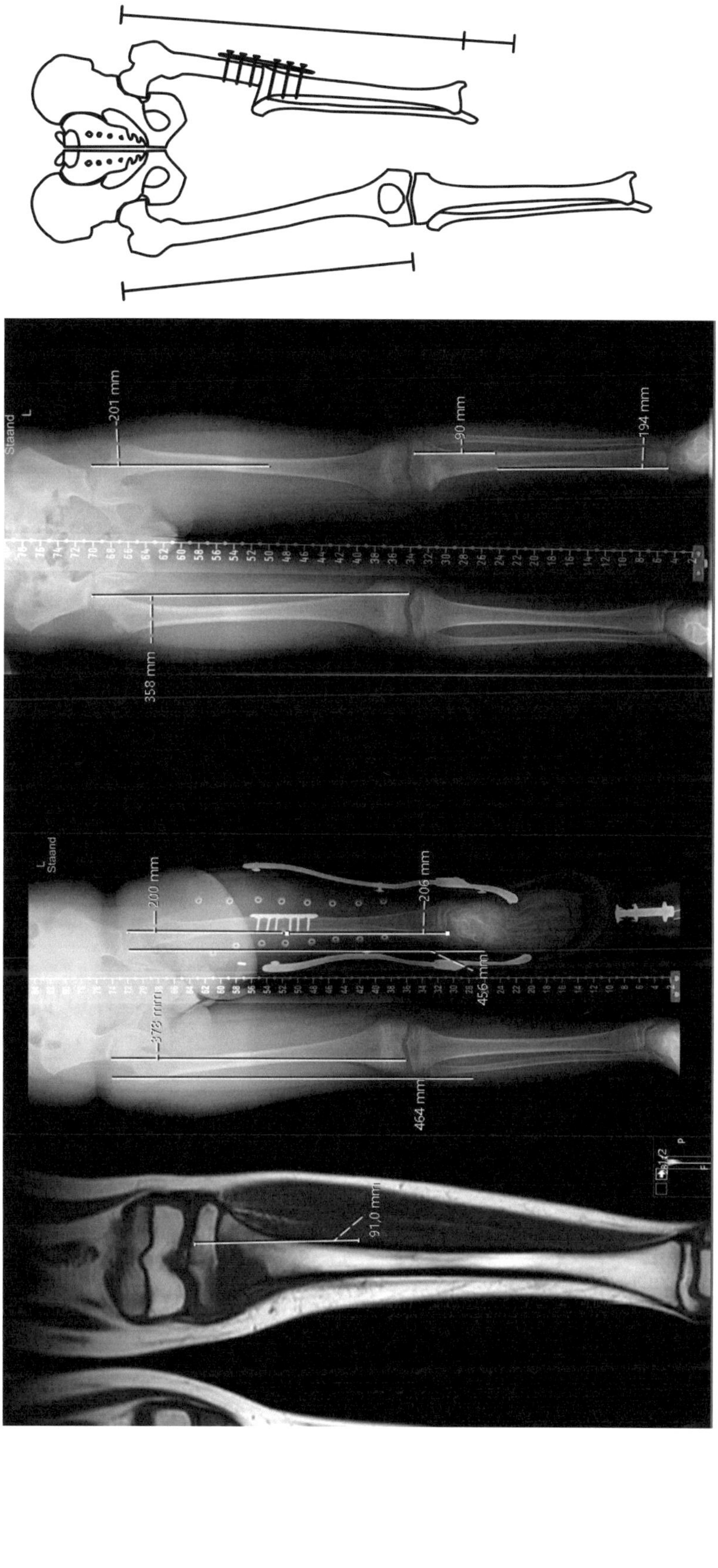

Figure 2.
Templating example for preoperative planning of rotationplasty.

The multiplier table can be used to calculate the expected leg length of the contralateral leg. In this example of a 10-year-old boy, the right femur is measured at 35.8 cm. At the end of growth, the femur is expected to be 35.8 × 1.310 (multiplier for a 10-year-old boy) = 46.9 cm. Taking into account the growth of the proximal femur and distal tibia, the sufficient leg length can be calculated. The height of the foot is generally 7 cm at the end of growth. Growth can also be arrested by epiphysiodesis of the growth plate to optimize leg length and symmetrical knee height. In the schematic drawing, an example of leg length measurements is shown.

4. Operative techniques

4.1 Surgical preparation

- Anesthesia: General anesthesia with a central line (or port-a-cath), arterial line, epidural analgesia catheter, and indwelling catheter (IDC).

- Positioning: Supine with a slight lateral tilt; consider placing the patient on a beanbag. Ensure there is adequate positioning and space for the image intensifier.

- Antibiotic prophylaxis: According to local protocols; we use intravenous cefazolin at induction and repeat it after 4 hours.

- Consider the use of intravenous tranexamic acid if there are no contraindications.

- Skin marking: Mark the preplanned osteotomy levels. Mark a circular incision at the preplanned level distal to the tip of the greater trochanter (GT). Mark a wavy incision at the knee joint to allow correction of the discrepancy in the circumference of the upper and lower legs. Finally, mark rotational alignment lines on the anterior and posterior sides of the upper and lower leg.

- Sterile prepping and draping: Colorless chlorhexidine for the entire limb, including the foot. Place the foot in a transparent foot bag for vascular evaluation during surgery. Apply sterile draping.

4.2 Rotationplasty procedures

4.2.1 Winkelmann A1 (distal femur resection)

4.2.1.1 Step 1 – Distal approach

- Wavy incision just above the knee to correct the discrepancy in circumference between the upper and lower leg. Incise the skin 1–2 cm more proximal than the tibial plateau, allowing for some additional skin for tension-free closure. Avoid incising the skin directly over the tibial tuberosity, as this area is at higher risk for wound healing problems.

- Further dissection circumferentially around the knee with diathermy effectively simulates a knee disarticulation. Preserve the length of the patellar tendon, lateral collateral ligament (LCL), and medial collateral ligament (MCL) for later reattachment.

- In the case of intra-articular tumor growth, an extra-articular resection can be performed, leaving the joint capsule closed.

- Identification of the biceps femoris tendon laterally. Opening of the peroneal and tibial compartments. Identifying the common peroneal nerve (CPN) and mobilizing it. Following the CPN proximally, subsequently identifying and mobilizing the tibial and sciatic nerves.

- Following the tibial nerve, the medial and lateral gastrocnemius heads are divided at the musculotendinous junction.

- Identify and dissect the distal popliteal artery and vein. In cases of vascular encasement or involvement, the artery and vein can be divided, and primary anastomoses of the popliteal and femoral arteries and veins can be performed, usually by vascular or plastic surgeons. In cases of free neurovascular structures and young, small children, the artery and vein can be preserved over their entire length, rolled up (without kinking), and stored in the adductor space.

- At this point, the knee is now nearly free: nerves (sciatic, tibial, peroneal) and popliteal vessels are mobilized; cruciate ligaments are still intact.

4.2.1.2 Step 2 – Medial thigh approach

- Longitudinal medial incision from the distal to the proximal incisions.

- Identify and mobilize the great saphenous vein (GSV) over its entire course. Preserving the GSV helps with venous outflow and reduces postoperative swelling, wound problems, and blister formation, as most of the other smaller (intramuscular) venous structures are divided. Depending on its diameter, one may choose between a primary anastomosis or rolling it up.

4.2.1.3 Step 3 – Posterior thigh approach

- Longitudinal posterior incision from the distal to the proximal incisions, with further dissection using diathermy down to the fascia.

- Subsequently, develop the muscular interval, identify the sciatic nerve, and mobilize it completely toward the proximal direction.

4.2.1.4 Step 4 – Proximal approach

- Circular incision made circumferentially at the preplanned proximal osteotomy level, distal to the tip of the greater trochanter.

- Dissection with diathermy down to the fascia.
- Identification and mobilization of the superficial and deep femoral vessels.
- Identification and mobilization of the sciatic nerve.
- Separate the sartorius, gracilis, quadriceps, adductors, and hamstrings muscles with LigaSure, harmonic scalpel, or diathermy to prevent bleeding, and leave them relatively short to provide space for the NV bundle.
- At this point, both the femur and the knee are completely mobilized circumferentially.

4.2.1.5 Step 5 – Osteotomies

- Perform the femoral osteotomy at the preplanned level distal to the greater trochanter, after elevating the periosteum, with an oscillating saw.
- Perform the tibial osteotomy just distal to the growth plate. The fibular head may be left in place but is often shortened.
- Occasionally, in very young children, preservation of the proximal tibia growth plate can be preferred. Remove the articular cartilage down to the subchondral bone, and K-wire fixation may be preferred over plate fixation to allow easy removal after bone healing, thereby preserving its growth potential.
- Resect the proximal fibular epiphysis to prevent regrowth, while carefully protecting the common peroneal nerve.
- Partially resect the medial tibial plateau with an oscillating saw to a flush level with the tibial shaft.
- Dissect the soft tissue cuff circumferentially around the medial and lateral tibial plateaus.
- Separate the remaining soft tissue attachments (ACL and PCL, if not an extra-articular resection).
- Resect the distal femur and knee as one specimen, and send it for histopathology.

4.2.1.6 Step 6 – Rotation and fixation

- Rotate the lower leg 180 degrees and position the proximal tibia end-to-end against the proximal femur.
- When preserving the neurovascular structures over their entire length, place them carefully within the adductor space, while making sure they are not twisted.

- Fixation is now achieved using a locking plate with bicortical locking screws on each side, after careful repositioning. Confirm adequate alignment in the coronal, sagittal, and axial planes with an image intensifier.
- In case of vascular involvement, the anastomoses are performed after the fixation in a mechanically stable environment to prevent traction on the newly formed anastomoses.

4.2.1.7 Step 7 – Closure

- Perform a thorough washout with saline or sterile water.
- Take time for good hemostasis.
- Approximate the muscles of the upper leg to the fascia of the lower leg using loose, interrupted Vicryl 1 sutures. Do not use running sutures to close the fascia. Ensure there is no excessive tension from the sutured structures on the neurovascular bundles.
- Subcuticular suture with running Vicryl 2-0.
- Skin suture with either intracutaneous or running mattress Monocryl 3-0, knots tied outside the skin. A V-shaped skin incision on the larger diameter may facilitate the difference in skin diameter.
- Silicone wound dressing, followed by non-compressive dressing.

4.2.2 Winkelmann A2 (proximal tibia resection)

4.2.2.1 Step 1 – Distal approach

- Wavy incision on the leg at the preplanned level proximal to the calcaneus, to correct the discrepancy in circumference between the upper and lower leg. Allow for some additional skin proximal to the planned osteotomy for tension-free skin closure.
- Further dissection with diathermy down to the fascia, circumferentially.
- The lower leg musculature is transected and tagged with Vicryl 1 stay sutures.
- Incise the periosteum at the preplanned osteotomy levels for the tibia and fibula.

4.2.2.2 Step 2 – Lateral approach

- Lateral incision over the femoral and fibular sides of the upper and lower leg.
- Identification of the biceps femoris tendon laterally. Opening of the peroneal and tibial compartments. Identifying the common peroneal nerve (CPN) and mobilizing it. Following the CPN proximally, subsequently identifying and mobilizing the tibial and sciatic nerves.

- Transection of the lateral gastrocnemius (with LigaSure).
- Identify and dissect the distal popliteal artery and vein.
- Via this lateral approach to the lower leg from the trifurcation, the fibular artery and vein, anterior tibial artery and vein, and posterior tibial artery and vein are identified and dissected distally, including the course of the tibial and deep peroneal nerves. To facilitate the dissection of the neurovascular bundles, the fibula may be removed if the tumor location and margins allow.
- When the anterior tibial artery runs too close to the tumor, according to preoperative planning, it can be ligated.
- Anastomosis of these vessels onto the popliteal artery is reported with a high risk of thrombosis due to the hourglass turbulence effect caused by the difference in diameter of these vessels and should, therefore, be avoided.
- The saphenous, sural, and superficial peroneal nerves are transected.

4.2.2.3 Step 3 – Posterior thigh approach

- Extend the lateral skin incision toward until reaching the preplanned proximal circular incision. Further dissection is performed with diathermy down to the fascia.
- Subsequently, develop the muscular interval, identify the sciatic nerve, and mobilize it completely toward the proximal direction.

4.2.2.4 Step 4 – Proximal approach

- Circular incision circumferentially at the preplanned osteotomy level, distal to the tip of the greater trochanter.
- Dissection with diathermy down to the fascia.
- Identification and mobilization of the superficial and deep femoral vessels.
- Separate the quadriceps, adductors, and hamstrings muscles using LigaSure, harmonic scalpel, or diathermy to prevent bleeding.
- At this point, both the femur and tibia are completely mobilized circumferentially.

4.2.2.5 Step 5 – Osteotomies

- Perform the femoral osteotomy at the preplanned level (providing the planned length of the rotationplasty), after elevating the periosteum with an oscillating saw.

- Perform the tibial and fibular osteotomies at the preplanned level proximal to the ankle joint, guided by sufficient margins and the planned length of the rotationplasty.
- Resect the proximal tibia and knee as one specimen, and send it for histopathology.

4.2.2.6 Step 6 – Rotation and fixation

- Using the preoperative skin markings on the tibia and femur, rotate the lower leg 180 degrees and position the distal tibia end-to-end against the proximal femur.
- Fixation is now achieved using a locking plate with bicortical locking screws on each side, after careful repositioning. Confirm adequate alignment in the coronal, sagittal, and axial planes with an image intensifier. If growth from the distal femoral physis is needed and anticipated, the tibia can be fixed using K-wires.
- Create space for the vessels within the hamstring compartment.

4.2.2.7 Step 7 – Closure

- Perform a thorough washout with saline or sterile water.
- Take time for good hemostasis.
- Suture the quadriceps muscle fascia to the (long) preserved gastrocnemius flap or Achilles tendon, depending on the level of the resection, with Vicryl.
- Suture the tibialis anterior tendon (TA), extensor hallucis longus (EHL), and extensor digitorum longus (EDC) to the hamstrings (semimembranosus, semitendinosus) and biceps femoris with Vicryl 1.
- Do not use running sutures to close the fascia. Make sure there is not too much tension on the sutured structures.
- Subcuticular suture with running Vicryl 2-0.
- Skin sutures with either intracutaneous or running mattress Monocryl 3-0, with knots tied outside the skin.
- Silicone wound dressing, followed by non-compressive dressing.

4.2.3 Winkelmann B3 (total femur resection)

4.2.3.1 Step 1 – Distal approach

- Wavy or U-shaped incision just above the knee to correct the discrepancy in circumference between the upper and lower leg. Incise the skin 1–2 cm more proximal than the tibial plateau, allowing for some additional skin for tension-free closure. Avoid incising the skin directly over the tibial tuberosity, as this area is at higher risk for wound healing problems. In selected cases, the anterior fascio-cutaneous skin flap overlying the quadriceps is preserved to facilitate skin closure over the gluteal musculature after rotation.

- Further dissection circumferentially around the knee with diathermy effectively simulates a knee disarticulation. Preserve the length of the patellar tendon, the circumferential capsule, including LCL and MCL, for later reattachment. Preserve the ACL for later attachment to the ligamentum teres.

- Identification of the biceps femoris tendon laterally. Opening of the peroneal and tibial compartments. Identifying the common peroneal nerve (CPN) and mobilizing it. Following the CPN proximally, subsequently identifying and mobilizing the tibial and sciatic nerves.

- Following the tibial nerve, the medial and lateral gastrocnemius heads are divided at the musculotendinous junction.

- Identify and dissect the distal popliteal artery and vein. In case of vascular encasement or involvement, the artery and vein can be divided, and primary anastomoses of the popliteal and femoral arteries and veins can be performed, usually by vascular or plastic surgeons. In the case of free neurovascular structures and young and small children, the artery and vein can be preserved over their entire length, rolled up (without kinking), and stored in the adductor space.

- At this point, the knee is now nearly free: nerves (sciatic, tibial, peroneal) and popliteal vessels are mobilized; cruciate ligaments are still intact.

- The deep femoral vein is ligated and transected posteriorly from the knee to facilitate anastomosis to the great saphenous vein (GSV), if the GSV cannot be reconstructed or left intact.

4.2.3.2 Step 2 – Medial thigh approach

- Longitudinal medial incision from the distal to the proximal incision.

- Identify and mobilize the GSV over its entire course. Preserving the GSV helps with venous outflow and reduces postoperative swelling, wound problems, and blister formation, as most of the other smaller (intramuscular) venous structures are divided. Depending on its diameter, one may choose between a primary anastomosis and rolling up.

- Identify the superficial femoral artery and vein, and dissect or transect them, leaving as long as the margins allow.

4.2.3.3 Step 3 – Posterior thigh approach

- Longitudinal posterior incision from the distal to the proximal incisions, with further dissection using diathermy down to the fascia.

- Subsequently, develop the muscular interval and identify the sciatic nerve, and mobilize this completely toward proximally.

4.2.3.4 Step 4 – Proximal approach

- Circular incision circumferentially at the groin level, from the anterior superior iliac spine (ASIS) through the gluteal crease.
- Dissection with diathermy down to the fascia.
- Identification and mobilization of the superficial and deep femoral vessels.
- Sartorius released from ASIS, rectus femoris from anterior inferior iliac spine (AIIS), adductors/pectineus from the superior pubic ramus.
- Gluteus maximus and tensor fascia lata insertions divided.
- Anterior hip capsule exposed; gluteus medius released from the greater trochanter.
- Iliopsoas divided at the lesser trochanter if margins allow.
- Identification and mobilization of the sciatic nerve.
- Proceed proximally by releasing the sartorius, rectus femoris, adductors, gluteal insertions, and iliopsoas while dissecting the femoral nerve and iliac vessels.
- Open the hip joint, divide the capsule and ligamentum teres, and remove the femur en bloc with associated lymph nodes.
- If margins allow, transect the hip capsule around the femoral neck.
- At this point, both the femur and knee are completely mobilized circumferentially. Resect the total femur/thigh as one specimen and send it for histopathology.

4.2.3.5 Step 5 – Rotation and fixation

For Winkelmann B3 rotationplasties, in which the entire femur and thigh are removed because of extensive femoral tumor involvement, there are two options for reconstruction.

4.2.3.6 Winkelmann B3A

In the youngest children below the age of five, there is good remodeling capacity of the lateral tibial plateau to a neo-femoral head when placed inside the acetabulum.

- Start with the preparation of the tibial plateau. Mobilize the soft tissue cuff of the lateral tibial plateau. The lateral meniscus can be left on the capsule or excised. Protect the articular cartilage of the lateral tibial plateau.
- The fibular head is dissected and removed; the course of the common peroneal nerve should be carefully preserved.
- The lower leg can now be rotated, and the lateral tibial plateau seated into the acetabulum.
- Soft tissue reconstructions:
    - ACL attached to the ligamentum teres.
    - MCL attached to the lateral labrum.
    - Medial capsule is attached to the lateral labrum.
    - Lateral gastrocnemius head fixation with transosseous sutures to the superior pubic ramus, if length allows.
    - Medial gastrocnemius head fixation to the cranial labrum, just below the rectus femoris origin.
    - Gluteal and psoas musculature is reinserted onto the tibial capsule.

4.2.3.7 Winkelmann B3B

In older children and adolescents, the remodeling capacity is lacking due to their advanced growth, and cementing a hip hemiarthroplasty in the tibia should be considered. Preoperative templating is crucial for determining the correct size of the implant and head.

- Start with the preparation of the tibial plateau. Mobilize the soft tissue cuff of the lateral tibial plateau. Remove the lateral meniscus.
- The fibular head is dissected and removed; the course of the common peroneal nerve should be carefully preserved.
- Prepare the tibia for the cemented hemiarthroplasty. It is advisable to use a modular implant with a straight stem to allow for the correction of rotation once the stem is cemented in place.
- Ream to the correct stem diameter. Place a cement restrictor in the tibial stem. Cement the definitive modular stem into the tibial shaft.
- Place the body of the prosthesis with the trunnion in the correct rotation, and place the ceramic head (preoperatively template the size to match the acetabulum).

- The lower leg can now be rotated, and the hemiarthroplasty reduced into the acetabulum.
- Soft tissue reconstructions:
  - MCL attached to the lateral labrum.
  - Medial capsule attached to the lateral labrum.
  - Lateral gastrocnemius head fixation with transosseous sutures to the superior pubic ramus, if length allows.
  - Medial gastrocnemius head fixation to the cranial labrum, just below the rectus femoris origin.
  - Gluteal and psoas musculature is reinserted onto the tibial capsule.
- In the case of vascular anastomoses, check for stability and rotation, as this may still be adjusted.

4.2.3.8 Step 6 – Vascular anastomoses (if needed)

- Typically, end-to-end anastomoses of the external iliac artery and vein to the popliteal artery and vein are performed by plastic or vascular surgeons (separate operation notes are available from the authors upon request).
- Additionally, the deep femoral vein and great saphenous vein can be anastomosed end-to-end to allow for adequate venous outflow of the lower leg.

4.2.3.9 Step 7 Closure

- Perform a thorough washout with saline or sterile water.
- Take time for good hemostasis.
- Suture the fascia of the lower leg to the fascia of the abdominal wall with interrupted Vicryl 1. Do not use running sutures to close the fascia to prevent vascular or neurological compression as a result of postsurgical swelling. Make sure there is not too much tension on the sutured structures.
- Subcuticular suture with running Vicryl 2-0.
- Skin sutures with either intracutaneous or running mattress Monocryl 3-0, with knots tied outside the skin.
- Silicone wound dressing, followed by non-compressive dressing.

5. Postoperative care and rehabilitation

5.1 Direct postoperative care

- Monitoring of capillary refill every hour for the first 24 hours. If not possible on a normal surgical ward, overnight ICU admission is advised.
- DVT prophylaxis, when indicated.
- Pain control: epidural analgesia catheter and IDC after checking neurological status; referral to the pain team.
- Positioning: foot elevated on a pillow, toes free from the mattress, to prevent decubitus and pressure sores whilst the epidural analgesia catheter is *in situ*.
- Antibiotics: as per local protocols; we continue cefazolin for 24 hours (3× daily, weight-adjusted).
- Imaging: postoperative conventional radiographs of the hip and lower limb.
- Wound: remove non-compressive dressing after 24–48 hours; leave silicone dressing on for 7 days or until wound inspection.
- Mobilization: directly start foot and ankle exercises to prevent postoperative swelling and reduce stiffness. Maintain bed rest while the epidural analgesia catheter is in place; once removed, begin non-weight-bearing mobilization under the supervision of physiotherapy. Early verticalization prevents contractures.

5.2 Rehabilitation and prosthetic management

- Days 1–3: Active toe and ankle mobilization.
- Days 4–7: Non-weight-bearing exercises and walking with a frame or two crutches.
- After three to four weeks: Temporary prosthesis fitting.
- After three to six months: Progressive gait training and sports reintroduction following bone healing.
- Final prosthesis: designed in ankle dorsiflexion to allow "full extension" in stance. Definitive sockets are fitted after union, typically without ischial tuberosity support.
- Patients benefit from energy-storing prostheses; gait analyses show lower energy expenditure compared to transfemoral amputees.
- Rehabilitation focuses on gait re-education, proprioception, and sports participation [4, 11, 12].

6. Complications

Early complications:

- Arterial occlusion and compromised venous outflow. Vessel-sparing techniques reduce the risks of problems with venous return; venous torsion must be avoided.
- Venous thrombosis (<1%)
- Infection: rare, but can lead to serious complications, requiring aggressive debridement.
- Wound healing problems may require surgical wound revision but can mostly be managed with vacuum-assisted closure (VAC) dressings.

Late complications:

- Nonunion: minimized by compression-stable fixation (<1%).
- Malrotation: requires corrective osteotomy if symptomatic.
- Fracture: especially tibial shaft, is mostly managed conservatively.
- Contracture of the ankle or hip: prevented by early physiotherapy and verticalization.
- Diffuse ankle osteopenia is common, but clinically significant arthritis is rare [4,5].

7. Functional outcomes, quality of life, and oncologic safety

7.1 Function and quality of life

Studies consistently show good-to-excellent long-term functional outcomes, including excellent participation in daily life activities and sports participation, such as high-impact and contact sports. Long-term series (>20 years) show MSTS scores >80% and LEFS within the normal range for age.

Compared with transfemoral amputation, rotationplasty has lower energy expenditure, better gait symmetry, and no phantom pain.

Quality of life is comparable to, or better than, amputation or endoprostheses [12–14]. The rate of sports participation (running, soccer, skiing) is high in rotationplasty.

7.2 Psychosocial impact

Psychosocial adaptation is favorable when adequate preoperative counseling is provided [2, 15]. Physical appearance and the esthetic concerns about rotationplasty are the main hurdles. With preoperative counseling, greater than 85% of patients and parents report satisfaction with function and lifestyle. Given the profound impact of procedures like rotationplasty, shared decision-making (SDM) is essential to ensure that patients and parents are fully informed and actively involved in choosing the most suitable treatment. This will contribute to patient-centered care and will increasingly empower patients and families in choosing their preferred reconstructive option.

Oncologic margins and survival are not compromised; outcomes reflect tumor biology and systemic therapy [16]. Follow-up studies over 30 years show durability without the revision burden typical of megaprostheses [17].

8. Practical pearls and checklist

8.1 Preoperative tips

- Multidisciplinary planning, including psychosocial counseling.
- Templating for predicted growth and length at skeletal maturity.
- In general, perpendicular osteotomies are preferred.
- For Winkelmann A1, generally aim for a relatively high osteotomy of the femur, about 5–7 cm below the trochanter minor or more distally if the femur is placed into the proximal tibia, to prevent a long rotationplasty at the end of growth.
- For Winkelmann A2, the femoral side is osteotomized depending on the resection length of the tibia.
- For Winkelmann B3b: template the modular hemiarthroplasty.

8.2 Intraoperative tips

- Skin marking, including orientation lines on the anterior and posterior sides of the thigh and lower leg, for orientation after rotation.
- Use a wavy incision distally for better skin closure.
- Protect venous drainage by preserving perforators and saving the great saphenous vein if possible.
- Confirm vascular pedicle orientation and preserve at least two out of three lower leg vessels.
- To identify the common peroneal nerve: open the fascia of the peroneus longus muscle, then cut fiber by fiber until the common peroneal nerve is exposed and can be freed.
- Laterally identify the common peroneal nerve, follow it to the sciatic nerve, and from there, find the tibial nerve.

- Early dissection of the lateral gastrocnemius significantly improves exposure to the neurovascular bundle.

- Perform the osteotomy below the proximal tibial growth plate to prevent tethered growth, resulting in a valgus of the leg.

- The fibula can be left intact or shortened to allow for a better fit and to correct size differences; perform epiphysiodesis if necessary.

- Verify kinematics and alignment, including rotation, before final fixation. Temporary short K-wires can be placed in the femur and tibia to test that dorsiflexion equals knee flexion and to assess rotation and angulation.

- Avoid under- or over-rotation, as it impairs gait or venous return.

- Fixation with lateral AO locking compression plate (LCP), small fragment for younger children, and large fragment for older children and adolescents.

- Fix the plate onto the lateral side of the femur first to add extra stability, allowing for easier medial fixation of the plate onto the tibia.

- Osteotomy of the medial side of the tibia to allow for the use of a straight plate and fixation under compression.

- For Winkelmann B3b: Check for rotation of the hip after temporary first fixation, as the modular implant can still be adjusted at this time.

- Before closing the fascia, photograph the location of the neurovascular bundle for future reference, in case of the need for reoperations.

8.3 Postoperative tips

- Directly postoperatively, perform a full neurovascular check before a complete motor block occurs due to the epidural.

- Hourly capillary refill and vascular checks; consider ICU monitoring if not available on the surgical ward.

- Elevation of the limb helps prevent swelling and promotes venous return.

- For faster recovery, start early range of motion exercises with ongoing physiotherapy to reduce swelling and progressive prosthetic fitting [4, 7].

9. Conclusion

Rotationplasty provides a durable, growth-compatible, and highly functional reconstructive option for children and young adults who require resection of malignant bone tumors around the knee. While cosmetic appearance remains challenging, oncologic safety, functional outcomes, and long-term patient satisfaction are consistently excellent. With proper patient selection, good preoperative counseling, meticulous surgical technique, and structured rehabilitation, rotationplasty remains one of the most successful biological reconstructions in pediatric orthopedic oncology, especially when durable function and quality of life are prioritized.

Author details

Lizz van der Heijden, Jonneke Kuperus and Michiel van de Sande*
Orthopedics, Princess Máxima Center, Utrecht, Netherlands

*Address all correspondence to: michielvds@me.com

References

[1] Bernthal NM, Monument MJ, Randall RL, Jones KB. Rotationplasty: Beauty is in the eye of the beholder. Operative Techniques in Orthopaedics. 2014;**24**:103–110

[2] Sawamura C, Hornicek FJ, Gebhardt MC. Complications and risk factors for failure of rotationplasty: review of 25 patients. Clinical Orthopaedics and Related Research. 2008;**466**:1302–1308

[3] Catani F, Capanna R, Benedetti MG, et al Gait analysis in patients after Van Nes rotationplasty. Clinical Orthopaedics and Related Research. 1993;**296**:270–277

[4] de Sande Maj V, Vochteloo AJH, Dijkstra PDS, Taminiau AHM. Van Nes-Borggreve Rotationplasty of the Knee. In Bentley G, editor. European Surgical Orthopaedics and Traumatology. Berlin: Springer; 2014. p. 4135–4147

[5] Krebbekx GGJ, Smithuis FF, Duivenvoorden MJC, et al. Good long-term functional outcomes after rotationplasty despite osteoarthritis in the (pseudo)knee. Osteoarthritis and Cartilage Open 2025;**7**:100644

[6] Fuller CB, Lichtblau CH, Paley D. Rotationplasty for Severe Congenital Femoral Deficiency. Children (Basel, Switzerland). 2021;**8**(6):462

[7] Gottsauner-Wolf F, Kotz R, Knahr K, Kristen H, Ritschl P, Salzer M. Rotationplasty for limb salvage in the treatment of malignant tumors at the knee. A follow-up study of seventy patients. The Journal of Bone & Joint Surgery. 1991;**73**:1365–1375

[8] Cammisa Jr FP, Glasser DB, Otis JC, Kroll MA, Lane JM, Healey JH. The Van Nes tibial rotationplasty. A functionally viable reconstructive procedure in children who have a tumor of the distal end of the femur. The Journal of Bone and Joint Surgery. American Volume. 1990;**72**:1541–1547

[9] Paley D, Bhave A, Herzenberg JE, et al. Multiplier method for predicting limb-length discrepancy. The Journal of Bone and Joint Surgery-American Volume 2000;**82**:1432–1446

[10] Anderson M, Green WT, Messner MB. Growth and predictions of growth in the lower extremities. The Journal of Bone & Joint Surgery. 1963;**45**:1–14

[11] Hillmann A, Rosenbaum D, Schroter J, Gosheger G, Hoffmann C, Winkelmann W. Electromyographic and gait analysis of forty-three patients after rotationplasty. The Journal of Bone and Joint Surgery-American Volume. 2000;**82**:187–196

[12] Gradl G, Postl LK, Lenze U, Stolberg-Stolberg J, Pohlig F, Rechl H, Schmitt-Sody M, von Eisenhart-rothe R, Kirchhoff C, et al Long-term functional outcome and quality of life following rotationplasty for treatment of malignant tumors. BMC Musculoskeletal Disorders. 2015;**16**:262

[13] Rödl RW, Pohlmann U, Gosheger G, Lindner NJ, Winkelmann W. Rotationplasty–quality of life after 10 years in 22 patients. Acta Orthopaedica Scandinavica. 2002;**73**:85–88

[14] Tigelaar LG, Haveman LM, Bekkering WP, et al. A multidisciplinary

and structured approach for comprehensive evaluation of functional outcomes, adverse events, psychosocial outcomes and health-related quality of life after local therapy for bone sarcoma in children: Protocol for a cross-sectional study. Frontiers in Pediatrics 2025; **45**:1534153

[15] van der Hoek H, Tigelaar LG, Maurice-Stam H, et al. Body image of patients in follow-up for pediatric bone sarcoma: Implications of tumor location and local therapy. Journal of Cancer Survivorship. 2025. DOI: 10.1007/s11764-025-01847-9

[16] Barr RD, Wunder JS. Bone and soft tissue sarcomas are often curable—But at what cost? Cancer. 2009; **115**:4046–4054

[17] Windhager R, Dominkus M, Krepler P, et al. Rotationplasty for malignant tumors of the proximal femur. The Journal of Bone and Joint Surgery. American Volume. 1996;**78**:593–602